Biomedical Library

Queen's University Belfast

Tel: 028 9097 2710

E-mail: BiomedicalLibrary@qub.ac.uk

For due dates and renewals:

QUB borrowers see 'MY ACCOUNT' at
http://library.qub.ac.uk/qcat
or go to the Library Home Page

HSC borrowers see 'MY ACCOUNT' at
www.honni.qub.ac.uk/qcat

This book must be returned not later
than its due date but may be recalled
earlier if in demand

Fines are imposed on overdue books

THE RISING TRENDS IN ASTHMA

The Ciba Foundation is an international scientific and educational charity (Registered Charity No. 313574). It was established in 1947 by the Swiss chemical and pharmaceutical company of CIBA Limited — now Ciba-Geigy Limited. The Foundation operates independently in London under English trust law.

The Ciba Foundation exists to promote international cooperation in biological, medical and chemical research. It organizes about eight international multidisciplinary symposia each year on topics that seem ready for discussion by a small group of research workers. The papers and discussions are published in the Ciba Foundation symposium series. The Foundation also holds many shorter meetings (not published), organized by the Foundation itself or by outside scientific organizations. The staff always welcome suggestions for future meetings.

The Foundation's house at 41 Portland Place, London W1N 4BN, provides facilities for meetings of all kinds. Its Media Resource Service supplies information to journalists on all scientific and technological topics. The library, open five days a week to any graduate in science or medicine, also provides information on scientific meetings throughout the world and answers general enquiries on biomedical and chemical subjects. Scientists from any part of the world may stay in the house during working visits to London.

Ciba Foundation Symposium 206

THE RISING TRENDS IN ASTHMA

1997

JOHN WILEY & SONS

Chichester · New York · Weinheim · Brisbane · Singapore · Toronto

© Ciba Foundation 1997
Published in 1997 by John Wiley & Sons Ltd,
Baffins Lane, Chichester,
West Sussex PO19 1UD, England

National 01243 779777
International (+44) 1243 779777
e-mail (for orders and customer service enquiries): cs-books@wiley.co.uk
Visit our Home Page on http://www.wiley.co.uk
or http://www.wiley.com

Other Wiley Editorial Offices

John Wiley & Sons, Inc., 605 Third Avenue,
New York, NY 10158-0012, USA

VCH Verlagsgesellschaft mbH
Pappelallee 3, D-69469 Weinheim, Germany

Jacaranda Wiley Ltd, 33 Park Road, Milton,
Queensland 4064, Australia

John Wiley & Sons (Canada) Ltd, 22 Worcester Road,
Rexdale, Ontario M9W 1L1, Canada

John Wiley & Sons (Asia) Pte Ltd, 2 Clementi Loop #02-01,
Jin Xing Distripark, Singapore 0512

Ciba Foundation Symposium 206
ix+280 pages, 30 figures, 16 tables

Library of Congress Cataloging-in-Publication Data

The rising trends in asthma.
    p.   cm.—(Ciba Foundation symposium ; 206)
    Edited by Derek Chadwick and Gail Cardew.
    Proceedings of a conference held at the Ciba Foundation, June
11–13, 1996.
    Includes bibliographical references and indexes.
    ISBN 0-471-97012-3 (alk. paper)
    1. Asthma—Congresses.   I. Chadwick, Derek.   II. Cardew, Gail.
III. Series.
    [DNLM: 1. Asthma—immunology—congresses.   2. Asthma—
epidemiology—congresses.   W3 C161F v.206 1997 / WF 553 R595 1997]
RC591.R56 1997
616.2′38—dc21
DNLM/DLC
for Library of Congress   96-40339
                                                            CIP

British Library Cataloguing in Publication Data

A catalogue record for this book is available from the British Library

ISBN 0 471 97012 3

Typeset in 10/12pt Garamond by Dobbie Typesetting Limited, Tavistock, Devon.
Printed and bound in Great Britain by Biddles Ltd, Guildford.
This book is printed on acid-free paper responsibly manufactured from sustainable forestation,
for which at least two trees are planted for each one used for paper production.

Contents

Participants

G. Anderson   Ciba-Geigy Limited, Pharma Division, K-125.10.15, CH-4–2, Basle, Switzerland

H. R. Anderson   Department of Public Health Sciences, St. George's Hospital Medical School, Cranmer Terrace, London SW17 0RE, UK

R. Beasley   Asthma Research Group, Department of Medicine, Wellington School of Medicine, PO Box 7343, Wellington South, New Zealand

E. R. Bleecker   University of Maryland School of Medicine, Division of Pulmonary and Critical Care Medicine, 10 South Pine Street, Suite 800, Baltimore, MD 21201, USA

H. A. Boushey   University of California, PO Box 0130, 505 Parnassus Avenue, San Francisco, CA 94143, USA

J. Britton   Division of Respiratory Medicine, University of Nottingham, The City Hospital, Hucknall Road, Nottingham NG5 1PB , UK

J. Brostoff   Department of Immunology, The University College London Hospitals, Arthur Stanley House, 40–50 Tottenham Street, London W1N 8AA, UK

P. Burney   Department of Public Health Medicine, UMDS, Block 8, South wing, St Thomas' Hospital, Lambeth Palace Road, London SE1 7EH, UK

W. W. Busse   University of Wisconsin Medical School, JS/220 Clinical Science Center, 600 Highland Avenue, Madison, WI 53792–3244, USA

P. A. Corris   Department of Respiratory Medicine, Freeman Hospital, High Heaton, Newcastle upon Tyne NE7 7DN, UK

P. Cullinan   Imperial College of Science, Technology & Medicine, National Heart & Lung Institute, 1b Manresa Road, London SW3 6LR, UK

C. Heusser   Ciba-Geigy Ltd, K-125.12.58, CH 4002, Basle, Switzerland

S. T. Holgate (*Chairman*)   School of Medicine, University of Southampton, Level D, Centre Block, Southampton General Hospital, Tremona Road, Southampton SO16 6YD, UK

P. G. Holt   TVW Telethon Institute for Child Health Research, Post Office Box 855, West Perth 6872, Western Australia

A. B. Kay   Allergy and Clinical Immunology, Imperial College School of Medicine at the National Heart & Lung Institute, Dovehouse Street, London SW3 6LY, UK

H. Magnussen   Zentrum für Pneumologie und Thoraxchirugie, Krankenhaus GroBhansdorf, Wohrendamm 80, D-22927 GroBhansdorf, Germany

F. Martinez   Respiratory Sciences Center, University of Arizona School of Medicine, 1501 North Campbell Avenue, Tucson, AZ 85724, USA

H. S. Nelson   National Jewish Center for Immunology and Respiratory Medicine, 1400 Jackson Street, Denver, CO 80206, USA

P. D. Paré   Respiratory Health Network of Centres of Excellence, University of British Columbia Pulmonary Research Laboratory, St. Paul's Hospital, Vancouver, Canada V6Z 1Y6

R. A. Pauwels   Department of Respiratory Disease University Hospital, De Pintelaan 185, B-9000 Ghent, Belgium

T. A. E. Platts-Mills   University of Virginia Asthma and Allergic Diseases Center, Box 225, Charlottesville, VA 22908, USA

P. C. Potter   Department of Clinical Science & Immunology, University of Cape Town, Medical School, Cape Town 7925, South Africa

M. R. Sears   Asthma Research Group, McMaster University, St Joseph's Hospital, 50 Charlton Avenue East, Hamilton, Ontario, Canada L8N 4A6

D. P. Strachan   Department of Public Health Sciences, St George's Hospital Medical School, Cranmer Terrace, London SW17 0RE, UK

J. Warner   Department of Child Health, University of Southampton, Level G, Centre Block, Southampton General Hospital, Tremona Road, Southampton SO16 6YD, UK

S. T. Weiss   Channing Laboratory, Department of Medicine, Harvard University Medical School, Brigham & Women's Hospital, 180 Longwood Avenue, Boston, MA 02115, USA

A. J. Woolcock   Institute of Respiratory Medicine, Royal Prince Alfred Hospital, Camperdown, Syndey, NSW 2050, Australia

C. Z.-A. Fromond (*Bursar*)   Institut Pasteur, Unité de Pharmacologie Cellulaire, 25 Rue du dr. Roux 75015, Paris, France

Introduction

Stephen T. Holgate

School of Medicine, University of Southampton, Level D, Centre Block, Southampton General Hospital, Tremona Road, Southampton SO16 6YD, UK

One of the most exciting prospects of this symposium is the opportunity to bring together people from different countries and different disciplines within the field of asthma. In particular, it's a pleasure to have epidemiologists, clinicians, pathophysiologists and geneticists sharing mutual experiences, exploring new ways of thinking about asthma and generating novel ideas about an 'old' disease.

I am particularly keen that we do not focus on drawing any specific conclusions too early in the symposium because they are often difficult to distil during the discussion periods. However, I hope we will be able to arrive at some principles relating to the possible causes of any rise in asthma trends that we will wish to pursue in the future.

In 1860 Henry Hyde Salter published a treatise on asthma, which was remarkably insightful considering that there was very little knowledge of pathophysiology of the disease at that time (Salter 1860). In this treatise he referred to narrowing of the airways in asthma as being due to smooth muscle contraction and that this was intimately involved in the mechanisms of episodic breathlessness in asthma. He also had ideas about the factors leading to airway narrowing in other forms of obstructive diseases that broadly fall into the category of chronic obstructive pulmonary disease, a debate that still continues.

The concept emerging from Salter's writings, and from two other Ciba Foundation symposia in 1959 and 1971 (Ciba Foundation guest symposium 1959, Ciba Foundation study group 1971), was that asthma was predominantly a disease of airway smooth muscle, which was altered so that it contracted too easily and too much. Following on from this concept, industry has responded by creating drugs such as the β2-agonists and cholinergic antagonists that relax the contracted airway smooth muscle and relieve the obstruction. However, thinking of asthma purely in terms of smooth muscle contraction hasn't been a very constructive exercise because somehow we have to explain why the smooth muscle around the airways contracts too easily and too much.

One reason why there has been so much interest in asthma is because of the view that over the last two decades it has been increasing in prevalence and possibly in severity. I am hoping that at the end of this symposium we will be able to make some clear statements about these trends in different parts of the world and come to some clear conclusions on the epidemiology of the disease. One can identify a range of markers that might be indicative of a rising trend in asthma: for example, between 1980 and

1993 in the UK there has been an increased prescribing of β2-agonists, inhaled corticosteroids and other anti-inflammatory drugs. I'm confident that we will be able to tease out whether this is being driven by an increased awareness of asthma by patients and doctors, and changes in the way asthma health care is delivered, or whether it is truly reflective of a change in the prevalence of asthma. We are also familiar with epidemics of asthma that have occurred in association with an increase in mortality. For example, in Barcelona asthma has been associated with the release of soybean allergens into the air around the storage silos of the harbour when soybean is off-loaded from ships (Synek et al 1996). An increased mortality has also been described in relation to possible adverse effects of treatment. For example, in New Zealand an association has been reported between increased asthma mortality and the prescribing of a particular type of β2-agonist (Crane et al 1989). This has fuelled an important debate on the consequences of relying too heavily on β2-agonists for relief of asthma symptoms (Beasley et al 1997, this volume).

Objective data on the prevalence of asthma in different countries have also been collected using questionnaires that have been well validated. These have been used on whole populations as well as on well-described subgroups of individuals over time. For example, the Finnish study of conscripts has demonstrated that there has been an increase in both the prevalence and severity of asthma (Haahtela et al 1990).

There is currently a view that any increase in the trends of asthma is accounted for by a parallel rise in allergy expressed in multiple organs (Lewis et al 1996). However, it appears that asthma has increased to a greater extent than other allergic manifestations, suggesting that other forces are operating in the lower airways.

Moving on to the causes of asthma, although we will hear about the importance of genetic factors in increasing the risk of acquiring asthma through interactions with the environment, most of this symposium will focus on the environment itself. This also includes the intrauterine environment because gestation is a period when the fetus is being programmed through the materno-fetal relationship influencing the developing immune system and lungs. The fact that the induction of asthma is so closely linked to aeroallergen exposure indicates the importance of this environmental aspect, especially in the first two to three years of life. Discussion relating to asthma will focus on the types of allergen and their marked geographical differences. House dust mites, cats, pollens and fungi in different parts of the world are all associated with specific sensitization of the lower respiratory tract and the induction of asthma. It would be helpful if a consensus were to emerge about the relative role of allergens, and if there are some that are more important than others. This would help in the design of allergen avoidance primary and secondary intervention studies.

Over the last half century there have also been substantial changes to our domestic and working environments. Allergens are important in our domestic environment, and we will probably hear about the increase in allergen load that has arisen as a consequence of sealing homes for air conditioning and heating. Poor ventilation of houses and work place environments leads not only to high concentrations of sensitizing allergens accumulating, but also to other pollutants such as combustion emissions and tobacco smoke, which could serve as adjuvants in the sensitization processes.

The public are presented with a very different view of the rising trends in asthma. Largely because of promotion by the lay press, they believe that external ambient pollutants, and especially emissions from motor vehicles, play a key role. However, there is little supporting evidence for this — at least in terms of new cases of asthma, rather than promoting attacks of asthma in those who already have the disease (COMEAP 1995). Studies in former East and West Germany have suggested that air pollution from industrial sources, as opposed to motor vehicles, may even be protective (von Mutius et al 1994). Cigarette smoking in pregnancy and the influence of inhalation of cigarette smoke by non-smokers are important causes of respiratory morbidity and may well contribute to the acquisition of asthma.

The role of viruses is presently a paradox and I'm not sure whether we will resolve the issues at this symposium. One fascinating observation is that children from one-child families seem to have more asthma and allergic disease than children from multiple sibling families (Strachan 1989). One explanation is that viruses have a protective role early in life by creating a stimulus that tilts the immune response away from the development of allergy and asthma. In contrast, other viruses such as the respiratory syncitial virus, and other infective organisms, such as *Chlamydia pneumoniae* or *Micoplasma pneumoniae*, might drive an asthmatic-type immunological response rather than protecting against it. A consideration of the roles of infection early in life will be particularly relevant, as will be the role of infection in exacerbating asthma. Although there is a strong emphasis on the role of allergens in triggering attacks of asthma, an important role of respiratory viruses in asthma morbidity is being increasingly recognized.

Much of this symposium will focus on the early life origins of asthma. There has been a change in the way we look at asthma, in that the infant and child are becoming the focus of novel exciting studies, which are not only epidemiological but also based on pathogenesis. By identifying possible genes that are important at increasing risks, by looking at vulnerable periods in life (especially early in life) and by identifying factors which through different mechanisms may be driving the immunological processes (amongst others) that lead to asthma, we will gain a better insight with which to make informed decisions regarding intervention studies. The crucial issues are whether early life interventions are truly effective, how to achieve interventions, what sort of interventions are most effective and what will be acceptable to patients. I would like to encourage you all to be as frank and as open as possible in your discussions so that we can expose some of the more controversial areas that will help take forward concepts in the origins and prevention of asthma.

References

Beasley R, Pearce N, Crane J 1997 International trends in asthma mortality. In: The rising trends in asthma. Wiley, Chichester (Ciba Found Symp 206) p 140–156

Ciba Foundation guest symposium 1959 Terminology, definitions and classification of chronic pulmonary emphysema and related conditions (a report of the conclusions of a Ciba guest symposium). Thorax 14:286–299

Ciba Foundation study group 1971 Identification of asthma. Churchill Livingstone, Edinburgh (Ciba Found study group 38)

COMEAP 1995 Asthma and outdoor air pollution. Committee on the medical effects of air pollutants report, Department of Health. HMSO, London, p 114

Crane J, Pearce N, Flatt A et al 1989 Prescribed fenoterol and death from asthma in New Zealand, 1981–83: case control study. Lancet I:917–922

Haahtela T, Lindholm H, Björksten F, Koskenvao K, Laitinen LA 1990 Prevalence of asthma in Finnish young men. Br Med J 301:266–268

Lewis S, Richard D, Bynner J, Butler N, Britton J 1996 Prospective study of risk factors for early and persistent wheezing in childhood. Eur Respir J 8:349–356

Salter HH 1860 On asthma: its pathology and treatment, 1st edn. Churchill, London

Strachan DP 1989 Hay fever, hygiene and household size. Br Med J 299:1259–1260

Synek M, Antó J, Beasley R et al 1996 Immunohistochemistry of soybean-induced fatal asthma. Eur Respir J 9:54–57

von Mutius E, Martinez FD, Fritzsch C, Nicolai T, Roell G, Thiemann HH 1994 Prevalence of asthma and atopy in two areas of West Germany and East Germany. Am J Respir Crit Care Med 149:358–364

Asthma: a dynamic disease of inflammation and repair

Stephen T. Holgate

School of Medicine, University of Southampton, Level D, Centre Block, Southampton General Hospital, Tremona Road, Southampton SO16 6YD, UK

Abstract. It is now widely accepted that asthma in its varied forms is an inflammatory disorder of the airways in which mediator release from activated mast cells and eosinophils plays a major role. T lymphocytes take a primary role in orchestrating these processes through their capacity to generate a range of cytokines of the interleukin 4 gene cluster encoded on the long arm of chromosome 5. Additional cytokines derived from mast cells and eosinophils also play a key role, especially tumour necrosis factor α, which is responsible for initiating the up-regulation of vascular adhesion molecules involved in the recruitment of eosinophils and other inflammatory cells from the circulation. The importance of C-X-C and C-C chemokines as local chemoattractants and activating stimuli is also recognized. In addition to releasing an array of pharmacologically active autacoids, the inflammatory response in asthma results in the generation of proteolytic activities from mast cells (tryptase, chymase), eosinophils (MMP-9) and the epithelium itself (MMP-2, MMP-9), which exert tissue-destructive and cell-signalling effects. The epithelium is also highly activated, as evidenced by the up-regulation of cytokine production, inducible enzymes and soluble mediators. Increased surface expression of the epithelial isoform of CD44 (9v) and subepithelial proliferation of myofibroblasts are indicative of a simultaneous active repair process and the laying down of new interstitial collagens. Together, inflammatory and repair processes create the complex phenotype that characterizes asthma and its progression.

1997 The rising trends in asthma. Wiley, Chichester (Ciba Foundation Symposium 206) p 5–34

In his classical treatise on asthma, published in 1860, Salter describes asthma as 'Paroxysmal dyspnoea of a peculiar character, generally periodic with healthy respiration between attacks.' (Salter 1860) He illustrates this in his book as being caused by contraction of airway smooth muscle, and separates it mechanistically from 'bronchial catarrh', 'recent' and 'old' bronchitis. Although he accepted 'nervous asthma', Salter made the important observation that there were other causes that precipitated attacks, including animal emanations, impure air, hay fever and foods. Among the many subjects covered in his book was a classification of asthma, which used the term 'intrinsic', and a description of cells characteristic of asthmatic sputum which Paul Ehrlich was later to identify as eosinophils (Ehrlich 1879). With this

5

historical background, it is of interest to see how much progress into asthma mechanisms has been achieved in the 100 years to follow.

There have been two previous meetings on asthma held under the auspices of the Ciba Foundation. These occurred in 1958 and 1971 and they focused on trying to agree a definition of various forms of airway obstruction (Ciba Foundation guest symposium 1959, Ciba Foundation study group 1971). From the conclusions drawn from the 1971 publication, it is clear that the participants were frustrated by the lack of knowledge on the underlying mechanisms of asthma and chronic obstructive pulmonary disease available at that time and a plea was made for further research. The clinical description of asthma that emerged from the 1959 publication of the symposium and later endorsed by the American Thoracic Society was a disease characterized by wide variation over short periods of time in resistance to flow in the airways of the lung. It is of interest to note that this description is almost identical to that of Salter's almost 100 years earlier.

The last decade has witnessed a dramatic increase in our understanding of the cellular and molecular basis of asthma, fuelled largely by the advent of fibreoptic bronchoscopy and its use to obtain airway surface fluid and mucosal biopsies. Since even in the mildest form of the disease airway inflammation was present, the World Health Organization/ National Heart, Lung and Blood Institute (WHO/NHLBI) combined working group described asthma as:

> A chronic inflammatory disorder of the airways in which many cells play a role, in particular mast cells, eosinophils and T lymphocytes. In susceptible individuals, this inflammation causes recurrent episodes of wheezing, breathlessness, chest tightness and cough particularly at night and/or early in the morning. These symptoms are usually associated with widespread but variable airflow limitation reversible either spontaneously or with treatment. The inflammation also causes an associated increase in airway responsiveness to a variety of stimuli (National Institutes of Health 1995)

By attaching primacy to airway inflammation, with disordered airway function following on from this, there emerged two important new principles concerning asthma. Firstly, the disease is a chronic (often lifelong) disorder which, like other chronic inflammatory diseases such as rheumatoid arthritis and inflammatory bowel disease, fluctuates in severity over time, sometimes with prolonged remissions. Secondly, therapy should be targeted towards preventing and/or reversing the inflammatory processes using appropriate environmental and pharmacological strategies. These principles have formed the basis of the national and international guidelines on asthma management, such as those produced by the WHO/NHLBI (National Institutes of Health 1995). Since airway inflammation is fundamental to modern thinking about asthma, it is worth reflecting on some of the common principles that underpin its importance to disease pathogenesis.

In all forms of asthma there appears to be a common set of local events leading to eosinophil-mediated airway injury. Irrespective of the underlying cause of asthma, much of the symptomatology results from the release of a wide range of biologically active molecules (mediators) with effects on airway smooth muscle, the microvasculature and nerves. For convenience these mediators can be divided into those released from primary effector cells and those secondary to the stimulation of other airway cells. The mast cell and eosinophil are thought to be the most important sources of autacoid mediators (i.e. those that have an effect distant from their site of release) although other cells, including monocytes and platelets, may contribute to the mediator pool in chronic forms of the disease. It seems reasonable to consider mast cells and eosinophils first and then those cells that are considered to orchestrate the inflammatory response.

Mast cells

Mast cells have long been known to play a key role in allergic tissue responses.

(1) They have a key role in allergic tissue responses by releasing bronchoconstrictors, such as histamine, prostaglandin D_2 (PGD_2) and leukotriene C_4 (LTC_4).
(2) They are derived from bone marrow precursor mononuclear cells in the tissue locality where they eventually reside.
(3) The differentiation/maturation of mucosal mast cells requires mast cell growth factors, such as stem cell factor (c-kit ligand) produced by mesenchymal cells including fibroblasts.
(4) There are two types of mast cell, differentiated on the basis of their neutral protease content: one found predominantly at mucosal sites containing tryptase alone (MC_T); and the other also containing chymase and carboxypeptidase A in connective tissue (MC_{TC}).
(5) The MC_T cell is thought to be the more important in asthma.
(6) Full maturation requires additional factors, some of which are produced by lymphocytes.

Increased concentrations of mast cell mediators are recovered from the airways of asthmatics by bronchoalveolar lavage (BAL). In the presence of specific allergen, mast cells in asthma are activated for mediator secretion by the cross linkage of IgE bound to high affinity receptors expressed on the cell surface. This sets into train a series of membrane and intracellular biochemical events that culminate in the release of intracellular calcium from microsomal stores, and the activation of protein kinases that initiate non-cytotoxic degranulation and the activation of phospholipases for the generation of the newly formed mediators (prostanoids, leukotrienes and platelet-activating factor). Once activated, mediator secretion occurs rapidly and explains the acute bronchoconstriction characteristic of acute allergen exposure.

The mast cell in asthma is also sensitive to other stimuli. It is widely thought that asthma provoked by exercise occurs through mast cell activation triggered by the hypertonic airway lining fluid (Makker & Holgate 1994). Hypertonicity results from increased water loss from the airway to condition the inspired air to body temperature and full humidity. In asthmatic but not in normal airways mast cells will respond to other stimuli including inhaled hypotonic aerosols, adenosine and, in susceptible subjects, non-steroidal, anti-inflammatory drugs.

Allergen provocation has frequently been used as a laboratory model of asthma, not so much because of the early bronchoconstrictor response, but because many patients also experience a second wave of bronchoconstriction, referred to as the late asthmatic reaction (LAR) (Pepys 1973). In being accompanied by an increase in airway responsiveness to a wide variety of stimuli, such as histamine, methacholine and cold air, the LAR is a particularly interesting model which is considered to be closer to clinical asthma than the early reaction. During the LAR, measurements of BAL and bronchial mucosal biopsy at different time points during evolution and recovery (2–24 h) shows that:

(1) it is dependent on the recruitment of leukocytes from the microvasculature (neutrophils at 1–6 h, eosinophils at 3–24 h);
(2) neutrophils and eosinophils are recruited following the sequential up-regulation of molecules that enhance adhesion of leukocytes to vascular endothelial cells; and
(3) endothelial adhesion molecules interact with specific receptors on the surface of passing leukocytes, resulting initially in rolling of the cells along the inside of the capillary walls, followed by tethering and cell activation.

Recent work suggests that mast cells are also an important source of cytokines — such as interleukin (IL)-4, IL-5, IL-6, IL-8 and granulocyte macrophage colony-stimulating factor (GM-CSF) (Bradding et al 1993) — that are important in the up-regulation of vascular adhesion molecules and the subsequent recruitment and activation of eosinophils (Casale et al 1996). With IgE triggering, these cells not only secrete preformed cytokines along with the more traditional mast cell products, but also produce newly formed cytokines which, in the case of IL-5 and tumour necrosis factor α (TNF-α), may persist for up to 72 h post-challenge (Okayama et al 1995, 1997). Acting in concert with other mast cell products, including the neutral protease tryptase, these cytokines most likely account for a major component of the LAR (Montefort et al 1994a). At the later time points the recruitment and activation of T helper (Th2)-type cells become increasingly important (Robinson et al 1993a). These mechanisms help explain the marked attenuation of antigen-induced late phase inflammatory responses in sensitized mice that are genetically mast cell deficient (Galli & Costa 1995).

Eosinophils

Although eosinophils at one time were thought to be protective in the allergic inflammatory response, they are now considered to be the cells that mediate much of the pathology and disordered airway function which characterizes atopic and non-atopic asthma (Gleich 1996).

Of the proteins secreted by eosinophils, major basic protein (MBP) (Frigas et al 1980) and eosinophil cationic protein (ECP) (Okayama et al 1995) seem particularly active in rendering the epithelium more fragile and unstable. Eosinophil-derived neurotoxin destroys ribonucleic acid, while eosinophil peroxidase is a prodigious generator of active free radicals (Ayars et al 1989). The mechanisms through which recruited eosinophils lead to epithelial damage in asthma are probably multiple. In addition to the direct cytotoxic effects of granule proteins on epithelial integrity, these cells also cause a non-cytotoxic loss of adhesion between the columnar (suprabasal) and basal cells of the epithelium (Montefort et al 1992a), probably due to a targeted attack on desmosomes and tight junctions, the adhesion structures that are largely responsible for maintaining epithelial integrity (Montefort et al 1992b). Explant and chamber studies indicate that eosinophils must enter into cell–cell contact with epithelial cells, probably involving an interaction between intercellular adhesion molecule (ICAM)-1 expressed on the surface of the eosinophil cell and a complementary ligand, called lymphocyte function antigen (LFA)-1, on the surface of the eosinophil (Herbert et al 1993). Chemokine production by epithelial cells also seems important in directing transepithelial leukocyte migration (Caralan & Casale 1996). In addition to releasing arginine-rich proteins with the capacity to neutralize heparin and heparan cell matrix proteoglycans, eosinophils also release a 92 kDa metalloprotease (MMP-9) with broad activity against proteins of the intercellular matrix, including epithelial adhesion proteins.

Although IL-5 plays a key role in eosinophil recruitment (Egan et al 1996), the mechanisms responsible for activating eosinophils in asthma are not well understood. Although they express a wide range of cell surface receptors, the precise process by which the eosinophil mediates tissue damage in asthma remains speculative. Priming of eosinophils for mediator secretion is important and results in a reduction in the threshold at which the cell responds to a range of activating stimuli. Cytokines such as IL-5 and GM-CSF seem particularly active in this regard and also prolong eosinophil survival by inhibiting programmed cell death (apoptosis) (Robinson et al 1993b, Wooley et al 1996). Chemokines are also important in eosinophil chemoattraction and priming, although they do not prolong eosinophil survival. A compelling hypothesis which is emerging is that IL-5, released from the airway cells into the circulation, recruits a population of eosinophils from the bone marrow which, when attracted into the lung, are especially susceptible to the chemoattractant properties of chemokines which then serve to direct their migration within the airways (Denburg 1996). Recent work also suggests that chemokines can induce eosinophils to generate their own cytokines, specifically IL-3, IL-5 and GM-CSF, which further prolong cell survival in an autocrine fashion.

Orchestration of airway inflammation: the role of T lymphocytes

Although it appears that all forms of asthma are characterized by mast cell- and eosinophil-mediated inflammation, it has become increasingly clear that the mucosal immune system, and particularly the T lymphocyte, plays a key role in orchestrating this inflammatory response (Anderson & Coyle 1994). Most asthma in later childhood and in adults occurs in association with atopy, which is defined as the predisposition to generate IgE against common environmental (usually airborne) allergens. Of particular relevance are allergens derived from domestic dust mites (*Dermatophagoides* sp), proteins from domestic pets (especially cats), cockroaches, fungal antigens and pollens. To initiate the synthesis of allergen-specific IgE, the subject must first become sensitized, which involves the participation of cells that recognize, process and in turn present allergens to the T cell effector arm of the immune system. For domestic allergens this may occur early in life (Sporik et al 1990) and it possibly starts prenatally (Warner et al 1994, 1996), whereas occupational asthma of later onset is initiated by exposure to the offending agent(s) in the work place. In those genetically at risk of developing allergic diseases such as asthma and eczema circulating allergen-specific T cells can be detected at birth. These cells are thought to take up residence in the specific organ and begin to express the disease phenotype over the following six to 12 months. Such findings indicate that the mother is able to present antigens to her offspring via the placenta; for occupational antigens, initial exposure is likely to occur through the lung. Additional factors may also be important in this initial sensitization, including the capacity of the fetus to generate IL-4, the cytokine responsible for the maturation of the T cell population associated with allergy (to become the so-called Th2 type) and the isotype switching of B cells from IgM to IgE synthesis. During development the amnion is a particularly important source of IL-4, and secretion into the amniotic fluid may be an important determinant of prenatal programming. Once sensitized, the level of allergen exposure during the first year or so of life is a major determinant of the later development of asthma.

Amplification of the inflammatory response

Allergen-specific responses occur locally in the airways through the recruitment of a network of professional antigen-presenting cells called dendritic cells. These processes are summarized below.

(1) Dendritic cells develop from mononuclear cell precursors in the presence of IL-3, stem cell factor and GM-CSF.
(2) Dendritic cells present antigen peptides to naive T cells in local lymphoid tissue (thereby sensitizing them).
(3) The clonal expansion of naive T cells directed towards the Th2 phenotype occurs in the presence of IL-4.
(4) Antigen presentation involves: intracellular processing of the allergen to peptides; presentation to the T cell receptor of peptides in the groove of major histocompatibility complex class II (HLA) molecules on the surface of the presenting cells; and engagement of a number of accessory adhesion molecules.

(5) Once committed and having returned to the airway mucosa, allergen-specific Th2-like cells respond to challenge with the generation of a number of cytokines encoded in the IL-4 cluster on the long arm of chromosome 5. The switching of B lymphocytes from IgM to IgE synthesis requires a cognate interaction with the T cells, contact between accessory molecules and the presence of specific cytokines (IL-4 or IL-13).

Once sensitized, the asthmatic airway will respond to further allergen exposure by rapid recruitment and expansion of the T cell population with elaboration of cytokines encoded in the IL-4 gene cluster (Robinson et al 1993b). Molecular-based techniques, including *in situ* hybridization, reverse transcriptase (RT)-PCR and direct cytokine measurement from T cell clones, indicate the importance of this cell type in generating cytokines that support the inflammatory response in asthma.

In occupational asthma and in late onset 'intrinsic' (non-allergic) asthma, $CD8^+$ T cells are also an important source of IL-4 and IL-5. Virus infection, an important cause of asthma exacerbations, also leads to expansion of both $CD4^+$ and $CD8^+$ T cells exhibiting the Th2-like phenotype (Fraenkel et al 1995, Coyle et al 1995).

Mechanisms of asthma severity and chronicity

There is overwhelming evidence to indicate that airway inflammation underlies the pathophysiology of asthma; however, its relationship to disease severity is less clear. Although the presence of eosinophils in the sputum, a persistent BAL fluid and blood eosinophilia with increased circulating levels of eosinophil granule proteins broadly relate to disease severity, these measures are too variable to provide clinically useful markers to predict the level of airway inflammation.

The selective recruitment of cells from the microvasculature with accompanying activation and enhanced survival underlies the ongoing inflammation in severe and chronic disease. Of considerable significance is the observation that asthma can be transferred to a non-asthmatic recipient by lung transplantation, even in the presence of sufficient immunosuppression to prevent lung rejection (Corris & Dart 1993). Since transplantation of normal lung into a previously asthmatic recipient fails to initiate asthma, it is likely that local factors in the lung, possibly immunological, are important in maintaining the chronic asthma phenotype.

Corticosteroids are highly effective anti-asthma drugs that act to reduce the inflammatory response. However, there are many patients in whom only partial relief is achieved, even when these drugs are taken by inhalation (and orally) at high doses. In a well-defined population of 'corticosteroid-resistant' asthmatics with preservation of β2-agonist bronchodilatation, abnormalities of circulating monocyte and T cell cytokine function have been described (Barnes & Adcock 1995). However, such patients represent only a minority of the 'difficult to control' asthmatics and the mechanisms underpinning corticosteroid refractoriness are probably multiple.

The majority of asthma occurs in association with atopy, the predisposition to generate IgE to common environmental allergens through a Th2 cell-dependent mechanism. In severe disease ongoing allergen-specific IgE production provides a rationale for allergen avoidance and high altitude treatment. However, environmental interventions have no effect on non-allergic asthma and many patients with severe atopic disease only partially or fail to respond (Djukanović et al 1995). Irrespective of atopy, powerful epidemiological studies have linked the total serum IgE to the presence of asthma and the level to disease progression (Burrows et al 1989). Moreover, there have been several long-term studies demonstrating that poorly controlled asthma progresses to an increasingly irreversible disorder (Peat et al 1987). Although airway inflammation has recently become accepted as an obligatory feature of asthma, increasingly, as with other chronic inflammatory diseases, tissue remodelling must now be considered as an integral component of the asthma phenotype.

It follows that the chronicity of asthma results from the dysregulation of cytokine networks leading to persistent inflammation, in structurally altered airways, which becomes refractory to treatment. Responsibility for disease progression does not lie with any single cellular element but embraces T and B cells, mast cells, eosinophils, endothelial cells, epithelial cells and myofibroblasts, which act co-operatively and also with the structural elements of the airway, including smooth muscle, matrix, microvasculature and nerves, leading to the variable phenotype characteristic of severe disease. This integrated view of asthma as a chronic disease of ongoing inflammation and repair leads us to incriminate a number of effector cells.

T cell activation and expression of mRNA for cytokines is a common feature of all types of asthma. In mild disease the level of T cell involvement in the airways is relatively low. The mast cell, with its capacity to respond to allergen provocation with mediator and cytokine release, alone is capable of recruiting and activating neutrophils and eosinophils. This might help explain why cromone-like drugs are more efficacious at the milder end of the asthma spectrum and in children with early disease (Barnes et al 1995). By contrast, a biopsy and lavage study of patients with severe asthma poorly controlled with corticosteroids reveals a vigorous ongoing T cell- and eosinophil-mediated inflammatory response in the absence of any known provoking factors (Djukanović et al 1995). Although in atopic asthmatics 24 h after allergen exposure there occurs a marked increase in IL-5 transcription in relation to T cell recruitment and activation (which supports the Th2 hypothesis) (Robinson et al 1993a,b, Shute et al 1995), in asthmatics of widely differing disease severity cloning studies have shown that airway T cells lavaged from the surface of the airways exhibit considerable heterogeneity of cytokine expression (Bodey et al 1997). At baseline, T cells from atopic asthmatic airways show strong expression of mRNA for IL-13, GM-CSF, γ-interferon (IFN-γ) and TNF-α; whereas upon allergen exposure there occurs a cytokine shift in favour of IL-3, IL-4, IL-5 and IL-13, and away from IFN-γ and TNF-α. Those factors that are responsible for the continuous T cell-mediated inflammation at baseline may be different from those brought into play on exposure to allergen. To explore this further, we have used a technique to evaluate the cytokine protein production by airway T cells stimulated with ionomycin and 12-O-tetradecanoylphorbol 13-acetate (TPA), in which monensin is used to inhibit Golgi-mediated cytokine transport, allowing flow cytometry to be used to quantify the population of CD3$^+$ cells expressing a particular cytokine (Jung et al 1993). Even in clinically active asthma, 60% of asthmatic BAL T cells produced IFN-γ and/or IL-2, whereas only 2–4% of the cells accumulated IL-4 or IL-5, an observation that was not found in blood T cells obtained from the same patients (Krug et al 1996). It is becoming clear that, while a Th2-like response explains the induction and some of the inflammatory components of asthma (especially that associated with allergen exposure), little is known about T cell responses influencing disease chronicity in asthma and how they may escape corticosteroid suppression.

The role of IgE in chronic asthma

Although the ability of IgE to bind to mast cells and to mediate antigen-induced degranulation is clear, its role in maintaining chronic asthma is not fully understood. However, patients with chronic disease have raised levels of allergen-specific IgE in serum, and IgE, particularly in complex form, is capable of mediating the release of a range of cytokines via Fc$_\varepsilon$R1, and Fc$_\varepsilon$R2 (CD23). Since both high and low affinity IgE receptors are up-regulated on eosinophils, mast cells, macrophages and dendritic cells in asthma, the opportunities for IgE to contribute to local inflammatory processes are numerous (Humbert et al 1996, Tunan-de-Lara et al 1996).

The question raised is whether the IgE is specific for allergens, or whether the spectrum of recognition widens during disease progression to include viral antigens and autoantigens, as recently described in chronic urticaria (Hide et al 1993). Past analysis of IgE specificities has been limited to serological investigation of mixed IgE but the new technology will allow the investigation of individual IgE molecules. It is also feasible to compare the molecular range of IgE found at the local sites of inflammation to that in the blood. Methods for amplifying the variable region genes used to encode IgE have been developed and already reveal an unexpected asymmetric usage of immunoglobulin V_H genes in patients with asthma (Snow et al 1995). In the inflammatory environment, where there may be local release of cytokines possibly exacerbated by viral infection, it is conceivable that autoantigens may be released. IgE antibodies could therefore be generated against allergens, viral antigens or autoantigens. The high levels of IgE characteristic of chronic asthma could also induce autoantibodies against IgE itself (Shakib et al 1994). These could have an additional role in inflammation, either by cross-linking IgE on the mast cell surface or by generating immune complexes that stimulate mononuclear phagocytes to release cytokines.

Leukocyte recruitment and the role of the microvasculature

Exposure of the asthmatic airway to a wide variety of environmental stimuli results in the recruitment of leukocytes to the airways involving a well co-ordinated and dynamic sequence of events in which several cell adhesion molecules and chemotactic cytokines play a role (Lawrence & Springer 1991). *In vitro* lines of evidence predict a multistep model involving: (1) initial low affinity selectin molecule-dependent 'vascular rolling' (margination); (2) leukocyte activation by endothelial-derived chemoattractants (e.g. IL-8, monocyte chemotactic peptide [MCP]-1); and (3) a transition to β-integrin-dependent high affinity leukocyte adherence cytokine-mediated up-regulation of the Ig superfamily of adhesion proteins, ICAMs and vascular cell adhesion molecules (VCAMs); followed by (4) transendothelial migration involving combinations of cell adhesion molecules.

Within 6 h of segmental allergen challenge of sensitized asthmatic airways, there occurs marked endothelial up-regulation of E-selectin and ICAM-1 accompanied by an influx of LFA-1[+] leukocytes comprising neutrophils and eosinophils (Montefort et al 1994a, Pilewski & Albeda 1995). By 24 h there is a marked increase in activated T cells and eosinophils present in BAL with variable expression of VCAM-1, an adhesion molecule not normally constitutively expressed. Because leukocyte recruitment occurs so rapidly, the first step most probably involves up-regulation of P-selectin (by histamine) and E-selectin (by TNF-α) released from activated mast cells which mediate rolling through a lectin interaction with the ligand sialyl Lewis X on the leukocyte surface (Bochner et al 1994). The IgE-dependent secretion of newly formed TNF-α increases ICAM-1 expression (Okayama et al 1997), while its interaction with mast cell-derived IL-4 induces and stabilizes VCAM-1 expression (Galli & Costa 1995). These cell adhesion molecules interact with the integrins LFA-1 and very late antigen (VLA)-4 to recruit T cells and eosinophils selectively. Immunohistochemical studies on biopsies from severe asthmatics have revealed a marked up-regulation of ICAM-1 and VCAM-1 in the absence of allergen exposure and while they are taking high doses of corticosteroids. Thus, in severe asthma there is continued expression of endothelial cell adhesion molecules to promote ongoing leukocyte recruitment and activation. Such a mechanism would explain the finding of elevated circulating and BAL levels of soluble cell adhesion molecules in symptomatic asthma (Montefort et al 1994b).

The expression of E-selectin, ICAM-1 and VCAM-1 is controlled by the nuclear transcription factor NFκB, a p50/p65 heterodimer of which both subunits contain the 300 amino acid NFκB/rel/dorsal (NRD) domain. The N-terminal end of the NRD domain is involved in specific binding to DNA, whereas the C-terminal end contains the nuclear localization signal (NLS), a cluster of positively charged amino acids necessary for translocation of NFκB across the nuclear membrane (Manning et al 1994). NFκB binds to the decameric DNA sequence $5'$- $GG^A_GNN^C_T{}^C_TCC$-$3'$ found in the promoters of a number of genes that are up-regulated in inflammation, especially in those that encode the cell adhesion molecules and specific cytokines (IL-2, IL-6, IL-8, members of the IL-4 gene cluster and TNF-α). Within the E-selectin promoter there are three closely spaced binding sites for NFκB clustered within a 40 bp segment and two additional regulatory elements, NF-ELAM-1 and NF-ELAM-2 (nuclear factors for the endothelial leukocyte adhesion molecule). Following cytokine exposure, all three NFκB sites are essential for maximal promoter activity. The promoter for the human ICAM-1 gene contains binding sites for Sp1, AP-1, AP-2, AP-3, NFκB and a putative silencer, whereas NFκB alone mediates VCAM-1 expression.

A range of factors have been shown to initiate activation of NFκB, including TNF-α, IL-1, IL-2, leukotriene B_4 (LTB$_4$) and viruses. Endothelial cells express a cytoplasmic inhibitor of NFκB activity, IκBα, the over expression of which inhibits E-selectin and VCAM-1 transcription. IκBα binds selectively to NFκB heterodimers and prevents its nuclear uptake by binding to the NLS (Manning et al 1994). A pathway of NFκB activation has been proposed that sequentially involves phosphorylation of IκBα, followed by its specific chymotryptic proteolysis, which reveals the previously masked NLS site and nuclear translocation signal (Baeurle & Henkel 1994). The activation is only transient as NFκB is also able to induce IκBα mRNA transcription resulting in re-accumulation of IκBα and its functional inhibition of cytoplasmic NFκB. Reactive oxygen intermediates serve as second messengers of NFκB activation, redox changes leading to activation of chymotryptic IκBα protease through modification of intracellular serpins (Manning et al 1994, Baeurle 1991). These intracellular events provide unique opportunities to investigate NFκB activation in severe asthma as it relates to increased cell adhesion molecules and cytokine expression, and to investigate pharmacological intervention with potential therapeutic significance. Activation of NFκB also provides one explanation for how air pollutant oxidants (O_3, NO_x, particulates, cigarette smoke) and respiratory viruses may exacerbate asthma by enhancing ongoing inflammatory pathways.

The bronchial epithelium

The bronchial epithelium has been viewed traditionally as a passive barrier that serves as a target for the inflammatory response. However, it is also an important source of inflammatory mediators including arachidonic acid products, endothelin-1, nitric oxide (NO) and cytokines which, along with altered adhesion molecule expression, participate directly in inflammatory cell recruitment and activation.

Arachidonic acid metabolism

The epithelium is a major source of 15-HETE (15-hydroxy-6,8,11,14-eicosatetraenioc acid) and, although expression of immunoreactive 15-lypoxygenase is unaltered (Bradding et al 1995), others have shown increased enzyme activity in severe disease (Shannon et al 1993). Although 15-HETE and 15-dihydroxy acids exhibit some mediator functions, more active oxidate products of arachidonic acid are the prostaglandins PGE_2 and PGF_{2a} with their opposite actions in bronchial smooth muscle. The epithelial expression of the inducible form of cyclooxygenase (Cox2) is enhanced over the constitutive form (Cox1), a change that is suppressed by corticosteroid treatment in parallel with their clinical efficacy (Springall et al 1995). Over expression of Cox2, NO and ET-1 molecules under the control of NFκB persists in asthma poorly controlled with corticosteroids.

Endothelin

Human endothelin comprises three structurally distinct 21 amino acid peptides, ET-1, ET-2 and ET-3, encoded on separate genes. In addition to its potent vasoconstricting property, ET-1 is a powerful spasmogen of airway smooth muscle mediated through the ETB receptor subtype (Mattoli et al 1990). ET-1 is also a mitogen for airway smooth muscle and in fibroblasts it is a chemoattractant, is mitogenic and provides an activating signal for collagen synthesis, again mediated through ETB receptors (Springall et al 1991). ET-1 induces collagenase production and is important in myofibroblast-mediated contraction of granulation tissue.

Human bronchial epithelial cells cultured from the airways of asthmatics secrete increased amounts of ET-1, which is sensitive to inhibition with corticosteroids (Mattoli et al 1990). ET-1 immunoreactivity *in vivo* is also increased in the epithelium (Springall et al 1991). In BAL, levels of ET-1 are increased in proportion to the resting level of airflow obstruction (Redington et al 1995a). The importance of ET-1 as a novel bronchoconstrictor is revealed by its capacity to reduce FEV_1 (forced expiratory volume in one second) by $\geqslant 20\%$ of baseline at inhaled concentrations of 10^{-10}–10^{-12} M. With effective corticosteroid treatment of asthma, both lavage ET-1 levels and ET-1 expression in the epithelium return to those found in normal subjects.

Nitric oxide

NO is a short-lived, highly soluble free radical that plays a major role in cell–cell communication. It is generated from L-arginine by NO synthase which exists in both constitutive and inducible isoforms (iNOS). Both enzymes require NADPH as a co-factor and are inhibited by L-arginine analogues such as N^G-nitro-L-arginine (L-NNA) and N^G-monomethyl-L-arginine (L-NMMA). The inducible form is also selectively inhibited by aminoguanidine (Barnes & Liew 1995), and it immunolocalizes strongly to the epithelium in bronchial biopsies from asthmatics but only rarely in those from normal controls (Hamid et al 1993). Consistent with enhanced NO generation in airway mucosal inflammation is the increased NO detected in exhaled air active asthma and rhinitis (Alving et al 1993, Kharitonov et al 1994). *In vitro* iNOS is induced in response to IFN-γ, IL-1β and TNF-α and it is inhibited by corticosteroids (Barnes & Liew 1995). In corticosteroid-responsive asthma iNOS in the epithelium is down-regulated and associated with a reduction in exhaled NO. Whilst NO produced by iNOS is a powerful vasodilator at nanomolar concentrations, it is also cytotoxic because it forms peroxynitrate and hydroxyl radicals and nitrosylating key mitochondrial enzymes. In severe asthma the epithelium is likely to be a major source of toxic levels of NO and as such may provide a novel surrogate marker of disease activity and response to treatment (Barnes 1995).

Cytokines

Human bronchial epithelial cells *in vitro* constitutively synthesize and release IL-1β, IL-6, IL-8 and GM-CSF, with greatly enhanced production occurring on exposure to IL-1β or TNF-α. Enhanced release of these cytokines has also been reported in asthmatic epithelial cells *in vitro*. Application of immunohistochemistry shows that the bronchial epithelium in asthma is a particularly rich source of IL-1β, IL-8 and GM-CSF.

IL-8, a member of the α(C-x-C) chemokine family, is particularly important in the expression of chronic and severe disease, although it is usually regarded as a neutrophil chemoattractant. IL-8 can induce human eosinophils from asthmatic subjects to secrete IL-3, IL-5 and GM-CSF. In a nasal polyp explant model of chronic mucosal inflammation, IL-8 and GM-CSF are the dominant cytokines produced (Park et al 1995).

In bronchial biopsies from asthmatics and in the peripheral circulation IL-8 binds strongly to IgA (Shute et al 1995). Despite clear immunostaining for IL-8 in the epithelium, no free IL-8 can be detected in detergent-extracted homogenates; however, IL-8–IgA complexes can be readily detected with significantly more being presented in allergic asthmatics. In patients with chronic severe asthma, both free and complexed forms of IL-8 are present in mucosal tissue, serum and sputum. Thus, although IL-8 can be formed by many cells in asthma, the bronchial epithelium seems to be the major site of production and concentration of this chemokine. Of particular interest is the finding that IL-8 co-localizes with secretory IgA in the epithelium. Secretory but not serum IgA is able to up-regulate the eosinophil chemotactic response to IL-8, reaching optimum at 10^{-10} M; whereas, under the same conditions, the neutrophil response is inhibited (Shute et al 1995). IL-8 is also known to complex carbohydrate residues of proteoglycans and glycoproteins, resulting in greatly enhanced eosinophil-specific properties. These include the secretory piece of IgA containing up to 20% N-linked oligosaccharides and proteoglycans, such as the granule products of mast cells and eosinophils, and CD44, which is expressed in greater amounts in the asthmatic epithelium (Peroni et al 1997, Lackie et al 1997). We hypothesize that IL-8 binding regulates the activity of and changes the target cell specificity for this cytokine, rendering it a potent attractant and activator of eosinophils.

Recently, a range of other chemokines belonging to the C-C class have been shown to be generated by human bronchial epithelial cells including RANTES (acronym for regulated on activation, normal T expressed and presumably secreted), MCP-1, macrophage inflammatory protein (MIP)-1α (Berkmann et al 1996) and a recently

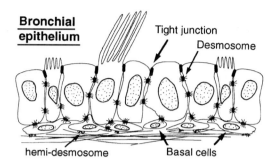

Bronchial epithelium

Tight junction

Desmosome

hemi-desmosome   Basal cells

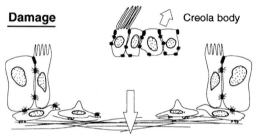

Damage   Creola body

Barrier loss: Macromolecular permeability +++

First response

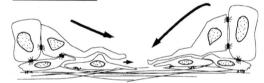

Interim repair

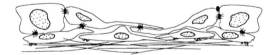

Differentiation

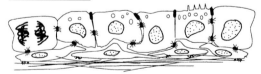

recognized eosinophil chemoattractant called eotaxin (Rothenburg et al 1996). Together with IL-5 and GM-CSF, these locally acting molecules will further promote eosinophil recruitment and activation at the mucosal surface (Saetta et al 1996). With allergen exposure BAL levels of RANTES, MCP-1 and MIP-1α markedly increase, suggesting that they are released selectively (Alam et al 1994, Holgate et al 1997). T cells are an important source of RANTES and MIP-1α but other cells including epithelial, endothelial, mast cells and eosinophils are other sources (Teran & Davies 1996).

Epithelial cell biology

Epithelial damage is a key feature of asthma, with the extent of damage being related to disease (Laitinen et al 1985). We have provided evidence that the major structural sites of damage are between the columnar and basal cells, and adjacent columnar cells, implicating disruption to the desmosomes (Montefort et al 1993a,b). The cause of increased epithelial dysfunction in asthma is not understood, although the arginine-rich basic proteins of the eosinophil and active radicals are considered to be important (Persson et al 1996). The level of damage may reflect either increased fragility or increased insult to the epithelium. To understand the importance of epithelial disruption in severe and chronic disease, we need to understand the processes of damage, repair and regeneration of the epithelium, and which normal functions of the epithelium are compromised. The following steps occur in epithelial damage and repair (Fig. 1).

(1) Immediate damage: selective cell loss due to injury with loss of barrier function.
(2) Immediate response: epithelial cells adjacent to areas of damage reduce cell substrate adhesion, increase cell migration and form a temporary squamous barrier.
(3) Proliferative response: division, differentiation and remodelling lead to re-formation of fully functional differentiated epithelium.
(4) Ongoing damage: asthma occurring during the above processes may further compromise epithelial integrity. Lack of appropriate down-regulation of the normal response may produce a similar effect.

FIG. 1.   (*opposite*) Bronchial epithelium consists of two cell layers: basal and columnar. Cells are linked by impermeable tight junctions at the luminal surface and desmosomes between cells. Hemidesmosomes link basal cells to the basement membrane (first panel). After epithelial damage, groups of epithelial cells are released and the barrier function of the epithelium is compromised (second panel). The first response of the remaining epithelial cells is to migrate into the damaged area (third panel) to provide an interim squamous barrier consisting of poorly differentiated and highly spread cells (fourth panel). After this interim barrier is formed, cells start to divide and differentiate to replace the cells which have been lost, and they return to the taller columnar phenotype (fifth panel).

Eosinophil–epithelial interactions

Cytokines

Like mast cells, eosinophils are a newly recognized source of cytokines (including IL-3, IL-4, IL-5, GM-CSF, IL-6, IL-8, TNF-α, MIP-1α, TGF (transforming growth factor)-α and TGF-β. Eosinophils exposed to these cytokines (especially IL-3, IL-5 and GM-CSF) have their life expectancy extended from days to weeks and are also more responsive to chemoattractant- and mediator-secreting stimuli. Additionally, since the three eosinophilopoietins antagonize the accelerating effect of corticosteroids on eosinophil apoptosis, their sustained production would serve to render the cells functionally 'corticosteroid resistant'. A plausible hypothesis is that the expression of eosinophil survival cytokines is increased in bronchial tissue in proportion to disease severity and that the intracellular cytokines are presented as a complex with proteoglycans of the eosinophil granules similar to the role of mast cell heparin in presenting IL-4.

Although it is likely that enzymes of the 5-lipoxygenase pathway are up-regulated in eosinophils in asthma, this has not yet been thoroughly investigated. However, increasing evidence exists for this in non-steroid anti-inflammatory drug (NSAID)-induced asthma, particularly involving LTC$_4$ synthase (Cowburn et al 1997). If accompanied by a decrease in PGE$_2$ production then an important autocrine cAMP-mediated inhibitory effect of this mediator on a number of eosinophil responses is removed, including the secretory IgA-induced release of basic granule proteins and generation of cytokines. Eosinophils in culture secrete PGE$_2$, which is increased in the presence of platelet-activating factor or IL-5 (Kroegel & Matthys 1993). Over 90% of the PGE$_2$ is released into the fluid phase and available for mediating negative feedback. Removal of PGE$_2$ inhibition of mast cell and eosinophil LTC$_4$ production has been suggested to occur in NSAID-induced asthma (Tenor et al 1996).

Eosinophils isolated from the airways are spontaneously cytotoxic towards alveolar epithelial cells. However, in the airways of asthmatics viable columnar cells are shed from the basal cells, which themselves remain firmly fixed to the basement membrane via hemidesmosome and fibronectin–integrin adhesion proteins. Using a bovine bronchial epithelial explant, activated eosinophils mediate epithelial detachment via a cognate interaction involving ICAM-1 and the subsequent release of metalloendoproteases, oxidants and arginine-rich proteins (Herbert et al 1993).

Metalloproteases

In BAL from patients with asthma we have shown increased concentrations of the 92 kDa metalloproteinase (MMP-9, gelatinase B) (Shute et al 1997a). In its active form, MMP-9 has to undergo cleavage into a 68 kDa component, a reaction brought about by the rich protease environment of the inflamed airways. Eosinophils are an important source of MMP-9, which has a broad substrate specificity in being able to degrade both basement membrane collagen type IV and interstitial matrix molecules

(Stahle-Backdahl & Parks 1993). Because of the extensive eosinophil infiltrate in severe asthma, this enzyme is important in infiltrating cell migration and matrix protein remodelling. MMP-9, along with the other metalloproteases, are inhibited by a specific tissue inhibitor (TIMP-1) which is produced by the bronchial epithelium and eosinophils (Shute et al 1997b).

Oxidants

The tissue-damaging effect of the products of eosinophil peroxidase are indicated by the effectiveness of antioxidants to inhibit eosinophil-mediated injury to lung epithelial cells and interstitial matrix *in vitro*. Eosinophil peroxidase is released asynchronously with ECP or MBP and, as with many highly charged proteins, remains largely cell associated. A closely coupled mechanism would also serve to exclude naturally occurring antioxidants, such as reduced glutathione, vitamins E and C or albumin, and concentrate the delivery of the oxidant injury.

Basic proteins

Considerable evidence exists for the disruptive effects of eosinophil cationic proteins (MBP, ECP, eosinophil-derived neurotoxin) on epithelial integrity in asthma. Their extreme cationicity renders matrix proteoglycans as susceptible targets. A number of proinflammatory cytokines, including IL-4, IL-8, IFN-γ and fibroblast growth factor (FGF)-2 are tightly bound to side chains of highly O-sulfated proteoglycans, which stabilize the cytokine, localize its activity and determine its specificity. IL-8 and IFN-γ localize to interepithelial clefts on account of their association with the glycosaminoglycans of CD44 and the N-sulfated carbohydrate moieties of secretory IgA. Similarly, IL-4 binds to heparan on mast cells, while FGF2 binds to heparan sulfate in basement membranes and TGF-α to decarin. Levels of IL-8, TGF-β and FGF2 are elevated in BAL from asthmatics with further increases occurring with allergen challenge (Teran et al 1996, Redington et al 1995b,c). An interaction of the eosinophil basic proteins with cytokine binding sites on matrix molecules would result in release of free cytokine so that a wider range of activity is achieved in severe disease.

Mast cell–epithelial interactions

In mucosal biopsies mast cells aggregate both within the epithelium and in relation to the connective tissue elements of the basement membrane and associated myofibroblasts. When assessed by flow cytometry on a human epithelial cell line (H292), human mast cell tryptase up-regulates the cell surface expression of ICAM-1 to a similar extent as TNF-α (Cairns & Walls 1996). A small increase in P-selectin and an apparent down-regulation of N-cadherin expression have also been observed as the activity of tryptase is increased. Tryptase also stimulates DNA synthesis in epithelial cells, as measured by ^{3}H-thymidine incorporation, and produces a dose-dependent release of IL-8. Inhibition of tryptase with leupeptin or benzamidine-HCl prevented these actions, indicating an obligatory requirement for the enzyme's catalytic sites (Cairns & Walls 1996). These observations suggest an important role for mast cells in epithelial repair, in the recruitment of granulocytes and in rendering the lower respiratory tract vulnerable to human rhinovirus infection, since the major type of human rhinovirus utilizes ICAM-1 to gain access to epithelial cells and up-regulates cytokine production (Papi et al 1996).

Epithelial cell–myofibroblast interactions

The apparent thickening of the subepithelial basement membrane in asthma is due to the deposition of collagen types III and V, tenascin and fibronectin being produced by proliferating myofibroblasts and epithelial cells (Brewster et al 1990, Wilson & Li 1997). The presence of tenascin in the lamina reticulosa indicates that this is a site of high matrix turnover and cell migration, towards which both epithelial cells and myofibroblasts contribute. In addition to their capacity to secrete matrix proteins, cultures of human subepithelial bronchial myofibroblasts produce GM-CSF, IL-6, IL-8 and stem cell factor constitutively, and the supernatant from cultures greatly extend eosinophil survival (Zhang et al 1996). GM-CSF transcription is greatly up-regulated in the presence of TNF-α, and it is accompanied by the secretion of GM-CSF, which accounts for the majority of the eosinophil survival capacity of the supernatants. These findings suggest that human myofibroblasts establish close contact with eosinophils and mast cells and as such play a critical role in maintaining the mucosal inflammation of chronic disease.

An integrated model of asthma

The complexities of human asthma as an inflammatory disorder are only just being appreciated. We have passed through the eras of believing that the disease is purely one of smooth muscle, mast cells, eosinophils or T cells to a picture where all these and other cells are involved in a co-operative fashion. Figure 2 attempts to demonstrate this by showing a close interrelationship between those factors responsible for inflammatory events and those involved in repair. Implicit in this model is an interdependency between the classical cells of inflammation and the formed elements of the airway. Varying contributions from each of these processes provide a rational basis for the variable clinical phenotype (Fig. 3) and responses to therapeutic interventions. This leads to the conclusions arrived at in the various national and international consensus reports on asthma management that, whenever possible, the inflammatory component of asthma should be treated early and effectively. It is equally important to recognize that those factors which may initiate asthma in those at genetic risk from the disease may be different from those which cause chronicity of the inflammatory response and lead to disease progression.

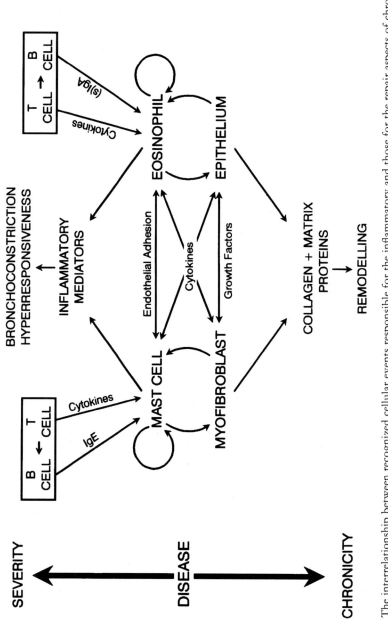

FIG. 2. The interrelationship between recognized cellular events responsible for the inflammatory and those for the repair aspects of chronic asthma.

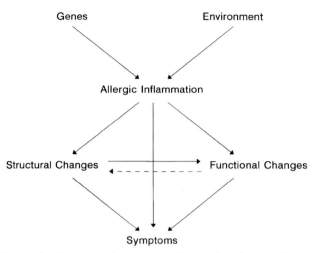

FIG. 3.   The interaction between inflammation and repair in asthma produces varying clinical phenotypes.

Acknowledgements

I thank the British Medical Research Council, the National Asthma Campaign and the British Lung Foundation for supporting the work that underpins this review, and Wendy Couper for help with the preparation of this manuscript.

References

Alam R, York J, Boyars M et al 1994 The involvement of chemokines in bronchial asthma. The detection of mRNA for MCP-1, MCP-3, RANTES and MIP-1α in the lavage fluid. Am J Respir Crit Care Med 149:951A

Alving K, Weitzberg E, Lundberg JM 1993 Increased amount of nitric oxide in exhaled air of asthmatics. Eur Respir J 6:1268–1270

Anderson GP, Coyle AJ 1994 TH2 and 'TH2-like' cells in allergy and asthma: pharmacological properties. Trends Pharmacol Sci 15:324–332

Ayars GH, Altman LC, McManus MM et al 1989 Injurious effect of the eosinophil peroxide-hydrogen peroxide-halide system and major basic protein on human nasal epithelium *in vitro*. Am Rev Respir Dis 140:125–131

Baeurle PA 1991 The inducible factor NFκB: regulation by distinct subunits. Biochem Biophys Acta 1072:63–80

Baeurle PA, Henkel T 1994 Function and activation of NFκB in the immune system. Ann Rev Immunol 12:141–179

Barnes PJ 1995 Nitric oxide and airway disease. Ann Int Med 27:91–97

Barnes PJ, Adcock IM 1995 Steroid-resistant asthma. Q J Med 88:455–468

Barnes PJ, Liew FY 1995 Nitric oxide and asthmatic inflammation. Immunol Today 16:128–130

Barnes PJ, Holgate ST, Laitinen LA, Pauwels R 1995 Asthma mechanisms, determinants of severity and treatment: the role of nedocromil sodium. Report of a Workshop held in Whistler, British Columbia, Canada, 18–19 May 1995. Clin Exp Allergy 25:771–787

Berkmann N, Robichaud A, Krishnan VL et al 1996 Expression of RANTES in human airway epithelial cells: effects of corticosteroids and IL-4, -10 and -13. Immunology 87:599–603

Bochner BS, Sterbinsky SA, Bickel CA, Werfel S, Wein M, Newman W 1994 Differences between human eosinophils and neutrophils in the function and expression of sialic acid containing counter-ligands for E-selectin. J Immunol 152:774–779

Bodey KJ, Semper AE, Redington AE et al 1997 Cytokine profiles of BAL T cells and T cell clones obtained from human asthmatic airways after local allergen challenge. Am J Respir Mol Biol, in press

Bradding P, Feather IH, Wilson S et al 1993 Immunolocalisation of cytokines in the nasal mucosa of normal and perennial rhinitic subjects: the mast cell as a source of IL-4, IL-5 and IL-6 in human allergic mucosal inflammation. J Immunol 151:3853–3865

Bradding P, Redington AE, Djukanović R, Conrad DJ, Holgate ST 1995 15-Lipoxygenase immunoreactivity in normal and asthmatic airways. Am J Respir Crit Care Med 151:1201–1204

Brewster CEP, Howarth PH, Djukanović R et al 1990 Myofibroblasts and subepithelial fibrosis in bronchial asthma. Am Rev Respir Cell Mol Biol 3:507–511

Burrows B, Martinez FD, Halonen M, Barbee RA, Cline MG 1989 Association of asthma with serum IgE levels and skin test reactivity to allergens. N Engl J Med 320:271–277

Cairns JA, Walls AF 1996 Human mast cell tryptase is a mitogen for epithelial cells. Stimulation of IL-8 production and ICAM-1 expression. J Immunol 156:275–283

Caralan EJ, Casale TB 1996 Neutrophil transepithelial migration is dependent upon epithelial characteristics. Am J Respir Cell Mol Biol 15:224–231

Casale TB, Costa JJ, Galli S 1996 TNFα is important in human lung allergic reactions. Am J Respir Cell Mol Biol 15:35–44

Ciba Foundation guest symposium 1959 Terminology, definitions and classification of chronic pulmonary emphysema and related conditions (a report of the conclusions of a Ciba guest symposium). Thorax 14:286–299

Ciba Foundation study group 1971 Identification of asthma. Churchill Livingstone, Edinburgh (Ciba Found study group 38)

Corris PA, Dart JH 1993 Aetiology of asthma: lessons from lung transplantation. Lancet 341:1377–1378

Cowburn AS, Sladek K, Adamek L et al 1997 Over expression of LTC$_4$ synthase in eosinophils accounts for cysteinyl-leukotriene over-production in aspirin-induced asthma. Respir Med, in press

Coyle AJ, Erard F, Bertrand C, Walti S, Pircher H, Le Gros G 1995 Virus-specific CD8$^+$ cells can switch to interleukin-5 production and induce airway eosinophilia. J Exp Med 181:1229–1233

Denburg JA 1996 The inflammatory response. Am J Respir Crit Care Med 153:511–513

Djukanović R, Howarth P, Vrugt B et al 1995 Determinants of asthma severity. Int Arch Allergy Immunol 107:389

Egan RW, Umland SP, Cuss FM, Chapman RW 1996 Biology of interleukin-5 and its relevance to allergic disease. Allergy 51:71–81

Ehrlich P 1879 Beiträge zur kenntnis der granulierten Bindegwebszellen und der eosinophilen leukocyten. Arch Anal Physiol A166

Fraenkel DJ, Bardin PG, Sanderson G, Lampe F, Johnstone SL, Holgate ST 1995 Lower airways inflammatory response during rhinovirus colds in normal and asthmatic subjects. Am J Respir Crit Care Med 151:879–886

Frigas E, Loegering DA, Gleich GJ 1980 Cytotoxic effects of the guinea pig eosinophil major basic protein on tracheal epithelium. Lab Invest 42:35–43

Galli SJ, Costa JJ 1995 Mast cell leukocyte cytokine cascades in allergic inflammation. Allergy 50:851–862

Gleich GJ 1996 Eosinophil granule proteins and bronchial asthma. Allergol Int 45:35–44

Hamid Q, Springall DR, Riveros-Moreno V et al 1993 Induction of nitric oxide synthase in asthma. Lancet 342:1510–1513

Herbert CA, Edwards D, Boot JR, Robinson C 1993 In vitro modulation of the eosinophil-dependent enhancement of the permeability. Br J Pharmacol 104:391–398

Hide M, Francis DM, Grattan CEH, Hakimi J, Kochan J-P, Greaves MW 1993 Auto-antibodies against the high affinity IgE receptor as a cause of histamine release in chronic urticaria. N Engl J Med 328:1599–1604

Holgate ST, Bodey KS, Janezic A, Frew AJ, Kaplan AP, Teran LM 1997 Release of the C-C chemokines RANTES, MIP-1α and MCP-1 into asthmatic airways following endobronchial allergen challenge. Am J Respir Crit Care Med, in press

Humbert M, Grant JA, Taborda-Barata L et al 1996 High affinity IgE receptor ($Fc_\varepsilon R1$)-bearing cells in bronchial biopsies from atopic and non-atopic asthma. Am J Respir Crit Care Med 153:1931–1937

Jung T, Schauer U, Heusser C, Neumann C, Rieger C 1993 Detection of intracytoplasmic cytokines by flow cytometry. J Immunol Methods 159:1381–1386

Kharitonov SA, Yates D, Robbins RA, Logan-Sinclair R, Shinebourne E, Barnes PJ 1994 Increased nitric oxide in exhaled air of asthmatic patients. Lancet 343:133–135

Kroegel C, Matthys H 1993 Platelet-activating factor-induced human eosinophil activation: generation and release of cyclooxygenase metabolites in human blood eosinophils from asthmatics. Immunology 78:279–285

Krug N, Madden J, Redington AE et al 1996 T-cell cytokine profile evaluated at the single cell level in BAL and blood in allergic asthma. Am J Respir Cell Mol Biol 14:319–326

Lackie PM, Baker JE, Gunther U, Holgate ST 1997 Expression of CD44 isoforms is increased in the airway epithelium of asthmatic subjects. Am J Resp Cell Mol Biol, in press

Laitinen L, Heind W, Laitinen A, Kava T, Haahtela T 1985 Damage of the airway epithelium and bronchial reactivity in patients with asthma. Am Rev Respir Dis 131:599–606

Lawrence MB, Springer TA 1991 Leukocytes role on a selectin at physiological flow rates: distinction from and pre-requisite for adhesion through integrins. Cell 65:859–873

Makker HK, Holgate ST 1994 Mechanisms of exercise-induced asthma. Eur J Clin Invest 24:571–585

Manning AM, Anderson DC, Bristol JA (eds) 1994 Transcription factor NFκB: an emerging regulation of inflammation. Annual reports in medicinal chemistry. Academic Press, San Diego, CA, p 235–244

Mattoli S, Mezzett M, Riva G, Allegra L, Fasoli A 1990 Specific binding of endothelin on human bronchial smooth muscle cells in culture and secretion of endothelin-like material from bronchial epithelial cells. Am J Respir Cell Mol Biol 3:145–151

Montefort S, Herbert CA, Robinson C, Holgate ST 1992a The bronchial epithelium as a target for inflammatory attack. Clin Exp Allergy 22:511–520

Montefort S, Roberts JA, Beasley CR, Holgate ST, Roche WR 1992b The site of disruption of the bronchial epithelium in asthmatics and non-asthmatics. Thorax 47:499–503

Montefort SL, Baker J, Roche WR, Holgate ST 1993a The distribution of adhesive mechanisms in the normal bronchial epithelium. Eur Resp J 6:1257–1263

Montefort S, Djukanović R, Holgate ST, Roche WR 1993b Ciliated cell damage in the bronchial epithelium of asthmatics and non-asthmatics. Clin Exp Allergy 23:185–189

Montefort S, Gratziou C, Goulding D et al 1994a Bronchial biopsy evidence for leucocyte infiltration and upregulation of leucocyte endothelial cell adhesion molecules 6 hours after local allergen challenge of sensitised asthmatic airway. J Clin Invest 93:1411–1421

Montefort S, Lai CKW, Kapahi P et al 1994b Circulating adhesion molecules in asthma. Am J Respir Crit Care Med 149:1149–1153

National Institutes of Health 1995 Epidemiology. In: Global Initiative for Asthma: global strategy for asthma management and prevention (National Institutes of Health, National

Heart, Lung and Blood Institute and World Health Organisation Workshop Report). NIH publication no. 95–3659

Okayama Y, Petit-Frére C, Kassel O et al 1995 Expression of messenger RNA for IL-4 and IL-5 in human lung and skin mast cells in response to FCε receptor cross-linkage and the presence of stem cell factor. J Immunol 155:1796–1808

Okayama Y, Lau LC-K, Church MK 1997 TNFα production by human lung mast cells in response to stimulation by stem cell factor and Fc$_ε$R1 cross-linkage. J Immunol, in press

Papi A, Wilson SJ, Johnston SL 1996 Rhinoviruses increase production of adhesion molecules (CAM) and NFκB. Am J Respir Crit Care Med 153:866A

Park H-S, Jung K-S, Shute J et al 1995 GM-CSF is the predominant cytokine which enhances eosinophil survival in nasal polyp tissue cultures with allergen. Am J Respir Crit Care Med 151:240A

Peat JK, Woolcock AJ, Cullen K 1987 Rate of decline of lung function in subjects with asthma. Eur J Respir Dis 70:171–179

Pepys J 1973 Disodium cromoglycate in clinical and experimental asthma. In: Austen KF, Lichtenstein CM (eds) Asthma: physiology, immunopharmacology and treatment. Academic Press, London, p 279–294

Peroni DG, Djukanović R, Bradding P et al 1997 Comparison of the expression of CD44 and integrins in bronchial mucosa of normal and mildly asthmatic subjects. Eur Resp J, in press

Persson CGA, Erjefält JS, Erjefält I, Korsgren MC, Nilsson MC, Sundler F 1996 Epithelial shedding restitution as a causative process in airway inflammation. Clin Exp Allergy 26:746–755

Pilewski JM, Albelda SM 1995 Cell adhesion molecules in asthma: homing activation and airway remodelling. Am J Respir Cell Mol Biol 12:1–3

Redington AE, Springall DR, Ghatei MA et al 1995a Endothelin in bronchoalveolar lavage fluid and its relationship to airflow obstruction in asthma. Am Rev Respir Crit Care Med 151:1034–1039

Redington AE, Madden J, Djukanović R, Roche WR, Howarth PH, Holgate ST 1995b Transforming growth factor-beta levels in bronchoalveolar lavage are increased in asthma. J Allergy Clin Immunol 95:377

Redington AE, Madden J, Frew AJ et al 1995c Basic fibroblast growth factor in asthma: immunolocalisation in bronchial biopsies and measurement in bronchoalveolar lavage fluid at baseline and following allergen challenge. Am J Respir Crit Care Med 15:702A

Robinson DS, Hamid Q, Bentley A, Ying S, Kay AB, Durham SR 1993a Activation of CD4$^+$ T cells, increased TH-2 type cytokine mRNA expression, and eosinophil recruitment in bronchoalveolar lavage after allergen inhalation challenge in patients with atopic asthma. J Allergy Clin Immunol 92:313–324

Robinson DS, Hamid Q, Bentley AM, Ying S, Kay AB, Durham SR 1993b CD4$^+$ T cell activation, eosinophil recruitment and interleukin-4 (IL-4), IL-5 and GM-CSF messenger RNA expression in bronchoalveolar lavage after allergen challenge in atopic asthmatics. J Allergy Clin Immunol 92:313–324

Rothenberg ME, Ownbey R, Melhop PD et al 1996 Eotaxin triggers eosinophil-selective chemotaxis and calcium flux via a distinct receptor and induces pulmonary eosinophilia in the presence of interleukin 5 in mice. Mol Med 2:1076–1551

Saetta M, Di Steffano A, Maestrelli P et al 1996 Airway eosinophilia and expression of interleukin-5 protein in asthma and in exacerbations of chronic bronchitis. Clin Exp Allergy 26:766–774

Salter HH 1860 On asthma: its pathology and treatment, 1st edn. Churchill, London

Shakib F, Sihoe J, Smith SJ, Wilding P, Clark MM, Knox A 1994 Circulating levels of IgG1 and IgG4 anti-IgE antibodies and asthma severity. Allergy 49:192–195

Shannon VR, Chanez P, Bousquet J, Holtzman MJ 1993 Histochemical evidence for induction of arachidonate 15-lipoxygenase in airway disease. Am Rev Respir Dis 147:1024–1028

Shute J, Lindley I, Piechl P et al 1995 Mucosal IgA is an important moderator of eosinophil responses to tissue-derived chemoattractants. Proc Coll Int Allergol, Nantucket 1994. Int Arch Allergy Appl Immunol 107:340–341

Shute JK, Howarth PH, Holgate ST 1997a A role of eosinophil-derived gelatinase B in tissue remodelling. Am J Respir Crit Care Med, in press

Shute JK, Parmar J, Holgate ST 1997b Urinary GAG levels are increased in acute severe asthma — a role for eosinophil-derived gelatinase B? Int Arch Allergy, in press

Snow RE, Chapman CJ, Frew AJ, Holgate ST, Stevenson FK 1995 Analysis of immunoglobulin (V_H) region genes encoding IgE antibodies in splenic B lymphocytes of a patient with asthma. J Immunol 154:5576–5581

Sporik R, Holgate ST, Platts-Mills TAE, Cogswell JJ 1990 Exposure to house dust mite allergen (Der p 1) and the development of asthma in childhood: a prospective study. N Engl J Med 323:502–507

Springall DR, Howarth PH, Counihan H et al 1991 Endothelin immunoreactivity of airway epithelium in asthmatic patients. Lancet 337:697–701

Springall DR, Meng Q-H, Redington AE, Howarth PH, Polak JM 1995 Inflammatory genes in asthmatic airway epithelium: suppression by corticosteroids. Eur Respir J (suppl 19) 8:44S

Stahle-Backdahl M, Parks WC 1993 92-Kd gelatinase is actively expressed by eosinophils and stored by neutrophils in squamous cell carcinoma. Am J Pathol 142:995–1000

Tenor H, Shute JK, Church MK, Hatzelmann A, Schudt C 1996 Endogenously released PGE_2 inhibits LTC_4 synthase in human eosinophils: a possible mechanism contributing to aspirin-induced asthma (AIA). Am J Respir Crit Care Med 153:684A

Teran LM, Davies DE 1996 The chemokines: their potential role in allergic inflammation. Clin Exp Allergy 26:1005–1019

Teran LM, Carroll M, Frew AJ et al 1996 Leukocyte recruitment after local endobronchial allergen challenge in asthma: relationship to procedure and to airway interleukin 8 release. Am J Respir Crit Care Med 154:469–476

Tunan-de-Lara JM, Redington AE, Bradding P et al 1996 Dendritic cells in normal and asthmatic airways: expression of the α subunit of the high affinity immunoglobulin E receptor ($Fc_\varepsilon R1_\alpha$). Clin Exp Allergy 26:648–655

Warner JA, Miles EA, Jones AC, Quint DJ, Colwell BM, Warner JO 1994 Is deficiency of interferon gamma production by allergen triggered cord blood cells a predictor of atopic eczema? Clin Exp Allergy 24:423–430

Warner JA, Jones AC, Miles EA, Colwell BM, Warner JM 1996 Maternofetal interaction and allergy. Allergy 51:447–451

Wilson JW, Li X 1997 The measurement of subepithelial and submucosal collagen in the asthmatic airway. Clin Exp Allergy, in press

Wooley KL, Gibson PG, Carty K, Wilson AJ, Twaddell SH, Wooley MJ 1996 Eosinophil apoptosis and the resolution of airway inflammation in asthma. Am J Respir Crit Care Med 154:237–243

Zhang S, Howarth PH, Roche WR 1996 Cytokine production by cultured bronchial subepithelial myofibroblasts. Eur Respir J 9:1839–1846

DISCUSSION

Paré: Do myofibroblasts originate from smooth muscle cells or from fibroblasts, or do they exist in the airway wall as myofibroblasts and simply proliferate?

Holgate: In normal airways they are present but in low numbers (Roche et al 1989). We have used a monoclonal antibody (PR2D3) against a marker originally identified on colonic myofibroblasts to identify them. We believe that these cells have the capacity to proliferate; however, we do not know whether they can originate from smooth muscle cells, although they do seem to have a high content of α-actin (Goulet et al 1996). In liver fibrosis myofibroblasts can differentiate from lipocytes or stellate cells, indicating that a cell designed to store vitamin A has the capacity to change into one that secretes collagen (Friedman 1993).

Paré: Could myofibroblast accumulation in asthma be analogous to atherosclerosis, in which the vascular smooth cells migrate towards the endothelium?

Holgate: That is a possibility.

Weiss: You presented an essentially linear model in that inflammation leads to airway hyper-responsiveness, which leads to asthma. However, you alluded to some difficulties with the model, i.e. that if asthmatics are treated the airway hyper-responsiveness phenotype doesn't disappear. There is also evidence to suggest that airway responsiveness has a complicated relationship with inflammation. Clearly, allergic inflammation will up-regulate airway responsiveness but airway responsiveness may also be part of the inflammatory phenotype. Could you comment on this?

Holgate: The concept I have is that the oedematous inflamed submucosa and the adventitial part of the airway undergo organization, which is the usual consequence of chronic inflammation at other mucosal sites such as the gastrointestinal tract. Under these conditions, a matrix is laid down containing fibronectin, collagens and proteoglycans, resulting in the conversion of a sol into a gel, with subsequent alterations in elastic properties. Thus, when the airway smooth muscle contracts the thickened submucosa produces a disproportionate reduction in the airway lumen (James et al 1989). Thickening of the adventitial aspect of the airway (outside the smooth muscle) increases the area over which the retractile elastin forces of the alveolar septae are distributed so that the elastic forces holding open the airways are reduced. Bronchial hyper-responsiveness will increase in parallel with increasing airway inflammation and wall remodelling.

Magnussen: In many patients with severe asthma we have been unable to identify an allergic cause of the disease. What are your views on the acceptance of this paradigm in non-allergic asthma?

Holgate: This question refers to the concept of intrinsic asthma. Barry Kay has done some interesting work on this, in which he has stained for IgE receptors. Could you describe your observations?

Kay: I will be elaborating on this further in my presentation, but briefly if one looks at the immunopathology of patients with classic 'intrinsic' asthma versus asthmatics who are skin test positive, one finds comparable expression of activated T cells (Bentley et al 1992) and the high affinity IgE receptor in both groups (Humbert et al 1996a). There were similar findings with respect to the mRNA and protein product for interleukin (IL)-4 and IL-5 (Humbert et al 1996b). This raised the possibility that in intrinsic and extrinsic asthma one is dealing with a final common pathway in terms of immunopathology, even though the initiation of these events may be quite distinct. So in a sense, we are 'lumpers' rather than 'splitters' when it comes to classification of these major variants of asthma. The question still remains, however, as to whether intrinsic asthma is an immunological process and if so what is the antigen involved.

Holgate: There has been some work which has demonstrated that in the nasal mucosa from atopic patients with severe allergic rhinitis local IgE synthesis takes place, as evidenced by germline and ε-chain transcription when assessed by reverse transcriptase PCR techniques (Durham et al 1996). We have also detected IgE transcription in the lower airways of patients with severe but not mild asthma. Therefore, it is possible that the source of IgE generation may move, and that in intrinsic asthma we're dealing a local IgE response rather than a systemic one.

Pauwels: How did you define severe asthma?

Holgate: Our definition was taken from the National Heart, Lung and Blood Institute/World Health Organization descriptions of mild, moderate and severe asthma (NHLBI/WHO 1993). The asthmatics that we did these biopsies on are moderate asthmatics, as defined by the WHO/NHLBI, whereas our most recent work investigating the contribution of growth factors has been undertaken on severe asthmatics who are taking high dose inhaled corticosteroids (Djukanović et al 1995). It is our belief and that of others that the phenotypic characteristics of the disease changes with severity (Kay 1996, Synek et al 1996).

Busse: It is difficult to differentiate between the responses of allergic non-asthmatics and allergic asthmatics. Do you have any observations concerning where these differences may lie? For example, do they differ in the response to antigen or does the resolution of response to antigen lead to the clinical characteristics of asthma?

Holgate: This is a fascinating and important question. If one matches people by skin tests or by serum IgE to specific antigens, there is a large difference in the expression of the phenotype in the form of asthma. For example, some individuals have large IgE responses to house dust mites but do not have asthma, whereas there are others who have minimal skin weal responses to house dust mites and yet their airways appear sensitive to inhalation of this antigen. One possibility is that the lower airways in asthma become selectively sensitized to domestic allergens, possibly from local IgE synthesis. The airways in asthma may differ from normal airways in other ways. The access of inhaled allergen to the responding cells may be increased in asthma on account of epithelial disruption. Finally, there may be completely separate factors intrinsic to the asthma process that go beyond allergy and in some way augment a final common pathway that leads to the contraction of airway smooth muscle. Examples might be alterations in the subtypes of myosin, or enzymes that phosphorylate myosin, to increase its contractile responsiveness.

Busse: What could this intrinsic differentiating factor be?

Holgate: I don't know. There is evidence in mice that there are specific genes which control airway responsiveness to contractile agonists. Whether such genes exist in human asthma is not known, although one study has linked a region of chromosome 5 to bronchial hyper-responsiveness independent of IgE responsiveness (Postma et al 1995).

Platts-Mills: If we consider an intrinsic asthmatic as a man of 45 who is not atopic and comes from a non-atopic family, and who suddenly starts coughing and develops severe asthma, then it becomes problematic to determine whether there is any evidence that the prevalence of intrinsic asthma has increased.

Holgate: In general, when one talks to the epidemiologists about this subject, they say that their data are not sufficiently sensitive to resolve such questions (Martinez et al 1989).

Martinez: There are very few subjects who suddenly become asthmatic at the age of 45. I am sure they exist clinically but they are not easily identified in epidemiological studies. It is possible that many of these so-called intrinsic asthmatics could have been allergic beforehand and what one is observing is the end of the natural progression of the disease.

Strachan: There are two issues here. One is whether atopy is a trait that persists over time, or whether people can gain and lose it with a simultaneous gain and loss of allergic inflammation of the airways. The second is to what extent people who have never had a history of any sort of atopic sensitization might be at risk of developing asthmatic airway inflammation. The epidemiological data only bear on asthmatic symptoms and not the definition of asthma that you offered, which is based both on pathology and symptoms. Both cross-sectional and longitudinal studies demonstrate that adults who smoke can develop symptoms which are similar to those experienced by asthmatics. Whether this is 'truly' asthma or whether it is better considered as one of Henry Salter's other airway diseases is at the moment a matter for intense debate. There is no strong evidence that this type of asthma is increasing worldwide because there aren't many serial prevalence studies of asthmatic-type symptoms in adults that adequately take into account the trends in cigarette smoking and all the nuances of smoking habit.

Weiss: The hard facts are that 85% of all childhood asthmatics are atopic and there is a tremendous effect of age on the modification of immunological phenotype, i.e. IgE levels peak in early adulthood and then both IgE levels and skin test reactivity decline. In any study that looks at older people for the first time, there will be a large detection bias with regard to prior events. When you're looking at a 45-year-old person who has a negative skin test result and low levels of IgE, you cannot say anything about what that person's immunological phenotype was when they were 12 or 14. They may not even remember whether or not they had asthma, so recall bias can be a major problem.

Sears: I would like to add some as yet unpublished data from our longitudinal study of New Zealand children followed to early adulthood. We found that among 18- and 20-year olds atopy had minimal or no effect on the development of new wheezing symptoms, suggesting that those who were atopic and were going to develop asthma had already developed it, and that the new asthma cases amongst this age group were caused by other factors. Smoking may be one of these factors because it is clearly one of the highest risk factors for respiratory symptoms.

Kay: What I particularly enjoyed about your presentation was the way in which inflammation, repair, resolution and organization were portrayed as a continuum. It is clearly a dynamic process in which there are various factors driving events in both directions. You mentioned the eosinophil and that matrix metalloproteases derived from this cell may be pro-inflammatory and responsible for some of the epithelial damage. You also touched on transforming growth factor (TGF)-β and collagen deposition. I would like to hear your views on the eosinophil as a repair cell with TGF-β and collagen deposition being critical to this cell's function in reorganization.

Holgate: The observation that eosinophils contribute to the repair process is established. For example, activated eosinophils possess VLA-4 that, in addition to interacting with vascular cell adhesion molecule-1 on the microvasculature, is able to interact with a specific sequence on fibronectin which primes the eosinophil and prolongs its survival (Lobb et al 1996).

Kay: Does this have a good or bad effect?

Holgate: This has a deleterious effect in augmenting eosinophil responses but it may promote repair by secreting TGF-α and TGF-β, for example.

Pauwels: Erjefält et al (1996) have removed the upper layer of the epithelium and have observed an influx of neutrophils and eosinophils, the release of eosinophil granular proteins and the complete restoration of the epithelium.

Busse: There are data which indicate that TGF-β down-regulates eosinophil function. Most of these studies have been performed on peripheral blood eosinophils and what needs to be done is to evaluate cells that have undergone migration, and determine whether the cells assume a different phenotype and fail to respond normally to those factors which down-regulate their function. The processes of cell regulation are not easy to resolve because the systems under which we study inflammatory cells are not similar to the conditions in which these cells exist *in vivo*.

Corris: People interested in the pathology of asthma have concentrated on large airway biopsies, and I would like to ask you whether you know anything about what's happening in the bronchioles. I ask this because I have an interest in obliterative bronchiolitis post lung transplantation. This is due to a T cell-orchestrated process associated with a later release of proliferative cytokines and myofibroblast recruitment and remodelling. These events take place in the smaller airways, so I'm therefore intrigued by the processes involved in remodelling the smaller airways in asthma.

Holgate: There have been few studies, and most of these have been based on post-mortem analysis. We have undertaken one study with Richard Martin in Denver in which we have examined inflammatory processes in trans-bronchial biopsies. We observed that the small airways and alveoli develop a vigorous eosinophil and T cell inflammatory reaction during periods of severe asthma associated with nocturnal symptoms (Kraft et al 1996). Our studies with Richard Beasley on post-mortem tissue from asthma deaths in the late 1970s and early 1980s in New Zealand, on the other hand, suggest that those who died from their disease, as opposed to those who had asthma and died of other causes, had T cell and eosinophil responses spreading proximally to involve the large airways. If the large airways are inflamed and therefore subject to narrowing then there will be a disproportionate effect on ventilation (Synek et al 1996). Studies that Gene Bleecker undertook with the fibreoptic bronchoscope using a biased airflow to measure small airway resistance revealed increased resistance in the peripheral airways that could not be reversed with a β2-agonist (Wagner et al 1990).

Paré: We have done a systematic analysis and found that, with the exception of the respiratory bronchioles, all the membranous bronchioles seem to be involved with inflammation and remodelling (Kuwano et al 1993). The effects of remodelling can be dramatic in small airways because their walls are thicker relative to their lumen size.

Corris: Have you observed myofibroblasts proliferating within the lumen?

Paré: No, we have not observed this in asthmatics.

References

Bentley AM, Menz G, Storz C et al 1992 Identification of T lymphocytes, macrophages and activated eosinophils in the bronchial mucosa in intrinsic asthma: relationship to symptoms and bronchial responsiveness. Am Rev Respir Dis 146:500–506

Durham SR, Gould JH, Thienes CP 1996 Local control of ε-gene expression in B cells of the nasal mucosa in hay fever patients following allergen challenge. J Allergy Clin Immunol 297:460 (abstr)

Djukanović R, Howarth P, Vrugt B et al 1995 Determinants of asthma severity. Int Arch Allergy Immunol 107:389

Erjefält JS, Sundler F, Persson CGA 1996 Eosinophils, neutrophils and venular gaps in the airway mucosa at epithelial removal–restitution. Am J Respir Crit Care Med 153:1666–1674

Friedman SL 1993 The cellular basis of hepatic fibrosis: mechanisms and treatment strategies. N Engl J Med 328:1828–1835

Goulet F, Boulet L-P, Chakir J, Tremblay N, Dubé J et al 1996 Morphologic and functional properties of bronchial cells isolated from normal and asthmatic subjects. Am J Respir Cell Biol 15:312–318

Humbert M, Grant JA, Taborda-Barata L et al 1996a High affinity IgE receptor ($Fc_\varepsilon R1$)-bearing cells in bronchial biopsies from atopic and nonatopic asthma. Am J Resp Crit Care Med 153:1931–1937

Humbert M, Durham SR, Ying S et al 1996b IL-4 and IL-5 mRNA and protein in bronchial biopsies from atopic and non-atopic asthmatics: evidence against 'intrinsic' asthma being a distinct immunopathological entity. Am J Resp Crit Care Med 154:1497–1504

Kay AB 1992 Identification of T-lymphocytes, macrophages and activated eosinophils in the bronchial mucosa in intrinsic asthma: relationship to symptoms and bronchial responsiveness. Am Rev Respir Dis 146:500–506

Kay AB 1996 Pathology of mild, severe and fatal asthma. Am J Respir Crit Care Med 154:66S–69S

James AL, Paré PD, Hogg JC 1989 The mechanics of airway narrowing in asthma. Am Rev Respir Dis 139:242–246

Kraft M, Djukanović R, Wilson S, Holgate ST, Martin RJ 1996 Alveolar tissue inflammation in asthma. Am J Resp Crit Care Med 154:1468–1472

Kuwano K, Bosken CH, Paré PD, Bai TR, Wiggs BR, Hogg JC 1993 Small airway dimensions in asthma and in chronic obstructive pulmonary disease. Am Rev Respir Dis 148:1220–1225

Lobb RR, Pepinsky B, Leone DR, Abraham WM 1996 The role of α_4 integrins in lung pathophysiology. Eur Respir J 9:104S–108S

Martinez FD, Haalonen M, Barbee RA, Cline MG 1989 Association of asthma with serum IgE
    levels and skin test reactivity to allergens. N Engl J Med 320:271–277
NHLBI/WHO 1993 Global initiative for asthma. Global strategy for asthma management and
    prevention. NHLBI/WHO workshop report. NIH, NHLBI publications no. 95-3659, p1–8
Postma DS, Bleecker ER, Amelung PJ et al 1995 Genetic susceptibility to asthma. Bronchial
    hyperresponsiveness coinherited with a major gene for atopy. New Engl J Med 333:894–900
Roche WR, Beasley R, Williams JH, Holgate ST 1989 Subepithelial fibrosis in the bronchi of
    asthmatics. Lancet I:520–523
Synek M, Beasley R, Frew AJ et al 1996 Cellular infiltration of the airways in asthma of varying
    severity. Am J Resp Crit Care Med 154:224–230
Wagner EM, Weinmann GG, Liu MC, Bleecker ER 1990 Comparison of peripheral airway
    resistive properties in normal and asthmatic subjects. Am Rev Respir Dis 141:584–588

Allergen recognition in the origin of asthma

P. G. Holt, A. Yabuhara*, S. Prescott, T. Venaille, C. Macaubas, B. J. Holt, B. Björkstén† and P. D. Sly

*TVW Telethon Institute for Child Health Research, Post Office Box 855, West Perth 6872, Western Australia, *Department of Pediatrics, Shinshu University School of Medicine, Asahi, Japan and †Department of Pediatrics, University of Linkoping, Sweden*

Abstract. Allergic respiratory diseases such as bronchial asthma are believed to result directly from the repeated local expression in airway tissues of T helper (Th) 2-polarized T cell immunity to inhaled allergens. Recent evidence suggests that these T cell responses are typically primed *in utero* and subsequently reshaped during postnatal allergen exposure via immune deviation, leading to the eventual emergence of stable allergen-specific T cell memory which is polarized towards the Th1 (normal) or Th2 (atopic) phenotype. The underlying Th1/Th2 switching process is influenced by a number of host and environmental factors that are poorly understood. Prominent amongst these are factors that affect the kinetics of maturation of immune competence during the early postnatal period. In particular, there is mounting evidence that the immunological milieu at the materno-fetal interface is naturally skewed towards the Th2 phenotype (possibly an evolutionary adaptation to protect the placenta against the toxic effects of Th1 cytokines). Furthermore, this bias appears to be preserved for varying periods into infancy, which may account for the presence of a high risk 'window' for allergic sensitization in early postnatal life. It is hypothesized that the principal impetus for postnatal development of a normal Th1/Th2 balance (and hence closure of the high risk sensitization window) is provided via contact with Th1-stimulatory commensal and pathogenic micro-organisms at the body's major mucosal surfaces.

1997 The rising trends in asthma. Wiley, Chichester (Ciba Foundation Symposium 206) p 35–55

Until comparatively recently, allergy to non-pathogenic environmental antigens (allergens) was ascribed primarily to defect(s) in the barrier functions of the respiratory and/or gastrointestinal mucosae, which in normal (non-atopic) individuals served to protect the immune system from contact with sensitizing doses of these allergens. This notion has been supplanted by the recognition that the immune system instead actively monitors virtually all of the antigens impinging on mucosal surfaces, even inhalant allergens to which annual exposure may be as low as in the nanogram range. The sequela of this allergen recognition process, in the form of the nature of immunological memory that develops and becomes imprinted (essentially

35

permanently) on the immune system, determines whether or not individuals will manifest allergic symptoms following re-exposure to the same allergens in later life.

Immunological basis for the allergen responder phenotype

The application of single-cell cloning technology to the analysis of allergen-specific T cell responses in atopic and non-atopic adult humans has proven to be a watershed in allergy research, in providing initial proof that allergen-specific T helper memory cells responsive to the major inhalant allergens occur with comparable frequency in both symptomatic atopic and non-symptomatic normal subjects (Halvorsen et al 1986). The key observation, which has set the research agenda in this field over the last 10 years, is that the respective T cell cytokine profiles differ markedly between these groups, being polarized towards the murine equivalent of a T helper (Th) 1 cell response (interleukin [IL]-2 and γ-interferon [IFN-γ]) in normal, versus a Th2 cell response (IL-4 and IL-5) in atopics (Wierenga et al 1990, Romagnani 1992). Although it is clear that the murine Th1/Th2 paradigm cannot be extrapolated to humans without reservation, it has nevertheless proven to be a useful experimental framework for relevant investigations in the human system.

One of the limitations of T cell cloning technology that is increasingly becoming evident is the plasticity of Th cell phenotypes in the face of changes in the *in vitro* cytokine milieu of growing clones, particularly when the cloning process takes several weeks (e.g. see Paliard et al 1991). The potential for inadvertent generation of artefactual data in such *in vitro* systems is self evident. However, the central observation of the differing polarities of allergen-specific cytokine profiles in atopics versus non-atopics has recently been confirmed employing a short-term T cell activation assay coupled with ultra-sensitive ELISA technology (Imada et al 1995). Furthermore, the universality of inhalant allergen-specific T cell responsiveness has also received independent confirmation, through the development of a sensitive serum-free T cell lymphoproliferation assay system that permits the demonstration of short-term *in vitro* responses to allergens such as the house dust mite (HDM) in nearly 100% of adults (Upham et al 1995).

In relation to the aetiology of allergic respiratory disease, the key issue is: what determines the polarity of T cell cytokine responses to inhaled antigens in different individuals?

Regulation of immune responses to inhaled antigens: insights from experimental animal models

The development of primary T cell immunity to inhaled antigens is now recognized to be controlled by events occurring in the airway mucosa and associated regional lymph nodes. The process is initiated by the acquisition of antigen by specialized dendritic cells within the airway epithelium, which in normal adults are present as a network comparable to the Langerhans' cell population in the epidermis (Holt et al 1989,

Schon-Hegrad et al 1991). The dendritic cells process antigens locally, but delay presentation of the antigen to the T cell system until their subsequent migration to the regional lymph nodes (Holt et al 1993). Dendritic cell traffic between the airway mucosa and the T cell system within the regional lymph nodes is heavy and continuous, with the intraepithelial dendritic cell population renewing every two to three days, even in resting tissue (Holt et al 1994). During inflammatory episodes, dendritic cell trafficking rapidly accelerates, further increasing the effectiveness of this antigen-surveillance mechanism (McWilliam et al 1994).

The generation of immunological memory to inhaled antigens can accordingly be viewed as the end result of a chain of cellular interactions that are initiated by the migration of antigen-bearing dendritic cells into the paracortical (T cell) areas of local regional lymph nodes. Insight into the nature of these interactions has been provided by experiments involving repeated exposure of aerosolized antigen to rats and mice. These studies (reviewed in Holt & McMenamin 1989, Holt 1994) have demonstrated that the normal response of healthy immunocompetent animals to inhaled antigen displays an inherent bias towards a Th1-like immunity, manifesting as selective suppression of IgE/IgG1 antibody responses, with the concomitant preservation of IgG2a/IgG2b and secretory IgA production and systemic Th1-like Th cell activity (Holt & McMenamin 1989, McMenamin & Holt 1993, McMenamin et al 1994).

The efficiency of this immune deviation process is determined to a significant extent by genetic factors, as revealed in dose–response studies demonstrating 1000- to 10 000-fold differences between animal strains in the threshold exposure levels of aerosolized antigen required for selective suppression of IgE antibody production — the latter occurs in low IgE-responder strains at (inhaled) antigen doses in the low nanogram range, whereas repeated exposure to doses in the high microgram range is required to elicit similar effects in animals expressing the high IgE-responder phenotype (Sedgwick & Holt 1984, Holt et al 1987, McMenamin & Holt 1993). It is of interest to note that a hallmark of this immune deviation process is the transient production of specific IgE antibody during the primary immune response (Holt & McMenamin 1989, McMenamin & Holt 1993; further discussion below).

A series of studies from our laboratory have demonstrated that in the rat and the mouse, immune deviation away from Th2-dependent IgE responses to inhaled antigen is mediated by major histocompatibility complex (MHC) class I-restricted CD8$^+$ T cells which secrete high levels of IFN-γ upon antigen stimulation *in vitro* (McMenamin & Holt 1993). The initial activation of these CD8$^+$ T cells is dependent upon IL-2 'help' from antigen-specific CD4$^+$ T cells; given that transient IgE production also occurs during these primary immune responses, it is logical to propose that the same CD4$^+$ T cells are the source of the initial IL-4 signal required to initiate this process (McMenamin & Holt 1993). As shown in Fig. 1, on the basis of current definitions this CD4$^+$ T cell can be designated as a Th0 (precursor) cell (Holt 1994). In this scheme, the eventual development of stable CD4$^+$ T cell memory that results from continual exposure to the inhaled antigen depends upon the equilibrium

Transient IgE response

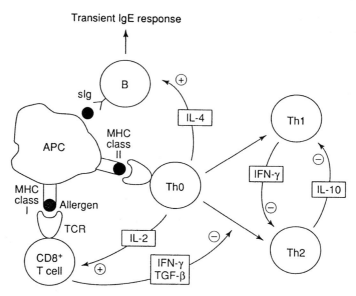

FIG.1. Immune deviation of CD4 T helper (Th) responses to inhaled allergen by class I major histocompatibility complex (MHC)-restricted CD8⁺ T cells. APC, antigen-presenting cell; IFN-γ, γ-interferon; IL, interleukin; sIg, surface immunoglobulin; TCR, T cell receptor; TGF-β, transforming growth factor β (Holt 1994, reproduced with permission).

that is established between the cross-regulating Th1 and Th2 progeny of these Th0 cells, the latter being influenced in turn by the cytokine products of the CD8⁺ T cells. In addition, this cytokine milieu may be influenced by a range of environmental factors, in particular bystander immune responses to local respiratory tract infections (Holt 1995; further discussion below).

Work is proceeding in our laboratory on the further characterization of these regulatory CD8⁺ T cells, in particular CD8⁺ γδ T cell receptor (TCR) cells, which appear to play an important role in Th1/Th2 switch regulation in immune responses to inhaled antigens (McMenamin et al 1994, 1995). Although it is not yet known precisely how these CD8⁺ cells mediate their effects on Th1/Th2 responses, it has been clearly established that their activity is generally restricted to the early phase of inhalant allergen exposure; once CD4⁺ T cell memory develops and becomes consolidated, further exposure to inhaled antigen, or even the parenteral administration of high doses of purified CD8⁺ T cells from pre-exposed (immune-deviated) animals, is no longer effective in down-modulating Th2-dependent immunity (Holt & McMenamin 1989, Holt 1994).

In relation to regulation of T cell immunity to inhaled allergens in humans, these experimental findings serve to focus attention on the life phase during which primary immune responses first develop.

IgE responses to inhalant allergens in humans: seroepidemiological studies in infants and children

The expectation that primary antibody responses to inhalant allergens would be triggered around the time the infant immune system first confronts the outside environment has been fulfilled by the results of prospective seroepidemiological studies on allergen-specific antibody responses in infants and children. Notably, IgG responses to major inhalant allergens such as the HDM are initiated in infants both with and without atopic family history within three months of birth, and they expand with continuing exposure during subsequent childhood (Mariani et al 1992, Devey et al 1993).

In contrast, IgE responses develop slowly over the ensuing one to two years (Rowntree et al 1985, Hattevig et al 1989, 1993). Employing low level IgE immunoassays, it has been demonstrated that these early inhalant allergen-specific IgE responses are common in both atopic and non-atopic children, being invariably biphasic in the latter but persistent in a subset of the former (Hattevig et al 1993, Holt 1994). Parallel IgE responses to common food allergens represent a microcosm of this process over a more compressed time-scale. Namely, these responses manifest in both atopic and non-atopic infants by around three months of age, attaining higher titres in the atopics which usually peak at nine to 12 months, before declining (in virtually all cases) towards baseline levels (Hattevig et al 1993, Holt 1994).

The hallmark of the primary immune response of both normal and atopic children to mucosally delivered allergens is thus transient IgE antibody production which (in most cases) spontaneously terminates with continued exposure, with the concomitant preservation of a low to moderate IgG subclass antibody response. This closely parallels the immune deviation process described above as the normal response of experimental animals to inhaled antigens.

Ontogeny of allergen-specific T cell responses in humans

The focus of research into the aetiology of allergic disease in humans is currently directed towards elucidation of: (i) the initial T cell priming process preceding antibody production, in which the naïve immune system receives its initial programming in relation to dietary and inhalant allergens; and (ii) the ensuing allergen-driven T cell selection process which determines the nature of relevant CD4$^+$ T cell memory that subsequently develops.

There is increasing evidence that, in many cases, initial allergen priming of the immune system occurs during fetal life. This conclusion derives from the results of studies demonstrating allergen-induced lymphoproliferation in samples of cord blood (Kondo et al 1992, Piccini et al 1993, Piastra et al 1994, Warner et al 1994, Holt et al 1995).

In a recent study from our laboratory, frequent responses were observed to panels of both inhalant and food allergens in cord blood, in contrast to the vaccine antigen

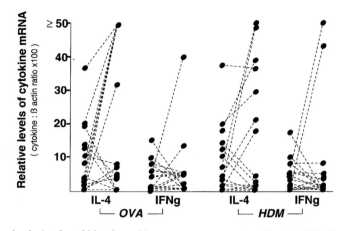

FIG. 2.   Analysis of cord blood cytokine responses to egg (ovalbumin [OVA]) and house dust mite (HDM) allergens by a semi-quantitative PCR technique. Cultures were sampled 24h post-allergen stimulation. Dotted lines link samples from individual cord blood samples incubated with (right) versus without (left) allergen. IFNg, γ-interferon; IL-4, interleukin 4.

tetanus toxoid which did not elicit responses in either cord blood or 10-week-old infant samples but (as predicted) did trigger lymphoproliferation in a high proportion of vaccinated infants up to six months old (Holt et al 1995). One possible explanation for the temporal differences in these T cell responses, as speculated earlier (Holt et al 1995), may be the presence or absence of relevant antigen in the fetal environment. Thus, the fetal circulation normally contains IgG subclass antibodies against all the major environmental allergens, and also against tetanus. In the case of dietary and inhalant allergens, exposure of the mother during pregnancy is unavoidable, leading to the possibility of transplacental leakage of allergen fragments with the potential to generate antigen–IgG complexes (nature's archetypal immunogen) in the fetus — this would occur only rarely in the case of tetanus, as vaccination is not normally carried out during pregnancy.

An alternative explanation is that these are not true primary responses against native allergens, but low level T memory responses against cross-reacting antigens. We are currently addressing these issues via a range of approaches, including analysis of patterns of cytokine production in late fetal/early postnatal T cell responses. Due to the extremely low precursor frequency of reactive cells in these early responses, it is not yet feasible to measure directly cytokine (protein) secretion by allergen-stimulated T cells, and instead we have been restricted to the detection of cytokine-specific mRNA by semi-quantitative reverse transcriptase PCR techniques.

As shown in Fig. 2, these early responses to both food and inhalant allergens are dominated by IL-4. This finding does not *per se* connote the initiation of Th2-skewed immunity, but may instead simply reflect the contribution of naïve T cells undergoing primary stimulation, which in humans (analogous to mice) has been shown to trigger a

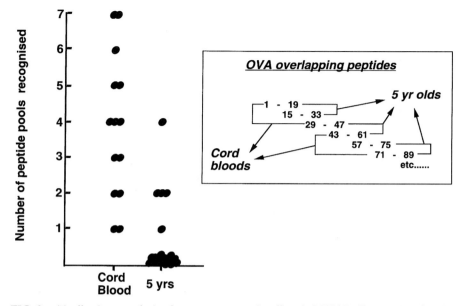

FIG. 3.   T cell epitope analysis of responses to egg (ovalbumin [OVA]) allergen. Overlapping 19mers spanning the ovalbumin molecule were pooled in groups of two or three as shown on the right, and added to cultures of T cells. Positive recognition of a pool was defined as a lymphoproliferative response with a skin reaction of $\geqslant 2.0$.

default IL-4 response (Demeure et al 1995). Further indirect evidence in support of the contention that these cord blood T cell responses are genuine primary immune responses directed at native allergen comes from ongoing cross-sectional studies involving epitope mapping of the response to egg (ovalbumin) allergen at different ages. This study employs a series of 28 overlapping peptides that span the ovalbumin molecule, pooled in groups of three. As shown in Fig. 3, at least 50% of cord blood T cell samples responded to four or more of the peptide pools, whereas T cells from five-year olds typically responded to less than one pool. The latter is consistent with a relatively mature immune response that has resulted in the selection of a restricted number of immunodominant T cell epitopes, in contrast to the heterogeneous cord blood response involving recognition of many regions throughout the ovalbumin molecule, as may be expected of a typical primary response.

How are these primary T cell responses shaped by direct environmental exposure to the allergens after birth, and what determines the ultimate direction of Th1/Th2 switching within individual immune responses?

Recent data on lymphoproliferation in response to different classes of antigens provide some clues. Thus, the typical pattern of T cell lymphoproliferation to the dietary ovalbumin allergen is that of an early peak in infancy, followed by a decline between infancy and adulthood (Holt et al 1995). This is consistent with the operation of regulatory mechanism(s) that include T cell deletion, presumably via high dose allergen exposure through the gastric mucosa (Holt 1994; note also the high frequency of non-responder five-year olds in Fig.3). An inverse pattern is observed with inhalant allergens such as the HDM, where (relatively) low level responses are seen in early life, progressively expanding into high level Th1 or Th2 responses in adulthood; the latter pattern is consistent with the operation of mechanism(s) analogous to immune deviation (Holt 1994).

It is interesting to note, in this context, the results of a recent study on HDM reactivity in Swedish infants, in a geographical setting where the prevalence of HDM allergy in children and adults is extremely low. As shown in Table 1, 80% of infants tested responded positively to crude and/or purified HDM allergens by lymphoproliferation, despite the fact that allergen levels in their home and day care environments were 10–100-fold lower than the proposed threshold level ($2\,\mu g$ allergen per gram house dust) for T cell sensitization (Björkstén et al 1996).

TABLE 1 T Cell proliferative responses to house dust mite (HDM) antigens in 18 children and the highest levels of HDM allergens (*Der p* 1 and *Der f* 1, μg/g dust) detected in either their homes or day care centres that they were regularly attending. Skin-prick test (SPT) results and allergic manifestations are also shown

			Lymphoproliferation			Allergen level (μg/g dust)	
Child	SPT	Symptom	HDM	Der p 1	Der p 2	Home	Day care
MB	—	E	8.7	4.5	<2	0.21	0.07
RM	Egg	E	4.0	<2	<2	0.08	<0.02
HE	Egg	E	4.6	<2	<2	0.18	0.18
AO	—	A	2.0	<2	<2	0.68	<0.02
JH	Birch	—	8.3	2.6	4.1	0.04	0.06
JE	—	—	4.6	<2	<2	0.18	0.08
FH	Milk	E	2.0	ND	ND	0.27	<0.02
GR	—	—	9.7	5.5	3.0	0.35	<0.02
JC	—	A,E	4.2	<2	<2	0.16	0.16
LP	—	E	6.2	2.5	<2	0.33	0.08
AL	Birch	—	4.4	<2	2.8	0.05	0.08
EJ	Birch	—	9.2	2.0	<2	0.10	<0.02
TB	—	—	17.1	<2	<2	0.09	<0.02
AE	—	—	150	139	77	0.08	0.10
SA	—	—	2.2	<2	ND	0.11	0.09
TEK	Birch, Timothy	E	7.5	ND	ND	0.12	0.05
GH	—	—	2.7	<2	<2	0.20	<0.02
EK	—	—	10.0	4.5	ND	0.06	0.02

A, asthma; E, eczema; ND, not determined due to insufficient cell numbers; —, negative.
Data derived from Björkstén et al (1996).

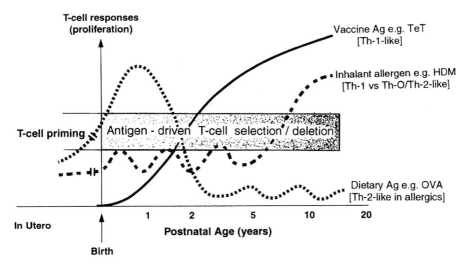

FIG. 4.   Development of T cell immunity to different classes of antigens: a working hypothesis. Ag, allergen; HDM, house dust mite; OVA, ovalbumin; TeT, tetanus toxoid; Th, T helper.

Collectively, these findings suggest a general working hypothesis for the regulation of T cell immunity to environmental allergens, as illustrated in Fig.4. This scheme envisages initial priming of T cell responses against both food and inhalant allergens *in utero*, with long-term T cell memory being determined postnatally via T cell selection processes that are driven by repeated exposure to the allergens.

Allergen-specific T cell priming and Th1/Th2 switch regulation: host and environmental factors influencing outcome

Much of the current progress in this area derives indirectly from epidemiological studies in the 1970s (reviewed in Holt et al 1990), linking early postnatal exposure to relatively high levels of inhalant allergens with subsequent allergic sensitization, particularly in subjects with a family history of atopy. These findings, which have been successfully reproduced in many subsequent studies, can still not be interpreted with confidence. What they infer is that certain key elements of the overall T cell regulatory process, which normally leads to successful immune deviation of allergen-specific T cell responses away from a Th2 response during infancy, are not fully developed at birth and remain dysfunctional for some period thereafter. Furthermore, the degree (and/or time-span) of this dysfunction during infancy is greatest in infants with a positive family history of atopic disease.

Precisely what are these 'key elements' of perinatal immune function? It appears increasingly likely that one may be perinatal T cell cytokine production. A recent study from our laboratory addressed the general hypothesis that the kinetics of postnatal maturation of immune competence may be slower in children who are genetically at high risk for atopy, compared to their low risk counterparts. This study, performed on children between the ages of two to four years, detected a markedly reduced frequency of immunocompetent T cell precursors in the blood of high risk children via limiting dilution analysis, and moreover demonstrated lower production of IL-4 and (particularly) IFN-γ in cloned cells from this group (Holt et al 1992). This finding has been confirmed, and importantly has been extended to cord blood, indicating that children at greatest risk for development of allergic disease are those with the lowest capacity for IFN-γ production (Rinas et al 1993, Tang et al 1994, Warner et al 1994, Martinez et al 1995), which may limit the efficiency of Th cell switching to Th1.

A further likely factor is perinatal antigen-presenting cell (APC) function. It is now generally believed that Th1/Th2 switching is to a significant extent controlled at the antigen presentation step in T cell activation. In the context of T cell responses to inhaled allergens, the relevant APC populations are the dendritic cells within the airway epithelium. During the early postnatal period, this cellular network is poorly developed in experimental animals both with respect to cell density, MHC class II expression (Fig. 5; Nelson et al 1994) and the capacity to respond to inductive cytokine signals (Nelson & Holt 1995). The kinetics of postnatal maturation of this network is accelerated by inflammatory stimuli, proceeding most rapidly at sites (in the airways) of maximal contact with inhaled particulates, in particular the nasal turbinates. It has not yet been determined if the human airway dendritic cell network displays a similar ontogenic profile, but on the basis of experience with other organ systems, this seems likely. If so, environmental factors that regulate the development of these dendritic cells may accordingly dictate quantitative and qualitative aspects of inhalant allergen signalling to the central immune system during early postnatal life, thus markedly influencing the T cell selection process underlying allergen-specific Th1/Th2 switch regulation.

Two likely candidates for such effects are air pollutants and respiratory infections. Epidemiological evidence indicates exposure to both these agents increases background levels of inhalant allergen sensitization (Björkstén 1994). Chemical irritants have been shown to increase airway dendritic cell density in adult rats (Schon-Hegrad et al 1991), and airborne microbial stimuli exert potent stimulatory effects on airway dendritic cell turnover (McWilliam et al 1994) in addition to their potential role in stimulating the release of Th1-selective cytokines within the respiratory tract regional lymph nodes (Holt et al 1995).

It is also feasible that microbial stimuli may exert significant systemic effects which influence the outcome of T cell responses to inhalant allergens. As noted above, sluggish postnatal maturation of T cell function appears to be associated with predilection to allergic sensitization, and environmental factors that influence T cell maturation are thus relevant to this discussion. Evidence from a variety of sources indicates that the principal drive for maturation of the adaptive immune system from

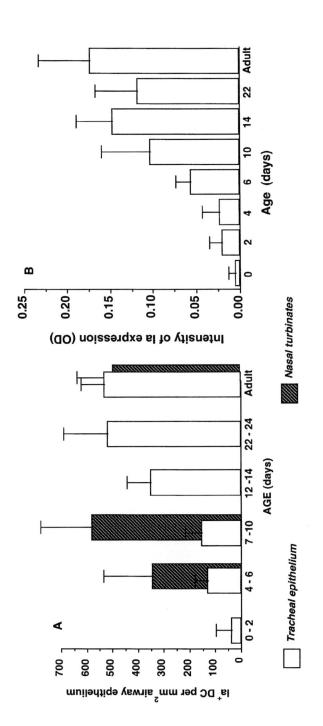

FIG. 5. Postnatal development of airway mucosal dendritic cell (DC) networks. Immunohistochemical analyses of class II major histocompatibility antigen (Ia)-bearing cells in the airway epithelium of rats (Nelson et al 1994; reproduced with permission). (A) Intraepithelial density. (B) Intensity of Ia expression.

the functionally deficient fetal phenotype into the adult-equivalent immunocompetent phenotype is confrontation with the microbial environment, particularly gastrointestinal tract commensals and pathogens, giving rise to the suggestion (Holt et al 1995) that variations in public health and hygiene practices (particularly as they relate to infants) may contribute to the marked differences in allergy prevalence being documented in different socioeconomic groups. It is pertinent to note in this context that the immunological milieu at the materno-fetal interface in experimental rats appears naturally skewed towards Th2 (Lin et al 1993), which may represent an evolutionary adaptation for protection of the placenta against the deleterious affects of Th1 cytokines (e.g. Krishnan et al 1996). Of further interest is the finding that this Th2 bias persists for variable periods into infancy (Chen et al 1995). The immunostimulating effects of the normal gastrointestinal flora during infancy may thus derive simply from their provision of lipopolysaccharide-related Th1-selective adjuvant signals, the effect of which is to hasten the establishment of a normal (adult-equivalent) Th1/Th2 balance.

An additional set of factors that should be considered are those which control the initial allergen-specific T cell priming events that occur in fetal life. Although the presence of these fetal T cell responses clearly does not *per se* connote risk for later allergy development, it has yet to be established whether qualitative aspects of the priming may increase the chances of subsequent skewing of Th1/Th2 responses in a particular direction. A precedent for the latter has recently been described in a novel model of neonatal tolerance, in which neonatal exposure to peptide was shown to prime the T cell system selectively for subsequent immune deviation towards Th2, in response to antigen re-exposure in adulthood (Holt 1996, Singh et al 1996). This phenomenon is due to a functional deficiency in neonatal APCs (Ridge et al 1996).

Clearly there is still much to learn before we obtain a full understanding of how allergic diseases such as bronchial asthma are initiated. However, it is equally clear that the recent developments in paediatric allergy provide an exciting and clear focus for future research in this area.

Acknowledgements

The authors' laboratories are supported by Glaxo Wellcome, the National Health and Medical Research Council of Australia, and the Western Australian Asthma Foundation.

References

Björkstén B 1994 Risk factors in early childhood for the development of atopic diseases. Allergy 49:400–407

Björkstén B, Holt BJ, Baron-Hay MJ, Munir AKM, Holt PG 1996 Low-level exposure to house dust mites stimulates T-cell responses during early childhood independent of atopy. Clin Exp Allergy 26:775–779

Chen N, Gao Q, Field EH 1995 Expansion of memory Th2 cells over Th1 cells in neonatal primed mice. Transplantation 60:1187–1193

Demeure CE, Yang L-P, Byun DG, Ishihara H, Vezzio N, Delespesse G 1995 Human naive CD4$^+$ T cells produce interleukin-4 at priming and acquire a Th2 phenotype upon repetitive stimulations in neutral conditions. Eur J Immunol 25:2722–2725

Devey ME, Beckman S, Kemeny DM 1993 The functional affinities of antibodies of different IgG subclass to dietary antigens in mothers and their babies. Clin Exp Immunol 94:117–121

Halvorsen R, Bosnes V, Thorsby E 1986 T cell responses to a *Dermatophagoides farinae* allergen preparation in allergics and healthy controls. Int Arch Allergy Appl Immunol 80:62–69

Hattevig G, Kjellman B, Sigurs N, Björkstén B, Kjellman NI 1989 Effect of maternal avoidance of eggs, cow's milk and fish during lactation upon allergic manifestations in infants. Clin Exp Allergy 19:27–32

Hattevig G, Kjellman B, Björkstén B 1993 Appearance of IgE antibodies to ingested and inhaled allergens during the first 12 years of life in atopic and non-atopic children. Ped Allergy Immunol 4:182–186

Holt PG 1994 Immunoprophylaxis of atopy: light at the end of the tunnel? Immunol Today 15:484–489

Holt PG 1995 Environmental factors and primary T-cell sensitization to inhalant allergens in infancy: reappraisal of the role of infections and air pollution. Pediatr Allergy Immunol 6:1–10

Holt PG 1996 Primary allergic sensitization to environmental antigens: perinatal T-cell priming as a determinant of responder phenotype in adulthood. J Exp Med 183:1297–1301

Holt PG, McMenamin C 1989 Defence against allergic sensitization in the healthy lung: the role of inhalation tolerance. Clin Exp Allergy 19:255–262

Holt PG, Britten D, Sedgwick JD 1987 Suppression of IgE responses by antigen inhalation: studies on the role of genetic and environmental factors. Immunology 60:97–102

Holt PG, Schon-Hegrad MA, Phillips, MJ, McMenamin PG 1989 Ia-positive dendritic cells form a tightly meshed network within the human airway epithelium. Clin Exp Allergy 19:597–601

Holt PG, McMenamin C, Nelson D 1990 Primary sensitization to inhalant allergens during infancy. Pediatr Allergy Immunol 1:3–13

Holt PG, Clough JB, Holt BJ et al 1992 Genetic 'risk' for atopy is associated with delayed postnatal maturation of T-cell competence. Clin Exp Allergy 22:1093–1099

Holt PG, Oliver J, Bilyk N et al 1993 Downregulation of the antigen presenting cell function(s) of pulmonary dendritic cells *in vivo* by resident alveolar macrophages. J Exp Med 177:397–407

Holt PG, Haining S, Nelson DJ, Sedgwick JD 1994 Origin and steady-state turnover of class II MHC-bearing dendritic cells in the epithelium of the conducting airways. J Immunol 153:256–261

Holt PG, O'Keeffe PO, Holt BJ et al 1995 T-cell 'priming' against environmental allergens in human neonates: sequential deletion of food antigen specificities during infancy with concomitant expansion of responses to ubiquitous inhalant allergens. Pediatr Allergy Immunol 6:85–90

Imada M, Estelle F, Simons R, Jay FT, Hayglass KT 1995 Allergen-stimulated interleukin-4 and interferon-γ production in primary culture: responses of subjects with allergic rhinitis and normal controls. Immunology 85:373–380

Kondo N, Kobayashi Y, Shinoda S et al 1992 Cord blood lymphocyte responses to food antigens for the prediction of allergic disorders. Arch Dis Child 67:1003–1007

Krishnan L, Guilbert LJ, Russell AS, Wegmann TG, Mosmann TR, Belosevic M 1996 Pregnancy impairs resistance of C57BL/6 mice to *Leishmania major* infection and causes decreased antigen-specific IFN-γ responses and increased production of T helper 2 cytokines. J Immunol 156:644–652

Lin H, Mosmann TR, Guilbert L, Tuntipopipat S, Wegmann TG 1993 Synthesis of T helper 2-type cytokines at the maternal–fetal interface. J Immunol 151:4562–4573

Mariani F, Price JF, Kemeny DM 1992 The IgG subclass antibody response to an inhalant antigen (*Dermatophagoides pteronyssinus*) during the first year of life: evidence for early stimulation of the immune system following natural exposure. Clin Exp Allergy 22:29–33

Martinez FD, Stern DA, Wright AL, Holberg CJ, Taussig LM, Halonen M 1995 Association of interleukin-2 and interferon-γ production by blood mononuclear cells in infancy with parental allergy skin tests and with subsequent development of atopy. J Allergy Clin Immunol 96:652–660

McMenamin C, Holt PG 1993 The natural immune response to inhaled soluble protein antigens involves major histocompatibility complex (MHC) class I-restricted CD8$^+$ T cell-mediated but MHC class II-restricted CD4$^+$ T cell-dependent immune deviation resulting in selective suppression of IgE production. J Exp Med 178:889–899

McMenamin C, Pimm C, McKersey M, Holt PG 1994 Regulation of IgE responses to inhaled antigen in mice by antigen-specific gamma delta T cells. Science 265:1869–1871

McMenamin C, McKersey M, Kuhnlein P, Hunig T, Holt PG 1995 γ/δ T-cells downregulate primary IgE responses in rats to inhaled soluble protein antigens. J Immunol 154:4390–4394

McWilliam AS, Nelson D, Thomas JA, Holt PG 1994 Rapid dendritic cell recruitment is a hallmark of the acute inflammatory response at mucosal surfaces. J Exp Med 179:1331–1336

Nelson DJ, Holt PG 1995 Defective regional immunity in the respiratory tract of neonates is attributable to hyporesponsiveness of local dendritic cells to activation signals. J Immunol 155:3517–3524

Nelson DJ, McMenamin C, McWilliam AS, Brenan M, Holt PG 1994 Development of the airway intraepithelial dendritic cell network in the rat from class II MHC (Ia) negative precursors: differential regulation of Ia expression at different levels of the respiratory tract. J Exp Med 179:203–212

Paliard X, de Vries JE, Spits H 1991 Comparison of lymphokine secretion and responsiveness of human T cell clones isolated in IL-4 and in IL-2. Cell Immunol 135:383–393

Piastra M, Stabile A, Fioravanti G, Castagnola M, Pani G, Ria F 1994 Cord blood mononuclear cell responsiveness to beta-lactoglobulin: T-cell activity in 'atopy-prone' and 'non-atopy-prone' newborns. Int Arch Allergy Immunol 104:358–365

Piccini M-P, Mecacci F, Sampognaro S et al 1993 Aeroallergen sensitization can occur during fetal life. Int Arch Allergy Immunol 102:301–303

Ridge SP, Fuchs EJ, Matzinger P 1996 Neonatal tolerance revisited: turning on newborn T-cells with dendritic cells. Science 271:1723–1726

Rinas U, Horneff G, Wahn V 1993 Interferon-γ production by cord blood mononuclear cells is reduced in newborns with a family history of atopic disease and is independent from cord blood IgE levels. Pediatr Allergy Immunol 4:60–64

Romagnani S 1992 Induction of T_H1 and T_H2 responses: a key role for the 'natural' immune response? Immunol Today 13:379–381

Rowntree S, Cogswell JJ, Platts-Mills TAE, Mitchell EB 1985 Development of IgE and IgG antibodies to food and inhalant allergens in children at risk of allergic disease. Arch Dis Child 60:727–735

Schon-Hegrad MA, Oliver J, McMenamin PG, Holt PG 1991 Studies on the density, distribution, and surface phenotype of intraepithelial class II major histocompatibility complex antigen (Ia)-bearing dendritic cells (DC) in the conducting airways. J Exp Med 173:1345–1356

Sedgwick JD, Holt PG 1984 Suppression of IgE responses in inbred rats by repeated respiratory tract exposure to antigen: responder phenotype influences isotype specificity of induced tolerance. Eur J Immunol 14:893–897

Singh RR, Hahn BH, Sercarz EE 1996 Neonatal peptide exposure can prime T cells and, upon subsequent immunization, induce their immune deviation: implications for antibody vs. T cell-mediated autoimmunity. J Exp Med 183:1613–1621

Tang MLK, Kemp AS, Thorburn J, Hill DJ 1994 Reduced interferon-γ secretion in neonates and subsequent atopy. Lancet 344:983–985

Upham JW, Holt BJ, Baron-Hay MJ et al 1995 Inhalant allergen-specific T-cell reactivity is detectable in close to 100% of atopic and normal individuals: covert responses are unmasked by serum-free medium. Clin Exp Allergy 25:634–642

Warner JA, Miles EA, Jones AC, Quint DJ, Colwell BM, Warner JO 1994 Is deficiency of interferon gamma production by allergen-triggered cord blood cells a predictor of atopic eczema? Clin Exp Allergy 24:423–430

Wierenga EA, Snoek M, de Groot C et al 1990 Evidence for compartmentalization of functional subsets of CD2+ T lymphocytes in atopic patients. J Immunol 144:4651–4656

DISCUSSION

Pauwels: Is it possible that beyond the neonatal period the dendritic cell function is modified, causing a shift towards a T helper (Th) 2 cell response?

Holt: Yes. We believe that in chronic disease there are factors in the epithelial milieu that can change the functional phenotype of the dendritic cells. We already know from kinetic studies that, at least in rodents (and I suspect it will also be true for humans), both in the gut epithelium and the airway epithelium there is a rapid turnover of the dendritic cell populations; in contrast with Langerhans' cells, which take 30 days to turnover, the gut and airway mucosal dendritic cells take only 72 h. This is quite a feat. They look like undifferentiated monocytes as they move from the bone marrow, through the basal lamina, into the airway epithelium. They mature within the epithelium and develop characteristic dendritiform morphology. They sample antigens that penetrate into the epithelium, but wait for a cytokine signal which mobilizes them, and eventually they present their antigens to T cells in the regional lymph node, after undergoing a final maturation step that is driven by cytokines (especially granulocyte macrophage colony-stimulating factor) produced in the node. However, theoretically, the cytokine milieu in the airway epithelium could change into one which is equivalent to that in the regional lymph node; as a consequence, the dendritic cells may then undergo complete functional maturation *in situ*, and therefore start to present powerful inductive signals to local T cells migrating through that epithelium. We have speculated that this might be the case in diseases such as atopic asthma, but there's no direct evidence for this yet. However, Moller et al (1996) have shown that the numbers of these cells increase in chronic asthma and also that their surface phenotype appears to change.

Holgate: And they also express the high affinity receptor for IgE (Fc$_\varepsilon$R1), which is another piece of evidence that supports this (Tunan-de-Lara et al 1996).

Boushey: Stephen Holgate has presented data on the regional production of IgE in the airways, and Patrick Holt has discussed what determines whether the dendritic cell presents an antigen locally or to a regional node. If certain allergens, for example house dust mite (HDM) allergens, are more likely to induce asthma than are others, the question then is whether the antigen determines the behaviour of the dendritic cell, directing its migration for antigen presentation.

Holt: Chemically active haptens can certainly pull all the strings. If such a hapten is painted on the skin a local cytokine response is generated (predominantly through keratinocytes), which immediately mobilizes local dendritic cells and drives them into the draining lymph node. We've looked for antigen preparations that can do this in the lung, but thus far without success; the only antigens that we have identified so far with such activity are microbial in origin. Microbial antigens invariably contain small amounts of contaminating bacterial lipopolysaccharide, which does precisely this, but simultaneously switches on the production of interleukin (IL)-12 by the dendritic cells and therefore directs responses towards Th1 cell immunity. Viral antigens behave similarly, but do so through triggering events in the epithelial cell. It has also been speculated that antigens which have proteolytic activity can also do this, but there's no direct evidence yet.

Busse: You mentioned that in premature babies there were increased numbers of eosinophils. Does this reflect a natural event or the consequence of an environmental exposure, or do the eosinophils, in this setting, have another role, such as antigen presentation?

Holt: This is not known.

Busse: Is there anything unusual about antigen presentation in asthmatics or atopics?

Holt: There is no firm evidence, but a number of people believe that there may be significant abnormalities, and there is active research going on in this area. We believe that the kinetics of maturation of antigen-presenting cell (APC) function is one of the factors regulating postnatal Th1/Th2 switching in allergen-specific immune responses.

Busse: Are the APCs driving the switch or do they promote sensitization because they fail to respond to down-regulation?

Holt: This is not known. However, the neonatal tolerance models may throw some light on this. The basis for neonatal tolerance has recently been shown to be the inability of the newborn immune system to generate effective Th1-skewed immunity. One can completely restore this function by priming newborn animals with genetically identical adult APCs that have been pulsed with antigen. This suggests that on an antigen-specific basis it is possible to bypass neonatal immune dysfunction by introducing functionally competent APCs. It remains to be proven whether the same applies to immune responses to environmental allergens, but this is an increasingly attractive proposition.

Kay: Parturition is, in a sense, a Th2 event, so is it possible that the failure to recover from the Th2 phenotype at parturition is the cause of allergic disease?

Holt: A failure to recover from the 'fetal' Th2 phenotype, perhaps best described as a 'delayed postnatal establishment of an appropriate Th1/Th2 balance', appears to be a factor in this process.

Holgate: There is also a high concentration of IL-4 in amniotic cells and encrypted on heparan sulfate in the amniotic basement membrane (Jones et al 1995). Therefore, the source of IL-4 in the uterine environment may not come from immune cells but from amniotic epithelial cells, the developing fetus thus gaining access to the cytokine by swallowing it.

Warner: I agree that the most important period in terms of the development of asthma is the period after birth. At the moment we're still unsure about the exact timing of 'the window of sensitization'. T cell migration studies have been performed at birth, up to 2.5 years post-partum and in adults. We have monitored systemic T cell reactions at birth, and at six and 12 months post-partum. We found that the presence of cells specific for an allergen depended on whether or not the children subsequently developed allergic disease. If they did, we observed a decrease in systemic T cell reactions at six months compared with birth, as though trafficking is already occurring to target organs. If they did not, we observed an increase in response similar to that seen in the general population. I'm not entirely sure what this tells us about the window of sensitization, but it is possible that the response could be changed by modulation of exposure or immune modulation.

Holt: We will not be able to answer that until we have prospective data on individual children that map cytokine responses on an allergen-specific basis throughout that period. My personal feeling is that the time window will prove to be reasonably large, of the order of three or four years at least, and that during this period allergen-specific immune responses will be highly plastic and easily manipulated. It will still be possible to manipulate them later on (i.e. desensitization), but it will become increasingly difficult to do so with increasing age.

Martinez: I can confirm that that there is a maturation process occurring early in life which seems to be delayed in those subjects who go on to develop allergic disease. We stimulated peripheral blood mononuclear cells non-specifically in subjects around the end of the first year of life. We found that those who develop allergic sensitization had extremely low γ-interferon (IFN-γ) responses (Martinez et al 1995a). However, by the time they had reached age 11, both those subjects who were sensitized to allergens and those who were not produced the same amount of IFN-γ when their peripheral blood mononuclear cells were stimulated non-specifically. These data support the idea that the abnormal Th2 phenotype present immediately after birth in children who later become atopic normalizes after the first few years of life. It is possible, therefore, that the interface between the mother and fetus may be important in determining cytokine reactions by Th cells in early life.

Platts-Mills: This whole conversation hinges on the evidence for sensitization at birth. I would like to raise two specific issues. First, has anyone looked at whether these T cell responses occur in children whose mothers have not been exposed to HDM allergens during gestation? Second, you showed the peptide data for ovalbumin but have you looked at HDM peptides?

Holt: Both of these types of experiment are currently being done, but we don't have the answers just yet. Initially, we were concerned by the possible contribution of cross-reacting antigens, which is one of the reasons why we decided to do peptide mapping. We looked at ovalbumin first because this was an easy response to study, being frequent and usually quite vigorous. We commonly observed cord blood T cell responses to multiple epitopes in the ovalbumin molecule, suggesting that it is unlikely that these responses were to cross-reacting antigens.

Woolcock: Could you please clarify the difference between sensitization and T cell immunity?

Holt: The development of T cell immunity to allergens may or may not lead to the development of allergic reactivity (i.e. sensitization). The latter will presumably occur only if T cell immunity is skewed towards the Th2 phenotype.

Brostoff: There are data which suggest that the fourth child in a family is less atopic than the first. Clearly, therefore, the idea of a Th1/Th2 switch in the neonatal period is perhaps a little too simplistic. Is it possible that the third and fourth siblings are more exposed to infection and that the bacterial flora in the gut affect the Th1/Th2 switch?

Holt: I believe that factors modulating the intestinal flora from birth to age four or five are likely to have a significant effect on the kinetics of the maturation of the Th1/Th2 compartment and the APC compartment. It's going to be difficult to quantitate this, although we are attempting to develop experimental models to answer some of the associated questions. Also, certain antibiotics administered in paediatric practices may create a semi-specified, pathogen-free environment in the gastrointestinal tract, which may upset the natural microbial balance and have downstream effects that we had not previously considered.

Holgate: Shaheen et al (1996) have produced some interesting data on measles in African children. They showed that children from Guinea-Bissau infected with measles in the first year of life have a third less positive allergen skin test reactivity when examined between the ages of 13 and 19 years than their uninfected siblings who had been immunized to measles later in childhood. One possible explanation for this is that measles injection in early life drives the T cell response strongly in the direction of Th1 cells with production of IFN-γ, which is inhibitory for the development of Th2 responses and IgE production.

Weiss: Over the past 30 years there has certainly been an increase, at least in the USA, in the amount of antibiotics paediatricians prescribe to children, so there would almost certainly be a positive correlation between this and the increase in asthma if one were to do such a study.

As a non-immunologist I'm curious as to what is the best way to tweak the system. One way could be to vaccinate children so that they produce a Th1-type response, but allergen exposure involves chronic low dose exposure, suggesting that a massive dose of HDM allergens would be required to induce tolerance.

Nelson: Another way could be to give the mother immunotherapy during pregnancy. Glovsky et al (1991) have found that children who had received immunotherapy *in utero* had fewer positive skin tests than their control siblings who had not.

Holt: There are theoretically two major classes of strategy: the immunologically specific approach involving attempts to down-regulate T cell responses against individual allergens during infancy; or a more general approach aimed at accelerating the postnatal development of a normal overall Th1/Th2 balance during infancy, thus redressing the skew towards the Th2 response that occurs during gestation. The latter would thus involve selective enhancement of Th1 immunity, perhaps employing microbial-derived stimuli of the type normally provided by the commensal flora of the gut, e.g. some form of oral microbial vaccine/adjuvant preparation. The former strategy involves the line of thought that in most cases nature successfully protects against food allergy, but it hasn't managed to cure inhalant allergy. Therefore, perhaps we should exploit the oral tolerance mechanisms that are responsible for suppression of Th2 immunity to food antigens. With this approach, however, one would have to define the timing and duration of the window of opportunity referred to earlier in this discussion, so that one doesn't jump through and push the immune response in the wrong direction.

Britton: Bearing in mind that nature seems to switch off food allergy effectively, but not inhalant allergy, and that Th2 cell-mediated immunity is bad in terms of asthma, but that in poor rural societies where the risk of parasitic infection is high Th2 immunity is vital, what are your views on the absence of parasitic infections in more affluent societies switching off inhalant allergy?

Holt: Neil Lynch has been working in Caracas in Venezuela for about 15 years. He and his colleagues treated parasitic diseases in slum-dwelling children in Caracas and they found that by doing so they created a new disease, which was inhalant allergy to HDM allergens. In these children, who were about seven years of age, there was no HDM allergy until after they had successfully eradicated their gut parasites. There are many possible explanations, which may involve 'blocking' IgE or IgG4.

Boushey: I would like to add that there has been some surprising work showing that in rats suppression of the IgE response by treatment with an anti-IgE antibody does not worsen the response to infection with *Schistosoma mansoni*. The IgE-depleted rats had a decreased worm burden and a decreased number of eggs produced per worm (Aimiri 1994). It thus appears from studies of some rodent models that Th2 cell-mediated immunity is not necessarily protective against parasitic infection.

G. Anderson: It depends on the pathogen. It is clear that some pathogens actually enhance Th2 immunity to their selective advantage. In such cases a Th2 response is an inappropriate immune response since it damages the host but does not clear infection. This diversity has been shown with a number of pathogens. However, the response to the pathogen may vary depending on the genetic background of the mouse strain. One has to bear in mind that the Th2 response to parasites (for example, the production of high titres of IgE) may be inappropriate and encouraged by the parasite for its selective advantage. This may also be true for certain viruses.

Weiss: One modifying factor, in terms of whether a child becomes parasitized or retains the parasite upon treatment, is the degree of nutrition. How might nutrition influence the immune paradigm that you've presented?

Holt: Nutrition is likely to be a factor, based on what's known from the experimental mouse literature. Many people have shown that it is possible to manipulate the maturation of murine immune function by severe malnutrition, but it is not possible to say whether this is also the case for humans — the mouse is not necessarily an ideal model because it has different dietary requirements.

Strachan: I have been puzzling for some years over what types of infection and what critical periods might be responsible for the epidemiological observations that we see. There does seem to be a fairly consistent association between small family size and increased risk of allergic sensitization in a number of communities in the developed world, and birth order is probably an independent risk factor, i.e. that the first born is at the highest risk. In these studies there weren't any parasitic infections that were common enough to account for that family size effect. In addition, diarrhoeal illnesses, and particularly those in the first year of life, tend not to be as strongly associated with family size as respiratory tract infection. Therefore, we should be looking at the effects of respiratory infections. There is also the intriguing observation that not only is the number of older children important, but also the number of younger siblings, which suggests that the critical period extends well beyond two years. It's interesting that the immunological basic science has moved to a position where at least two coherent explanations are now being offered as to how an infection might protect against allergy, which is a completely different situation to where we were five years ago.

Holt: I would like to suggest that we shouldn't use the word infection quite so loosely as we do. For example, the drive from the microbial flora in the gastrointestinal tract has a maturational effect on postnatal immune function, but this doesn't have to be caused by pathogens; it may be due entirely to commensals. If this were the case, and one was using diarrhoea as a marker, then one would be looking for the wrong thing.

Martinez: Last year we published a paper in which we described a study of children with non-wheezing illnesses such as pneumonia or severe laryngo-bronchitis (Martinez et al 1995b). We have been following these children for 10 years. The children with these illnesses had a significantly higher level of IFN-γ, half the amount of IgE and half the prevalence of asthma at age six, and the same was true at age 10. These children were born and raised in Tucson, Arizona and the only difference between the two groups is that one had a more severe non-wheezing infection. These results suggest that viral infections may influence the way in which the immune system matures. An interesting observation was that this effect of viral infections could occur up to the age of three, suggesting that the window of opportunity extends beyond the period of infancy.

Paré: What are the current views on respiratory syncytial virus (RSV) infection being a risk factor for the development of asthma?

Martinez: By the age of two every child develops an RSV infection, but the issue is how they react to the virus. We are trying to understand why 30% of the population reacts with a lower respiratory illness and the other 70% does not. It's not infection itself that is the issue, but the nature of the immune response, which may be depend on the maturation of the immune system.

Boushey: Are there any data to suggest that some viruses are more 'asthmagenic' than others?

Martinez: In our studies it was not possible to distinguish between the severities of the disease in terms of the viruses that they were infected with because children who went on to develop asthma after a wheezing lower respiratory illness were infected by the same viruses that infected those who did not go on to develop asthma after such illnesses.

References

Amiri P, Haak-Frendscho M, Robbins K, McKerrow JH, Stewart T, Jardieu P 1994 Anti-immunoglobulin E treatment decreases worm burden and egg production in *Schistosoma mansoni*-infected normal and interferon-γ knockout mice. J Exp Med 180:43–51

Glovsky MM, Ghekiere L, Rejzek E 1991 Effect of maternal immunotherapy on immediate skin test reactivity, specific rye IgG and IgE antibody and total IgE of the children. Ann Allergy 67:21–24

Jones CA, Williams KA, Finlay-Jones J, Hart PH 1995 Interleukin-4 production by human amnion epithelial cells and regulation of its activity by glycosaminoglycan binding. Biol Reprod 52:839–847

Martinez FD, Stern DA, Wright AL, Holberg CJ, Taussig LM, Halonen M 1995a Association of interleukin-2 and interferon-γ production by blood mononuclear cells in infancy with parental allergy skin tests and with subsequent development of atopy. J Allergy Clin Immunol 96:652–660

Martinez FD, Stern DA, Wright AL, Taussig LM, Halonen M 1995b Association of non-wheezing lower respiratory tract illnesses in early life with persistently diminished serum IgE levels. Thorax 50:1067–1072

Moller GM, Overbeek SE, van Heldenmeeuwsen et al 1996 Increased numbers of dendritic cells in the bronchial mucosa of atopic asthmatic patients: down-regulation by inhaled corticosteroids. Clin Exp Allergy 26:517–524

Shaheen SO, Aaby P, Hall AJ et al 1996 Measles and atopy in Guinea-Bissau. Lancet 347:1792–1796

Tunan-de-Lara JM, Redington AE, Bradding P et al 1996 Dendritic cells in normal and asthmatic airways: expression of the α subunit of the high affinity immunoglobulin E receptor ($FC_\varepsilon R1_\alpha$). Clin Exp Allergy 26:648–655

T cells as orchestrators of the asthmatic response

A. B. Kay

Allergy and Clinical Immunology, Imperial College School of Medicine at the National Heart & Lung Institute, Dovehouse Street, London SW3 6LY, UK

Abstract. The T cell hypothesis of asthma, particularly chronic asthma, is based around the concept that the disease is driven and maintained by the persistence of a specialized subset of chronically activated T memory cells sensitized against an array of allergenic, occupational or viral antigens which home to the lung after appropriate antigen exposure or viral infection. Allergens induce a $CD4^+$ T helper (Th) cell response, whereas viruses recognize $CD8^+$ T cytotoxic (Tc) cells. In the asthmatic airway there appears to be both $CD4^+$ and $CD8^+$ cells with a type 2 cytokine phenotype (i.e. Th2 and Tc2 type). These cells produce: interleukin (IL)-5, IL-3 and granulocyte macrophage colony-stimulating factor, which recruit, mobilize and activate eosinophils for subsequent mucosal tissue damage; and IL-4, an essential co-factor for local or generalized IgE production. This in turn leads to eosinophilic desquamative bronchitis, with epithelial shedding, mucus hypersecretion and bronchial smooth muscle contraction. Thus, although the eosinophil is largely responsible for airway symptoms, its function appears to be under T cell control. Support for this hypothesis includes: the observations that activated T cells and their products can be identified in biopsies from the major variants of the disease (atopic, non-atopic [intrinsic] and occupational asthma); the co-localization of mRNA for type 2 cytokines to $CD4^+$ and $CD8^+$ cells in atopic and non-atopic asthma; the presence of chronically activated cytokine-producing T cells in corticosteroid-resistant asthma; the association of disease severity with type 2 cytokines, especially IL-5; and the efficacy of cyclosporin A in chronic steroid-dependent disease. Inhibitors and/or antagonists directed against more precise T cell-associated molecular targets hold promise for the future treatment of chronic asthma.

1997 The rising trends in asthma. Wiley, Chichester (Ciba Foundation Symposium 206) p 56–70

Up to the mid-1980s there was a fairly general consensus that the mast cell was central in the pathophysiology of asthma. At the 3rd International Symposium on Asthma (Kay et al 1984) it was suggested that 'perhaps asthma is no more than physical allergy of the mast cells of the lung' the analogy being made with urticaria where it was established that allergic and non-allergic triggers could release histamine (and presumably other mediators) from mast cells, which in turn produced the urticarial lesion. Thus asthma, which was characterized clinically as intermittent airway narrowing, was believed to result, in atopic asthma, from intermittent type I (immediate-type hypersensitivity) reactions by IgE-dependent mast cell mediator release, or by mast cell degranulation due to physical or other stimuli in non-atopic (intrinsic) asthma. The hypothesis explained both atopic and non-atopic asthma, as well as the mode of action of drugs such as sodium cromoglycate considered at that time to work principally through the stabilization of mast cells. Set against the 'leaky mast cell' theory was the observation that corticosteroids, a mainstay in asthma treatment since the 1950s, had no effect on histamine release from dispersed mast cells from human lung tissue. Furthermore, agents such as antihistamines, which antagonize the effects of mast cell mediators, were shown to have little effect in asthma. In addition, the mast cell hypothesis did not explain why only a proportion of atopic subjects are asthmatic, since mast cell degranulation might be expected to produce similar symptoms in any sensitized individual. Most importantly was the realization that even between acute attacks the asthmatic airways were hyper-responsive to non-specific stimuli such as histamine even when the patient was asymptomatic, and thus the concept of asthma as a chronic inflammatory disease emerged. This was given greater currency by the application of fibreoptic bronchoscopy and the ability to study the inflammatory infiltrate in the airway mucosa of asthmatics. This advance in the early 1980s soon established that an eosinophilic and mononuclear cell infiltrate was a feature of asthmatic airways even in the absence of symptoms. By 1987, asthma definitions included eosinophilic airway hyper-responsiveness, airway inflammation and desquamative bronchial eosinophilia as characteristics of the disease.

There were several reasons for turning to the T cell for clues as to what drives the asthma process — not the least being the exquisite sensitivity of T cells to the antiproliferative action of corticosteroids (a drug that remains the mainstay of treatment of the disease). Also, at this time, there had been a considerable increase in the understanding of the allergic response in terms of the essential role of T cells in both antibody-mediated as well as cell-mediated hypersensitivity reactions.

The T cell hypothesis of asthma

The T cell hypothesis of asthma, particularly chronic asthma, is based around the concept that the disease is driven and maintained by persistence of a specialized subset of chronically activated T memory cells sensitized against an array of allergenic, occupational and viral antigens which home to the lung after appropriate antigen exposure or viral infection (Fig. 1). Allergens induce a $CD4^+$ T helper (Th) cell response whereas $CD8^+$ T cytotoxic (Tc) cells recognize virally infected cells. In the asthmatic airways $CD4^+$ and $CD8^+$ cells have a type 2 (Th2/Tc2) cytokine profile producing interleukin (IL)-5, IL-3 and granulocyte macrophage colony-stimulating factor (GM-CSF), which mobilize and activate eosinophils for subsequent mucosal tissue injury, as well as IL-4, which is an essential co-factor for local or general IgE production. These events lead to an eosinophilic desquamative bronchitis, with epithelial shedding, mucous hypersecretion and bronchial smooth muscle

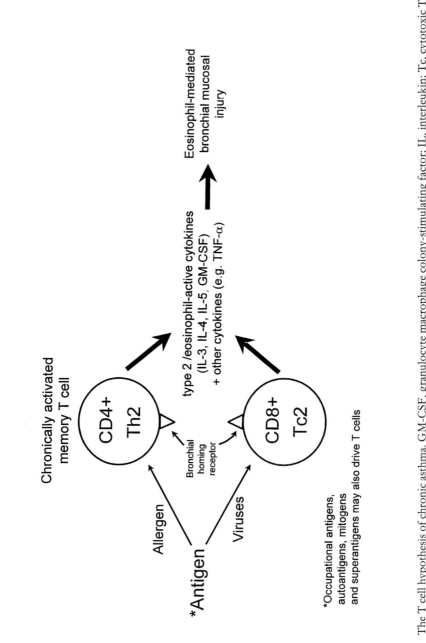

FIG. 1. The T cell hypothesis of chronic asthma. GM-CSF, granulocyte macrophage colony-stimulating factor; IL, interleukin; Tc, cytotoxic T cell; Th, T helper cell; TNF-α, tumour necrosis factor α.

contraction. Thus, although the eosinophil is largely responsible for asthma symptoms, its function is under T cell control.

This hypothesis has been tested in several ways and has included the identification of activated T cells and T cell products: (1) in baseline asthma compared to relevant controls; (2) after provoked asthma; (3) in relation to clinical features; (4) after other successful treatment of asthma; (5) in corticosteroid-resistant asthma; and (6) in atopic and non-atopic (intrinsic) asthma. Most of these studies have addressed the interrelationships among activated T cells (and their products), the eosinophil and disease severity.

Of particular interest are recent genetic studies of atopy and asthma which have linked inheritance to candidate genes in either the 5q31.1 locus, which encodes many type 2 cytokines (Marsh et al 1994), or the T cell receptor genes (Moffat et al 1994).

Activated T cells

Strong support for the hypothesis initially came from the observation that, compared to controls, the numbers of activated $CD4^+$, $CD25^+$ Th cells in peripheral blood were markedly elevated in patients admitted to hospital with acute severe asthma (status asthmaticus) (Corrigan et al 1988). There was also a direct correlation between the numbers of activated peripheral blood T cells and airway narrowing as measured by the peak expiratory flow rate. Jeffery et al (1989) identified a striking increase in the number of irregularly shaped lymphocytes in the lamina propria and submucosa of endobronchial mucosal biopsies from symptomatic asthmatics. Immuno-histochemical studies suggested that these irregularly shaped cells were probably activated T cells (Azzawi et al 1990). There was also the expected increase in the numbers of eosinophils in asthma compared to controls. By double immunofluorescence the majority ($> 85\%$) of $CD25^+$ cells were $CD3^+$ T cells (Hamid et al 1992) and by flow cytometric analysis of bronchoalveolar lavage (BAL) cells Robinson et al (1993a) found a correlation between $CD4^+$, $CD25^+$ lymphocytes and eosinophils, with the majority of $CD4^+$ cells being of the memory ($CD45RO^+$) phenotype.

Some studies have suggested increases in $CD8^+$ cells in biopsies from occupational asthma (Frew et al 1995, Maestrelli et al 1993) and in a mouse model it was shown that virus-specific $CD8^+$ cells can switch to IL-5 production and induce airway eosinophilia (Coyle et al 1995). One interpretation of this finding is that some variants of asthma are a form of autoallergic disease, in which viruses or chemical haptens modify intrinsic antigens, which in turn are targeted by $CD8^+$ cytotoxic cells. Determining the frequency of usage of TCR V (T cell antigen receptor variable) gene families and junctional analysis among T cells isolated from asthmatic airways may also provide indirect evidence for T cell responsiveness to as yet unidentified antigens.

Cytokines

IL-5, of which the T cell is an important source, promotes terminal differentiation of the committed eosinophil precursor, as well as enhancing the effector capacity of the mature eosinophil (reviewed in Wardlaw et al 1996). IL-5 also prolongs the survival of eosinophils *in vitro* and anti-IL-5 antibody inhibits allergen-induced bronchial hyper-responsiveness and eosinophilia in a primate model of asthma. In order to strengthen the hypothesis that products of activated T cells regulate local eosinophilia in asthma, Hamid et al (1991) identified elevated numbers of IL-5 mRNA-positive cells in endobronchial mucosal biopsies from asthmatics compared with controls. Within the subjects who demonstrated detectable IL-5 mRNA there was a correlation between IL-5 mRNA expression and the number of $CD25^+$ and $EG2^+$ cells and total eosinophil counts. Again, this study supported the concept that in the bronchial mucosa of asthmatics T cell-derived cytokines regulate eosinophil accumulation and function.

In a study examining the wider cytokine profile in atopic asthma, Robinson et al (1992) showed that, compared with cells from non-atopic control subjects, there were increased numbers of BAL cells encoding mRNA for IL-3, IL-4, IL-5 and GM-CSF, a pattern compatible with predominant activation of the Th2-type T cell population. mRNA for IL-4 and IL-5 was localized to T cells within the BAL cell population. These findings were confirmed using $CD4^+$- and $CD8^+$-enriched peripheral blood T cells isolated from patients with severe asthma (Corrigan et al 1995). These individuals, but not controls, showed spontaneous expression of mRNA for Th2-type cytokines localized to $CD4^+$ but not $CD8^+$ cells. This was accompanied by spontaneous elaboration of the eosinophil-active cytokines IL-3, IL-5 and GM-CSF.

Conversely, prednisolone treatment in asthmatics was associated with reduction in BAL cells expressing mRNA for IL-4 and IL-5 (Robinson et al 1993b, Bentley et al 1996). This was accompanied by decreased BAL eosinophils and clinical improvement, as shown by an increased methacholine PC_{20}. Interestingly, there was an increased number of cells expressing mRNA for γ-interferon (IFN-γ), indicating that prednisolone treatment favours enhancement of a cytokine which down-regulates IgE production.

In situ hybridization techniques showed that in a group of atopic asthmatics with a range of disease severity, there were significant associations between the numbers of cells expressing mRNA for IL-4, IL-5 and GM-CSF, and airflow restriction, bronchial hyper-responsiveness and asthma symptom score (Robinson et al 1993c). These results have recently been confirmed (in the case of IL-5) using a more precise semi-quantitative reverse transcriptase (RT)-PCR technique (Humbert et al 1996a). Furthermore, Virchow et al (1995), using segmental allergen challenge, found a correlation between IL-5 concentration, and numbers of eosinophils and activated T cells, again supporting the hypothesis that T cell-derived IL-5 is involved in tissue eosinophilia in allergic asthma.

Although several authors have now confirmed that asthma is characterized by elevated expression, at either the mRNA or protein levels, of several cytokines including IL-4 and IL-5, there has been some debate as to the principal cellular source of these cytokines. Our experience using double *in situ* hybridization/immunohistochemistry is that T cells are the major source of mRNA encoding IL-4 and IL-5 in asthmatics compared with controls (Ying et al 1995). Eosinophils and mast cells also contribute to the overall cytokine profile, although there are fivefold more mRNA-positive CD3$^+$ T cells. Furthermore, we have been able to establish, using a combination of semi-quantitative PCR analysis, *in situ* hybridization and immunohistochemistry that the amount and cellular origin of IL-4 and IL-5 expression were similar in bronchial biopsies taken from atopic and non-atopic asthmatics with, in general, IL-5 being significantly higher in asthmatics compared to atopic non-asthmatic normal controls, whereas IL-4 was elevated in asthmatics and atopic non-asthmatics compared to normal non-atopic controls (Humbert et al 1996a). The detection of cells with elevated levels of IL-4 mRNA in atopic non-asthmatic bronchial mucosal biopsies by the sensitive RT-PCR technique raises the possibility that, in general, IL-5 is related more closely to the clinical expression of asthma, whereas IL-4 is related to the overproduction of IgE. In both atopic and non-atopic asthmatics mRNA for IL-4 and IL-5 co-localized predominantly to CD4$^+$ cells but also to CD8$^+$ T cells (Ying et al 1996), which is in agreement with Till et al (1995), who found that CD8$^+$ as well as CD4$^+$ T cell lines derived from asthmatic BAL cells elaborated the IL-5 protein. These findings are compatible with the concept of Tc2 lymphocytes. Our finding of elevated IL-4 expression at both the mRNA and protein levels in intrinsic asthma was in contrast to that of Walker et al (1992), who measured the levels of cytokine proteins in concentrated BAL fluid. These authors detected increased concentrations of IL-2 and IL-5 (but not IL-4) in BAL fluid from non-atopic asthmatics compared with control subjects, whereas IL-4 and IL-5 were increased in atopic asthmatics. There is, at present, no satisfactory explanation for these apparent discrepancies. The role of Th2-type cells in intrinsic asthma, as well as that of local IgE-dependent mechanisms as suggested by Humbert et al (1996b), is unlikely to be resolved until the putative antigen(s) have been identified.

In contrast to the expression patterns of the IL-4 and IL-5 mRNAs, the IL-4 and IL-5 proteins in bronchial biopsies from atopic and non-atopic asthmatics appeared to be associated more with eosinophils and mast cells rather than T cells (Bradding et al 1992, Ying et al 1996). There are difficulties in demonstrating the intracytoplasmic staining of cytokines in non-granular cells such as T cells, presumably because of the limitations of sensitivity of current immunostaining methods. On the other hand, the eosinophil appears to concentrate several cytokines in its cell granule with granule-associated cytokines being readily detectable by immunocytochemistry (Levi-Schaffer et al 1995, Moqbel et al 1995). Despite these limitations of immunocytochemical detection of cytokines, it seems likely that T cells are an important source of IL-4 and IL-5 in asthma, although the relative contribution of the different cell types to the overall cytokine profile remains uncertain.

Recent examination of IL-12 mRNA expression in bronchial biopsies from asthmatic subjects and controls suggests that there may be a defective IL-12 response in asthma: this might also favour a Th2 environment (Naseer et al 1995). This would be in keeping with the observation of increased IL-12 mRNA-encoding cells in cutaneous late responses after immunotherapy, when it was suggested that induction of an IL-12 response might be protective (Hamid et al 1996).

T cell homing receptors

It is known from work with mice that the traffic of lymphocytes to lymph nodes and Peyer's patches is controlled in part by the interaction of lymphocyte adhesion molecules called homing receptors. These bind to tissue-selective endothelial ligands known as vascular addressins. For example, in the gut, $\alpha_4\beta_7$ integrin and L-selectin (both expressed on T cells) are involved in complex interactions with mucosal addressin cellular adhesion molecule 1 (MAdCAM-1), vascular cell adhesion molecule 1 (VCAM-1), GlyCAM-1 and CD34 expressed on vascular endothelium (Michie et al 1995). $\alpha_4\beta_7$ integrin ligates predominantly with VCAM-1 and MAdCAM-1, whereas L-selectin binds to MAdCAM-1, GlyCAM-1 and CD34. Similarly, the cutaneous lymphocyte antigen (CLA) is believed to represent a skin-homing receptor for T cells through the interaction with E-selectin on endothelial cells. Santamaria et al (1995a,b) observed that CLA^+, $CD45RO^+$ (memory/effector) (but not CLA^-, $CD45RO^+$) T cells from the blood of patients with allergen contact dermatitis or atopic eczema specifically proliferated in response to specific antigen . In contrast, peripheral blood CLA^-, $CD45RO^+$ cells from asthmatics proliferated in response to allergen, suggesting that there may be an as yet unidentified bronchial homing receptor in defined memory T cell subsets (Santamaria et al 1995b).

Glucocorticoid resistance in asthma

Glucocorticosteroids are remarkably effective in the majority of asthmatics in controlling symptoms. In vitro very low doses inhibit T cell proliferative responses to mitogens, concentrations of methylprednisolone as low as 10^{-10} M being effective in inhibiting human T cell expansion. A small proportion of asthmatic subjects do not show clinical improvement with glucocorticoid treatment (reviewed in Kay et al 1997). Formal definitions vary, but most would encompass failure to show a 10% or more increase in forced expiratory volume in one second (FEV_1) after two weeks treatment with 40 mg/day prednisolone or equivalent in subjects with asthma symptoms and demonstrated reversibility of airflow obstruction of at least 15% to inhaled β-agonists. It is not clear whether this is a distinct group or a continuum of clinical responsiveness, but glucocorticoid resistance is also seen in other inflammatory diseases. Peripheral blood mononuclear cells from patients with corticosteroid-resistant asthma proliferated in response to phytohaemagglutinin in the presence of relatively high doses of methylprednisolone, and a clear relationship was shown between clinical responsiveness to steroids and the in vitro effect of steroids on mitogen-driven colony counts. This adds support to the T cell hypothesis of asthma, since both T cell proliferation and cytokine production are exquisitely sensitive to steroid inhibition, and the in vitro responsiveness of T lymphocyte proliferation and cytokine production was closely correlated with clinical response to glucocorticoids.

The mechanisms of steroid resistance are unclear. It has been suggested that steroid resistance might arise from the cytokine environment of the T cell. Sher et al (1994) found that the majority of patients with steroid-resistant asthma had a reversible defect in glucocorticoid receptor binding affinity which could be sustained *in vitro* by the addition of IL-2 and IL-4 combined, but not individually. Furthermore, *in vitro* incubation of normal T cells with the combination of IL-2 and IL-4, in the absence of IFN-γ, reduced their glucocorticoid receptor binding affinity to the levels seen in steroid-resistant asthma. On this basis they suggested two types of glucocorticosteroid resistance: a reduced affinity of glucocorticoid receptor binding confined to T lymphocytes which reverted to normal after 48 h in culture, and a much less common reduction in glucocorticoid receptor density (in only two of 17 steroid-resistant patients) which did not normalize with prolonged incubation. This supported the concept that there may be different types of steroid resistance in asthma. These *in vitro* data suggested that the pattern of cytokine gene expression may play a role in determining steroid resistance. For this reason Leung et al (1995) used the technique of *in situ* hybridization to examine whether airway cells from steroid-resistant asthmatics versus steroid-sensitive asthmatics expressed different patterns of mRNA for cytokines, particularly after treatment with oral steroids. They confirmed that steroid-sensitive asthmatics responded well to glucocorticoids and this was accompanied by a decreased number of cells expressing mRNA for IL-4 and IL-5 and increased IFN-γ transcripts. In contrast, after prednisolone therapy, steroid-resistant asthmatics had no significant changes in the number of BAL cells expressing mRNA for IL-4 or IL-5. Furthermore, instead of a decrease there was an increase in the numbers of IFN-γ mRNA-positive cells. These findings suggested that steroid-resistant asthma is associated with a dysregulated expression of the genes encoding Th2/Th1 cytokines in airway cells and it is compatible with the concept that a combination of IL-2 and IL-4 induce glucocorticoid receptor binding affinity and T cell responsiveness to glucocorticoids.

Studies by Adcock et al (1995) have suggested a dysregulated expression of transcription factors in glucocorticoid-resistant asthma, with increased expression of the proinflammatory AP-1 molecule interfering with steroid actions by cytoplasmic binding to the glucocorticoid receptor. Small alterations in glucocorticoid pharmacokinetics and ligand binding affinity are also seen in these subjects, but they are probably insufficient to account for the clinical features.

Cyclosporin A

It is generally accepted that the primary mode of action of cyclosporin A is through the inhibition of T cell activation secondary to the blocking of early calcium-dependent transcription of mRNAs encoding several cytokines. In a group of severe steroid-dependent asthmatics, treatment over a 12-week period with cyclosporin A at low dosage (5 mg/kg per day) was associated with improvement in lung function and a reduction in the numbers of disease exacerbations requiring an increased corticosteroid dosage (Alexander et al 1992). Two further studies (Lock et al 1996, Nizankowska et al 1995) have shown a corticosteroid-sparing effect of cyclosporin A in steroid-dependent asthmatics. In both studies lung function concurrently improved despite the reduction in corticosteroid dose, although in one study this improvement was small.

It is generally accepted that the late asthmatic reaction (LAR) provoked by inhaled allergen represents a model of asthmatic airway inflammation, since the pathogenesis of the disease is, at least in part, believed to involve the mobilization and local influx of eosinophils subsequent to the release of IL-5, IL-3 and GM-CSF from activated T cells. In contrast, mediators released from IgE-sensitized mast cells have been implicated in the pathogenesis of the allergen-induced early asthmatic reaction (EAR). Since cyclosporin A inhibits both cytokine mRNA transcription by T cells and mast cell degranulation *in vitro*, it might be expected to inhibit both the EAR and LAR as well as the associated elevation in blood eosinophils. Sihra et al (1996) have recently demonstrated in a double-blind, placebo-controlled, randomized crossover trial that, compared to placebo treatment, cyclosporin A reduced the magnitude of the LAR but not the EAR following allergen challenge. This provides strong indirect evidence that cyclosporin A is effective in this model of asthmatic allergic inflammation through its effects on the T cell as opposed to mast cells and basophils.

Further developments

There is now persuasive evidence to support the hypothesis that activation of Th2 cells and/or Tc2 cells is pivotal to the asthma process. The hypothesis is supported by numerous lines of evidence, particularly in studies of BAL and bronchial biopies from asthmatic subjects, in treatment studies and in studies of experimental animal models.

The T cell hypothesis of chronic asthma has led to the possibility of a number of novel therapeutic approaches (reviewed in Kay et al 1997). These include: (1) a range of immunosuppressive drugs, including FK506, rapamycin and mycophenalate mofetil, all of which are active in inhibiting mitogen-driven T cells from corticosteroid-resistant asthmatics *in vitro;* (2) humanized antibodies against CD4 (shown to have efficacy in rheumatoid arthritis); (3) anti-cytokine antibodies, particularly against IL-4 and IL-5; (4) cytokine receptor antagonists (e.g. the IL-1 receptor antagonist has been shown to modulate human cutaneous late responses to allergen); (5) agents that modulate the Th2 response, e.g. IL-12; and (6) strategies to inhibit co-stimulatory pathways, e.g. CTLA4 Ig and anti-B7-2 antibody.

A number of important questions still remain unanswered. (i) What initiates the Th2/Tc2 response in asthma and allergy? (ii) How does asthma differ from atopy alone at the immunopathological level, because not all atopics have asthma? (iii) What proportion of activated T cells in the bronchial mucosa are allergen (or antigen)-specific? (iv) What is the role of CD8$^+$ T cells in asthma? (v) What is the role of other cell types in modifying the T cell response and in perpetuating airway inflammation in asthma? It is anticipated that with advances in molecular pathological techniques and more precise and selective therapy many of these questions can be answered.

Acknowledgements

Much of this work was supported by a Medical Research Council programme grant and the National Asthma Campaign. I also thank D. S. Robinson, C. J. Corrigan, A. J. Frew, Sun Ying, N. C. Barnes, Q. Hamid, P. K. Jeffery, M. Humbert, A. M. Bentley, O. M. Kon and B. S. Sihra.

References

Adcock IM, Lane S J, Brown CR, Lee TH, Barnes P J 1995 Abnormal glucocorticoid receptor–activator protein I interaction in steroid-resistant asthma. J Exp Med 182:1951–1958

Alexander AG, Barnes NC, Kay AB 1992 Trial of cyclosporin A in corticosteroid-dependent chronic severe asthma. Lancet 339:324–328

Azzawi M, Bradley B, Jeffery PK et al 1990 Identification of activated T lymphocytes and eosinophils in bronchial biopsies in stable atopic asthma. Am Rev Respir Dis 142:1407–1413

Bentley AM, Hamid Q, Robinson DS et al 1996 Prednisolone treatment in asthma. Reduction in the numbers of eosinophils, T cells, tryptase-only positive mast cells, and modulation of IL-4, IL-5, and interferon-gamma cytokine gene expression within the bronchial mucosa. Am J Resp Crit Care Med 153:551–556

Bradding P, Feather IH, Howarth PH et al 1992 Interleukin 4 is localized to and released by human mast cells. J Exp Med 176:1381–1386

Corrigan C J, Hartnell A, Kay AB 1988 T lymphocyte activation in acute severe asthma. Lancet I:1129–1132

Corrigan C J, Hamid Q, North J et al 1995 Peripheral blood CD4, but not CD8 T lymphocytes in patients with exacerbation of asthma transcribe and translate messenger RNA encoding cytokines which prolong eosinophil survival in the context of a Th2-type pattern: effect of glucocorticoid therapy. Am J Resp Cell Mol Biol 12:567–578

Coyle A J, Erard F, Bertrand C, Walti S, Pircher H, Le Gros G 1995 Virus-specific CD8$^+$ cells can switch to interleukin 5 production and induce airway eosinophilia. J Exp Med 181:1229–1233

Frew A J, Chan H, Lam S, Chan-Yeung M 1995 Bronchial inflammation in occupational asthma due to western red cedar. Am J Resp Crit Care Med 151:340–344

Hamid Q, Azzawi M, Ying S et al 1991 Expression of mRNA for interleukin-5 in mucosal bronchial biopsies from asthma. J Clin Invest 87:1541–1546

Hamid Q, Barkans J, Robinson DS, Durham SR, Kay AB 1992 Co-expression of CD25 and CD3 in atopic allergy and asthma. Immunology 75:659–663

Hamid QA, Schotman E, Jacobson MR, Walker SM, Durham SR 1996 Increases in interleukin-12 (IL-12) messenger RNA$^+$ (mRNA$^+$) cells accompany inhibition of allergen-induced late skin responses following successful grass pollen immunotherapy. J Allergy Clin Immunol, in press

Humbert M, Durham SR, Ying S et al 1996a IL-4 and IL-5 mRNA and protein in bronchial biopsies from atopic and non-atopic asthmatics: evidence against 'intrinsic' asthma being a distinct immunopathological entity. Am J Resp Crit Care Med 154:1497–1504

Humbert M, Grant J A, Taborda-Barata L et al 1996b High affinity IgE receptor (Fc$_\varepsilon$R1)-bearing cells in bronchial biopsies from atopic and nonatopic asthma. Am J Resp Crit Care Med 153:1931–1937

Jeffery PK, Wardlaw A J, Nelson FC, Collins J V, Kay AB 1989 Bronchial biopsies in asthma: an ultrastructural, quantitative study and correlation with hyperreactivity. Am Rev Respir Dis 140:1745–1753

Kay AB, Austen KF, Lichtenstein LM (eds) 1984 Asthma. Physiology, immunopharmacology and treatment. Academic Press, London

Kay AB, Frew A J, Corrigan C J, Robinson DS 1997 The T cell hypothesis of chronic asthma. In: Kay AB (ed) Allergy and allergic diseases. Blackwell Science, Oxford, in press

Leung DYM, Martin R J, Szefler S J et al 1995 Dysregulation of interleukin 4, interleukin 5, and interferon-γ gene expression in steroid-resistant asthma. J Exp Med 181:33–40

Levi-Schaffer F, Lacey P, Severs N J et al 1995 Association of granulocyte macrophage colony-stimulating factor with the crystalloid granules of human eosinophils. Blood 85:2579–2586

Lock SH, Kay AB, Barnes NC 1996 Double-blind, placebo-controlled study of cyclosporin A as a corticosteroid-sparing agent in corticosteroid-dependent asthma. Am J Resp Crit Care Med 153:509–514

Maestrelli P, Del Prete GF, de Carli M et al 1993 Activated CD8$^+$ T lymphocytes producing interferon-gamma and interleukin-5 in bronchial mucosa of subjects sensitised to toluene diisocyanate. J Allergy Clin Immunol 91:220

Marsh DG, Neely JD, Breazeale DR et al 1994 Linkage analysis of IL-4 and other chromosome 5q31.1 markers and total serum IgE concentrations. Science 264:1152–1156

Michie SA, Streeter PR, Butcher EC, Rouse RV 1995 L-selectin and $\alpha_4\beta_7$ integrin homing receptor pathways mediate peripheral lymphocyte traffic to AKR mouse hyperplastic thymus. Am J Pathol 147:412–421

Moffatt MF, Hill MR, Cornelis F et al 1994 Genetic linkage of T-cell receptor alpha/delta complex to specific IgE responses. Lancet 343:1597–1600

Moqbel R, Ying S, Barkans J et al 1995 Identification of mRNA for interleukin-4 in human eosinophils with granule localization and release of the translated product. J Immunol 155:4939–4947

Naseer T, Leung DYM, Song Y, Martin R, Hamid Q 1995 Expression of IL-12 mRNA in baseline asthma and in response to steroid therapy. Am J Resp Crit Care Med 151:701A

Nizankowska E, Soja J, Pinis G et al 1995 Treatment of steroid-dependent bronchial asthma with cyclosporin. Eur Resp J 8:1091–1099

Robinson DS, Hamid Q, Ying S et al 1992 Predominant T$_H$2-type bronchoalveolar lavage T-lymphocyte population in atopic asthma. New Engl J Med 326:298–304

Robinson DS, Bentley AM, Hartnell A, Kay AB, Durham SR 1993a Activated memory T helper cells in bronchoalveolar lavage from atopic asthmatics. Relationship to asthma symptoms, lung function and bronchial responsiveness. Thorax 48:26–32

Robinson DS, Hamid Q, Ying S et al 1993b Prednisolone treatment in asthma is associated with modulation of bronchoalveolar lavage cell interleukin-4, interleukin-5 and interferon-gamma cytokine gene expression. Am Rev Resp Dis 148:401–406

Robinson DS, Ying S, Bentley AM et al 1993c Relationships among numbers of bronchoalveolar lavage cells expressing messenger ribonucleic acid for cytokines, asthma symptoms, and airway methacholine responsiveness in atopic asthma. J Allergy Clin Immunol 92:397–403

Santamaria LF, Soler MTP, Hauser C, Blaser K 1995a Allergen specificity and endothelial transmigration of T cells in allergic contact dermatitis and atopic dermatitis are associated with the cutaneous lymphocyte antigen. Int Arch Allergy Immunol 107:359–362

Santamaria LF, Picker LJ, Soler MTP et al 1995b Circulating allergen-reactive T cells from patients with atopic dermatitis and allergic contact dermatitis express the skin-selective homing receptor, the cutaneous lymphocyte-associated antigen. J Exp Med 181:1935–1940

Sher E, Leung DYM, Surs W et al 1994 Steroid-resistant asthma. Cellular mechanisms contributing to inadequate response to glucocorticoid therapy. J Clin Invest 93:33–39

Sihra BS, Durham SR, Walker S, Kon OM, Barnes NC, Kay AB 1996 Inhibition of the allergen-induced late asthmatic response by cyclosporin A. Thorax, in press

Till S, Li B, Durham S et al 1995 Secretion of the eosinophil-active cytokines interleukin-5, granulocyte/macrophage colony-stimulating factor and interleukin-3 by bronchoalveolar lavage $CD4^+$ and $CD8^+$ T cell lines in atopic asthmatics, and atopic and non-atopic controls. Eur J Immunol 25:2727–2731

Virchow JC Jr, Walker C, Hafner D et al 1995 T cells and cytokines in bronchoalveolar lavage fluid after segmental allergen provocation in atopic asthma. Am J Resp Crit Care Med 151:960–968

Walker C, Bode E, Boer L, Hansel TT, Blaser K, Virchow JC Jr 1992 Allergic and non-allergic asthmatics have distinct patterns of cytokine production in peripheral blood and bronchoalveolar lavage. Am J Resp Dis 146:109–115

Wardlaw AJ, Moqbel R, Kay AB 1996 Eosinophils: biology and role in disease. Adv Immunol 60:151–266

Ying S, Durham SR, Corrigan CJ, Hamid Q, Kay AB 1995 Phenotype of cells expressing mRNA for TH2-type (interleukin-4 and interleukin-5) and TH1-type (interleukin-2 and interferon-γ) cytokines in bronchoalveolar lavage and bronchial biopsies from atopic asthmatics and normal control subjects. Am J Resp Cell Mol Biol 12:477–487

Ying S, Humbert M, Barkans J et al 1996 Expression of IL-4 and IL-5 mRNA and protein product by $CD4^+$ and $CD8^+$ T cells, eosinophils and mast cells in bronchial biopsies obtained from atopic and non-atopic (intrinsic) asthmatics. J Immunol, in press

DISCUSSION

Busse: You indicated that you have found interleukin (IL)-5 in eosinophils. Have you been able to demonstrate IL-5 secretion by eosinophils?

Kay: IL-5 can be extracted from eosinophils by freeze-thaw methods and it co-elutes with granule proteins when passed over Nicodenz columns. IL-5 is not so easy to release with secretagogues.

Busse: Is the difficulty to detect IL-5 because some of the cytokine that is released binds to the IL-5 receptor and is not detected in the supernatant?

Kay: I'm not sure. It is difficult to detect intracellular IL-5 by flow cytometry using permeabilized cells, whereas γ-interferon (IFN-γ) and IL-4 are much easier to detect. This seems to be the experience of several groups and probably reflects the efficiency of the reagents currently available.

Paré: Do the peripheral eosinophils show differential expression of the spliced and alternatively spliced IL-5α receptor?

Kay: We are currently looking at this, but do not yet have the answer.

Paré: What is the function of the soluble IL-5α receptor?

Kay: Apart from the demonstration of inhibitory activity in an IL-5-dependent eosinophil differentiation assay (Tavernier et al 1992), I believe this is largely unknown.

Magnussen: You showed that the level of IL-5 was correlated with airway hyper-responsiveness. Do you recommend that IL-5 should be used as an inflammatory marker of disease activity?

Kay: If it were possible to measure IL-5 reliably in peripheral blood it could well be a useful marker of asthmatic inflammation. However, present assays are not sensitive enough.

Pauwels: You showed that the production of IL-4 in both intrinsic and extrinsic asthmatics was increased compared to non-asthmatics, but did you also look at the local levels of IgE in those subjects?

Kay: The concept of a local IgE response in intrinsic asthma against, for example, viral antigens is interesting and is supported by other data (Frick 1986). Also the high affinity IgE receptor is up-regulated on inflammatory cells in intrinsic and extrinsic asthmatics (Humbert et al 1996).

Holgate: One might be able to investigate this by looking at the signature of the IgE V_H gene sequence, for example, i.e. by exploring the situation in reverse. It would appear that an immune response for the production of IgE against house dust mites selects specific clusters of responses in the V_H region such as V_H5 (Snow et al 1995). Selection of V_H sequences is also a characteristic feature of autoimmunity and a signature for the involvement of superantigens (Pascual et al 1992).

Busse: Have you looked for differences in cytokine patterns secreted by lymphocytes in the airway and those in the mucosa?

Kay: The cytokine profiles of cells in bronchoalveolar lavage and bronchial biopsies are very similar (Robinson et al 1993, Bentley et al 1993).

Busse: Did you also evaluate the levels of IFN-γ? Because, in terms of the difference between the acute allergic inflammatory response and the persistent response, one wonders whether the cells that are trapped in the matrix interact with adhesion proteins to cause activation and consequently the expression of either a different cytokine profile or global cytokine pattern.

Kay: We have always found that mRNA encoding IFN-γ is expressed at low levels in bronchoalveolar lavage and cells from asthmatic bronchial biopsies. However, these subjects have mild disease and therefore IFN-γ may be expressed to a greater extent in the more severe cases.

Holgate: We are talking about two roles of IFN-γ: first, its role in infancy in orchestrating the balance between T helper (Th) 1- and Th2-like lymphocyte responses; and second, in driving a granulomatous response and associated tissue reorganization. The interesting relationship between eosinophils and IFN-γ tends not to be discussed very much. In chronic inflammation there may be a IFN-γ response superimposed on top of a Th2 response, as has been described in schistosomata granulomatosis (Kelso 1995). Chronic severe asthma may be closer to a granulomatosis-like disease, involving both Th2 and Th1 cytokines with eosinophila and fibrosis.

Kay: This is an interesting concept, but what evidence is there to support it? Granulomas are essentially discrete collections of macrophages not usually associated with the asthma process.

Holgate: I agree for the types of asthma we've used for these biopsy studies. However, at the more severe end of the disease spectrum there are strong monocyte and macrophage signals involving a different array of cytokines including IFN-γ (Jeffery 1996). We should be careful not to restrict ourselves by drawing conclusions based on mild forms of asthma.

Kay: I am not sure that granulomas are a feature even in asthma deaths.

Holgate: We have recently examined post-mortem tissue from patients who have died from asthma using oligonucleotide *in situ* hybridization. Within the airway wall and in lumen secretions there are strong Th1 signals with IFN-γ transcription occurring in both mononuclear cells and eosinophils. We believe that under these conditions eosinophils themselves are capable of generating IFN-γ. Clearly, further work is warranted in this area of cytokine production in severe asthma.

Woolcock: I would like to ask a basic question. It has been estimated by measurements of skin test reactivity and IgE levels that 50% of the population are atopic but only some have asthma. I can imagine that these atopic subjects have Th2 cells sitting in the airway wall that are capable of making IL-5 when stimulated. Why do only a small number of these cells become activated to produce eosinophils and thus the inflammation of asthma? Is it related to the amount of IL-5 that the Th2 cells produce and therefore the type or number of T cells present?

Kay: There are no differences between the total numbers of bronchial T cells in normal and atopic controls. The interesting point is that in asthmatics there are increased numbers of Th2-like cells, independent of whether they are skin test positive or skin test negative.

Busse: We've done segmental antigen challenges, and we have found that eosinophils can be attracted to the airway in any allergic subject if a sufficient dose of antigen is given. Furthermore, the amount of IL-5 secreted parallels the number of eosinophils that come to the airway, and the intensity of the eosinophil response depends on the dose of antigen given.

Martinez: In other words, anyone who is sensitized but has never had an asthmatic attack could have an attack if enough of the antigen is introduced into the airway.

References

Bentley AM, Meng Q, Robinson DS, Hamid Q, Kay AB, Durham SR 1993 Increases in activated T lymphocytes, eosinophils and cytokine messenger RNA for interleukin 5 and granulocyte macrophage colony-stimulating factor in bronchial biopsies after allergen inhalation challenge in atopic asthmatics. Am J Resp Cell Mol Biol 8:35–42

Frick OL 1986 Effect of respiratory and other virus infections on IgE immunoregulation. J Allergy Clin Immunol 78:1013–1018

Humbert M, Grant JA, Taborda-Barata L et al 1996 High affinity IgE receptor (Fc$_\varepsilon$R1)-bearing cells in broncial biopsies from atopic and nonatopic asthma. Am J Resp Crit Care Med 153:1931–1937

Jeffery P 1996 Bronchial biopsies and airway inflammation. Eur Respir J 9:1583–1587

Kelso A 1995 Th1 and Th2 subsets: paradigms lost? Immunol Today 16:374–379

Pascual V, Victor K, Spellenberg M, Hamblin TS, Stevenson FK, Capra JD 1992 V_H restriction among human cold agglutinins: the V_H4–21 gene segment is required to encode anti-I and anti-i specificities. J Immunol 149:2337–2342

Robinson DS, Hamid Q, Bentley A, Ying S, Kay AB, Durham SR 1993 Activation of CD4[+] T cells, increased Th2-type cytokine mRNA expression, and eosinophil recruitment in bronchoalveolar lavage after allergen inhalation challenge in patients with atopic asthma. J Allergy Clin Immunol 92:313–324

Snow RE, Champman CJ, Frew AJ, Holgate ST, Stevenson FK 1995 Analysis of immunoglobulin (V_H) region genes encoding IgE antibodies in splenic B lymphocytes of a patient with asthma. J Immunol 154:5576–5581

Tavernier J, Tuypens T, Plaetinck G, Verhee A, Fiers W, Devos R 1992 Molecular basis of the membrane-anchored and two soluble isoforms of the human interleukin 5 receptor alpha subunit. Proc Natl Acad Sci USA 89:7041–7045

The structural and functional consequences of chronic allergic inflammation of the airways

P. D. Paré, Tony R. Bai and Clive R. Roberts

Respiratory Health Network of Centres of Excellence, University of British Columbia Pulmonary Research Laboratory, St. Paul's Hospital, Vancouver, Canada V6Z 1Y6

Abstract. Although asthma is generally considered a form of reversible airway obstruction, there is evidence that chronic allergic inflammation can lead to structural changes in the airway and a degree of progressive fixed airway obstruction. More importantly, these structural changes can lead to airway hyper-responsiveness. The structural consequences of chronic allergic inflammation are secondary to cellular proliferation and reorganization of the connective tissue constituents of the airway wall. Smooth muscle proliferation and hypertrophy may increase the potential for smooth muscle shortening against the elastic loads provided by lung parenchymal recoil and airway mucosal folding. Resident airway cells, as well as inflammatory cells, produce mediators, cytokines and growth factors that stimulate production of connective tissue proteins and proteoglycans that cause airway remodelling and altered mechanical function. Thickening of the airway wall internal to the smooth muscle layer can amplify the effect of smooth muscle shortening on airway calibre, and it could also stiffen the airway making it less distensible. Thickening of the airway wall external to the muscle can uncouple the airway from the distending force applied by the lung parenchyma. Early and aggressive anti-inflammatory medication may alter the natural history of asthma by preventing the structural changes that are a consequence of chronic allergic inflammation.

1997 The rising trends in asthma. Wiley, Chichester (Ciba Foundation Symposium 206) p 71–89

There is increasing evidence that the chronic nature of asthma is significantly influenced by changes to the structure of the airways which occur as a consequence of episodic and ongoing allergic inflammation. Allergic inflammation is the chronic inflammatory response, usually accompanied by elevated IgE levels, which is the most prevalent inflammatory process associated with asthma. Although asthma is characterized, indeed defined, by a significant reversible component, there can be an element of fixed obstruction, especially in those patients who have a long history of symptoms. In addition, the airway hyper-responsiveness to non-specific stimuli that accompanies asthma is persistent even in periods of symptomatic remission and after

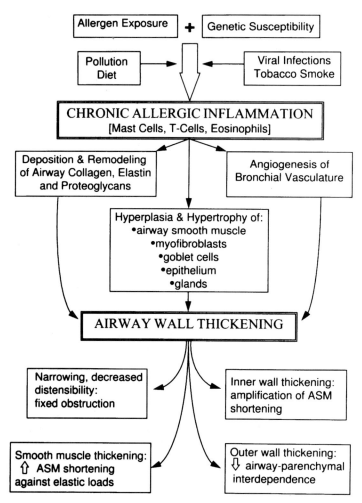

FIG. 1.   This schema illustrates the pathogenetic mechanisms which can cause airway wall thickening and the functional consequences of the structural changes. ASM, airway smooth muscle.

optimal anti-inflammatory therapy. Figure 1 shows an overview of the pathogenetic mechanisms that lead to persistent functional and structural changes. Sufficient allergen exposure, particularly in the first few years of life, can lead to the development of chronic allergic inflammation in the airways of genetically susceptible individuals; co-risk factors for the development of asthma are respiratory viral infection, a diet low in antioxidants, and exposure to environmental tobacco smoke and atmospheric pollution.

The structural changes that occur in the airways are caused by the deposition and remodelling of connective tissue components, hypertrophy and hyperplasia of tissue cells and new vessel formation in the bronchial vasculature. These alterations combine to produce airway wall thickening. Airway wall thickening can have profound effects on airway function. Airway mechanics may be changed because of quantitative changes in airway wall compartments and/or by changes in the biochemical composition or material properties of the various constituents of the airway wall.

Structural changes in the airway walls in asthma

Figure 2 shows a diagram of an intra-parenchymal airway cut in cross-section. The wall can be divided into three compartments: (1) the inner wall, consisting of epithelium, basement membrane, lamina reticularis and loose connective tissue between the lamina reticularis and the airway smooth muscle; (2) the outer wall, consisting of the loose connective tissue between the muscle layer and the surrounding parenchyma (the adventitia); and (3) the smooth muscle layer (Bai et al 1994). Figure 3 shows a schematic mechanical model of the forces and dimensions of the airway wall and illustrates how changes in dimensions can alter airway narrowing in response to smooth muscle stimulation. Panel A depicts the normal situation at equilibrium. The horizontal bars represent the airway walls; airway narrowing is simulated by an approximation of the bars. The springs outside the bars represent the lung elastic recoil which tends to dilate the airways; the tension in these springs is balanced by the tension in the springs parallel to the airway smooth muscle, which represent the connective tissue elements in the airway wall. The smooth muscle cell between the bars represents the airway smooth muscle; when stimulated to contract it narrows the airway (approximation of the bars) until the maximal force generated by the muscle is balanced by lung elastic recoil. Panel B shows the effect of thickening of the inner airway wall. In addition to narrowing the airway lumen, thickening of this layer will exaggerate the effect of any smooth muscle shortening. An increased volume of intraluminal secretions could also amplify the effects of smooth muscle shortening in addition to decreasing baseline airway luminal area. Panel C shows the effect of thickening of the outer wall area. Thickening of this layer causes a relaxation in the springs representing the lung parenchyma, i.e. a decrease in parenchymal tethering. When stimulated, the smooth muscle in such an airway will shorten more before the elastic load provided by the parenchymal recoil prevents further narrowing. Panel D shows the effect of increased airway smooth muscle thickness. If the force-generating capacity of the muscle increases in parallel with its mass, the muscle will be able to shorten more against the elastic load provided by parenchymal recoil.

Although it has been recognized for some time that the airway walls of asthmatic subjects are thickened (Huber & Koessler 1922, Houston et al 1953), it was not possible to perform a systematic study of the quantitative changes in airway wall dimensions because a yardstick of airway size was not available to allow a valid comparison between control and asthmatic subjects. The demonstration by James et

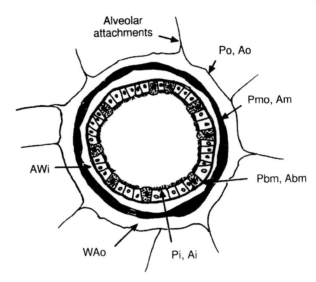

FIG. 2.   Schematic of a cross-section through a membranous airway. The three layers of the airway wall are illustrated. Abm, area within basement membrane; Ai, inner area; Am, muscle area; Ao, outer area; AWi, inner wall area; Pbm, basement membrane perimeter; Pi, internal perimeter; Pmo, outer muscle perimeter; Po, outer perimeter; WAo, outer wall area.

al (1988a,b) that the airway basement membrane perimeter is relatively constant after smooth muscle contraction or changes in lung volume has allowed a number of investigators to examine the relationship between airway wall compartment areas and airway size (James et al 1989, Bosken et al 1990, Kuwano et al 1993, Tiddens et al 1995). This is most easily done by examining the relationships between airway internal perimeter (Pi) or basement membrane perimeter (Pbm) and the areas occupied by the respective tissue components. The slopes and intercepts of these relationships can be constructed and compared using valid techniques for pooling data (Wiggs et al 1992). These results confirm that patients with fatal asthma show a marked increase in airway wall thickness that involves all layers of the airway wall. There are fewer data on patients who have had asthma but who died for other reasons or had a lobectomy. However, the available data suggest that the airway wall dimensions in these subjects are intermediate between the fatal asthmatics and the control or normal subjects (Kuwano et al 1993, Carroll et al 1993). Thus, an increase in airway wall dimensions does not simply reflect a terminal event in patients with severe asthma.

   Airway wall thickening in asthma involves increased collagen deposition. Roche et al (1989) have shown that the thickened subepithelial 'basement membrane' in asthma consists of a dense layer rich in fibrillar collagens, under a normal sub-epithelial basal lamina. This distinct collagenous matrix layer is typically doubled in thickness from

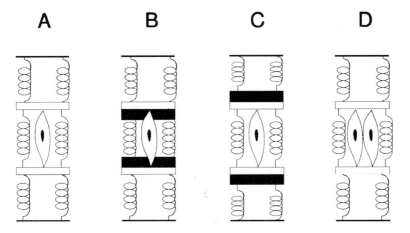

FIG. 3.   A mechanical model of airway wall structures and forces to illustrate how the structural alterations can cause exaggerated narrowing in response to stimulation of airways smooth muscle contraction. (A) Normal situation at equilibrium. (B) Effect of inner airway wall thickening. (C) Effect of outer wall area thickening. (D) Effect of increased airway smooth muscle thickness. (See text for details.)

5–8 μm (normal) to 10–15 μm (asthma) and contains types I, III and V collagen and fibronectin (Roche et al 1989), but not basal lamina components (type IV collagen, laminin). This collagenous matrix may be synthesized by its associated myofibroblasts, since myofibroblast number correlates with the magnitude of subepithelial thickening (Brewster et al 1990). Similar structural changes have been observed in patients with mild asthma and in occupational asthma associated with exposure to a variety of chemicals (Boulet et al 1994). In some individuals with toluene di-isocyanate-induced asthma, cessation of exposure to toluene di-isocyanate leads, after six to 20 months, to decreased subepithelial collagen thickness, and decreased numbers of subepithelial fibroblasts associated with decreased numbers of mast cells and lymphocytes (Saetta et al 1995). This suggests that these changes are potentially reversible, but the mechanism of this reversal is unknown.

The mechanical effects of changes in abundance of collagen types in the subepithelial matrix are unknown but they are likely to depend on the precise architecture and chemistry of the collagens deposited. The collagen fibrils in the subepithelial collagen layer in the airways of asthmatics appear to be more densely packed than normal (Roche et al 1989) and although the significance of this is unknown, it is probable that both increased collagen fibril density and thickening of this layer would increase both the tensile stiffness and resistance to deformation of the airway wall, thus tending to oppose smooth muscle contraction and airway narrowing. Airway distensibility has been shown to be decreased in asthmatics (Colebatch et al 1979, Wilson et al 1993) and this could be explained by excess collagen deposition in the sub-epithelial layer.

In addition to collagen, the adhesive glycoprotein fibronectin and the anti-adhesive glycoprotein tenascin appear to be deposited in the airway wall in asthmatics (Laitenen & Laitenen 1994). These may be synthesized by epithelial cells in response to inflammatory mediators; fibronectin synthesis by bovine bronchial epithelial cells is stimulated by transforming growth factor β (TGF-β) (Romberger et al 1992), and tenascin synthesis by transformed human bronchial epithelial cells is stimulated by tumour necrosis factor α and interferon-γ (Harkonen et al 1995).

The airway walls contain proteoglycans with their characteristic polysaccharides, the glycosaminoglycans. Specific proteoglycans and glycosaminoglycans of the extracellular matrix influence tissue biomechanics, fluid balance, cellular functions and growth factor and cytokine biological activities. Changes in glycosaminoglycan metabolism occur early in a number of animal models of inflammation (Blackwood et al 1983).

We have localized hyaluronan and the proteoglycans versican and decorin in surgical and post-mortem lung samples from individuals with normal lung function and individuals in whom asthma was the cause of death. Hyaluronan and versican were localized in and around the smooth muscle bundles in the airways (Roberts & Burke 1995). Decorin was found in areas rich in type I collagen. In airways from asthmatics, staining for the proteoglycans was particularly prominent around smooth muscle cells and in the layer between the smooth muscle and the epithelial layer. The matrix of thickened airway walls in fatal asthma contains abundant versican and hyaluronan, especially between and around the smooth muscle bundles, areas that appear to be 'space' following routine formalin fixation and paraffin embedding. These 'spaces' appear to be hydrated, proteoglycan-rich domains *in vivo* (Roberts & Burke 1995).

Although the functional correlates of proteoglycan deposition in the airway wall are unknown, hydrated proteoglycans may contribute to the increased volume of the submucosa in asthmatics (Kuwano et al 1993) and to altered airway mechanics. Hyaluronan–versican aggregates could influence the compressive stiffness of the airway wall, and they may have an effect on airway interstitial fluid balance, through their osmotic activity. The reversible redistribution of glycosaminoglycan-bound water may contribute to compressive stiffness of airway walls in a similar manner to that in which proteoglycans influence cartilage mechanical properties. The deposition of a versican–hyaluronan complex in the inner wall between the muscle and basement membrane could contribute to exaggerated airway narrowing as depicted in Fig. 3. Conversely, deposition of hyaluronan and versican between the smooth muscle and epithelium may increase tissue turgor and thus increase the resistance of the airway wall to deformation under loading. In addition, accumulation of a relatively incompressible matrix around smooth muscle cells in the airways might provide a parallel elastic afterload and decrease smooth muscle shortening.

The mechanisms underlying changes in extracellular matrix composition in asthma are incompletely understood but they are the subject of intense investigation. A number of growth factors and cytokines released by inflammatory or epithelial cells during the inflammatory process have the capacity to drive altered extracellular matrix metabolism by mesenchymal cells in the airway wall. Eosinophil and mast cell numbers are increased in asthma, which is driven by a T helper cell type 2 response. Both inflammatory cells and stimulated epithelial and mesenchymal cells (including smooth muscle cells) have the capacity to release TGF-β1, a growth factor that induces matrix deposition, and to release the potent fibroblast mitogens, including platelet-derived growth factor (PDGF) and insulin-like growth factor 1 (IGF-1). This combination of mitogens and growth factors is known to induce matrix synthesis in other systems and it is a potentially powerful mechanism for remodelling the architecture of the airway wall in asthma.

Aubert et al (1994a) showed that steady-state mRNA levels for TGF-β1, as well as the pattern of expression of the latent precursor and mature forms of TGF-β1, were similar in lung tissue from individuals with asthma, a group of individuals with chronic obstructive pulmonary disease (COPD) and a control group of cigarette smokers who had normal lung function. Similarly, there were no clear differences among these same groups of patients in the expression of mRNA for the collagen-associated proteoglycan decorin, a putative regulator of TGF-β1 biological activity (C. R. Roberts & A. Burke, unpublished results 1996). The precursor protein for TGF-β1 was detected in epithelial cells, implying epithelial cell synthesis of this growth factor. The observation that abundant mRNA and protein for TGF-β1 was found in the 'control' group is of questionable significance since individuals in the control group were chronic smokers, albeit without airflow obstruction. TGF-β1 mRNA levels in mononuclear cells from the bronchoalveolar lavage of asthmatics and normals have been shown to be similar (Deguchi 1992). Eosinophils also express TGF-β1, and their abundance in asthma would be expected to contribute to increased local, if not total, tissue levels of this growth factor. Another potential contributor to increased matrix synthesis is PDGF. Eosinophils from asthmatics express higher levels of PDGF-β mRNA than normals (Ohno et al 1995) and this growth factor is mitogenic for mesenchymal cells, including fibroblasts and smooth muscle cells. Aubert et al (1994b) examined the presence and distribution of PDGF and PDGF receptor mRNA and protein in the lungs and airways of a small group of patients with fatal asthma, as well as controls and patients with COPD. PDGF mRNA levels tended to be greater in asthmatics than in normals and lower in patients with COPD than in normals. The PDGF mRNA levels were significantly greater in patients with asthma compared to patients with COPD. In addition, there was a significant association between PDGF mRNA levels and PDGF receptor mRNA levels, suggesting that there is a link between the expression of this growth factor and its receptor.

Human airway epithelial cells have been shown to secrete fibroblast mitogenic activity, at least 50% of which is attributable to IGF-1 (Cambrey et al 1995). This growth factor stimulates collagen production by dermal fibroblasts *in vitro* (Ghahary et al 1995), suggesting a further mechanism by which epithelial cells might stimulate collagen production and cell proliferation in the underlying matrix.

Corticosteroids have multiple effects but may prevent remodelling both by decreasing influx of inflammatory cells (perhaps without decreasing the amount of mediators such as TGF-β1 per cell [Khalil et al 1993]) and by exerting specific inhibitory effects on synthesis of matrix molecules including collagen (Hamalainen et al 1985).

The airway wall remodelling that occurs in chronic asthma must be accompanied by degradation of matrix components in addition to synthesis and deposition of new matrix. Ultrastructural evidence for elastin degradation in some individuals with asthma has been reported (Bousquet et al 1992). We have observed structural changes in the cartilage in airways of 1 to 5 mm diameter, consistent with cartilage proteoglycan degradation and cartilage remodelling in each of six fatal asthma cases studied in detail. These changes may be specific to cartilage proteoglycans, and they may have effects on lung function resulting from softening of airway cartilage. Conversely, the changes in cartilage may be indicators of a much more general process of cleavage of structural elements, with even more far-reaching effects. The proteinase(s) responsible for the cartilage changes are unknown and there are a number of possibilities. Neutrophil elastase, cathepsin G and lysosomal cysteine proteinases such as cathepsins B and L are able to degrade collagen, elastin and proteoglycans. Latent cathepsin B is present in the sputum of patients who have chronic bronchitis (Buttle et al 1991). Latent cysteine proteinases can be activated by a number of means, including direct activation by neutrophil proteinases (Buttle et al 1991) and activation by a cartilage-specific mechanism that is not yet understood (C. R. Roberts, personal communication 1996). Indirect mechanisms for cartilage destruction include interleukin 1-driven resorption of airway cartilage by chondrocytes mediated by matrix metalloproteinases (Saklatvala & Sarsfield 1988), as has been described in cartilage destruction in inflammatory joint diseases. Proteinases released by mast cells, including tryptase, may also be responsible for degradation of a range of matrix macromolecules in asthma.

Degradation of airway cartilage could contribute to airflow obstruction by decreasing airway wall stiffness, which would decrease maximal expiratory flow rates from the lung. Cartilage degradation could also decrease the force required for the smooth muscle to constrict the airways.

Degradation of elastin, as shown by Bousquet et al (1992), and possibly degradation of other matrix molecules, may have similar effects on airway wall mechanics. Matrix degradation and increased proteoglycan synthesis are associated with tissue swelling during development (Toole 1991), and proteolysis in the airway wall matrix may facilitate oedema in asthma. Mast cell degranulation is associated with oedema of the airway wall and an acute decrease in interstitial pressure (Koller et al 1993). Proteoglycan synthesis, in concert with matrix degradation, may influence tissue swelling.

As previously discussed, the force required to deform the matrix constitutes an afterload that must be overcome by the smooth muscle during shortening. Degradation of matrix elements could increase the deformability of the airway wall and thus decrease its ability to act as a load on the muscle. Consistent with this hypothesis, *in vitro* studies by Bramley et al (1995) suggest that mild proteolysis in the extracellular matrix associated with airway smooth muscle allows increased force generation and shortening by strips of human airway smooth muscle. Degradation of smooth muscle-associated matrix as a consequence of chronic inflammation has been postulated to induce the increased smooth muscle contractility in asthma (Bramley et al 1994, 1995).

Since tethering of the parenchyma to both the smooth muscle and perichondrium is believed to limit smooth muscle shortening, we suggest that degradation of collagen connected to smooth muscle bundles is a prerequisite for the uncoupling of airway smooth muscle from parenchymal tethering, which has been suggested by Macklem (1995) and Robinson et al (1992) to be an important component of asthma.

A number of studies show that the airway smooth muscle layer is markedly thickened in patients with chronic asthma (Dunnill et al 1969, Heard & Hossain 1973). Part of this thickening could have been artefactual, since the airways of asthmatic subjects are often contracted and narrowed. However, correction of airway smooth muscle area for basement membrane perimeter indicates that in patients with fatal asthma, peripheral airway smooth muscle area is approximately doubled, whereas in patients who have asthma but die of other causes, lesser degrees of airway smooth muscle thickening are observed. There is evidence that the increase in smooth muscle is due both to hypertrophy of existing airway smooth muscle cells, as well as hyperplasia. Ebina et al (1990, 1993) have reported two patterns of airway smooth muscle hypertrophy and hyperplasia: in type 1 asthmatics, airway smooth muscle mass was increased only in central bronchi where hyperplasia predominated; and in type 2 asthmatics, there was increased muscle throughout the tracheobronchial tree, which was characterized by hyperplasia as well as hypertrophy, especially in peripheral airways. Thomson et al (1997) suggested that the increased airway smooth muscle area that has been reported in asthma could have been overestimated. These investigators measured the airway smooth muscle area at high magnification in the large central airways of five asthmatic subjects and showed no significant difference compared to a control group of chronic smokers. They used 1.5 mm sections of plastic-embedded tissue and they discriminated between smooth muscle cells and their surrounding matrix. They reasoned that the plane of section, the use of thick sections and a failure to distinguish between smooth muscle cells and their associated extracellular matrix could explain an overestimation of smooth muscle area in other studies. However, Thomson and co-workers studied only large central cartilaginous airways, and most of the increase in smooth muscle area that has been reported is in peripheral airways.

The increase in airway smooth muscle mass in asthma can have a simple geometric effect on airway narrowing, much like the effect of thickening of the submucosal region of the airway wall, and it can also narrow the airways as well as amplifying the effect of smooth muscle shortening. However, an increase in smooth muscle mass, if associated with a parallel and concomitant increase in force-generating ability of the muscle, will have the additional effect of allowing the airway smooth muscle to shorten excessively against the elastic loads provided by the lung parenchyma and parallel elastic elements.

Unfortunately, there have been few studies in which the functional properties of airway smooth muscle from asthmatic subjects have been measured and corrected for the amount of smooth muscle in the preparation. Schellenberg (1992) has reported increased maximal isotonic shortening and increased isometric force generation in a single asthmatic bronchial smooth muscle specimen, despite a normal amount of smooth muscle. de Jongste et al (1987) have reported increased maximal force generation in a single specimen from an asthmatic subject. However, they did not correct for the force of the smooth muscle mass. Bai & Prasad (1990) found increased force generation and decreased relaxation in the tracheal smooth muscle obtained from patients with fatal asthma, even after correction for tissue weight. No studies have shown increased airway smooth muscle sensitivity in asthmatic subjects compared to controls.

Although one might expect that an increased airway smooth muscle mass would be accompanied by an increased force, this is not necessarily the case. Vascular smooth muscle proliferation induced in rabbits by hyperoxia produces an increased smooth muscle mass, but a decreased maximal stress-generating ability of the vascular smooth muscle (Coflesky et al 1987). *In vitro*, when airway smooth muscle is stimulated to proliferate, the muscle differentiates from a contractile to a more motile phenotype, concomitant with decreased smooth muscle α-actin content and increased γ-actin and non-muscle myosin content with increasing time in culture (Halayko et al 1996). Similar de-differentiation of vascular smooth muscle occurs in vascular remodelling associated with atherosclerosis (Karnovsky & Edelman 1994), and it is possible that chronic stimulation by cytokines and growth factors in the inflamed airway walls of asthmatic subjects results in proliferation and de-differentiation of the airway smooth muscle, making it less contractile.

In summary, structural changes in the airway walls involving extracellular matrix remodelling are prominent features of asthma. These changes are likely driven by mediators released as a consequence of chronic allergic inflammation. It is clear that changes in matrix have the capacity to influence airway function in asthma. However, it is not clear how each of the many changes that occur in the airway wall contribute to altered airway function in asthma. Collagen deposition in the subepithelial matrix, and hyaluronan and versican deposition around and internal to the smooth muscle, would be expected to oppose the effect of smooth muscle contraction. Conversely, geometric considerations would result in exaggerated airway narrowing for a given degree of smooth muscle shortening, as the airway wall is thickened by the deposition of these molecules internal to the smooth muscle. Elastin and cartilage degradation in the airway walls would be expected to result in decreased airway wall stiffness and increased airway narrowing for a given amount of force generated by the smooth muscle. Degradation of matrix associated with the smooth muscle may both decrease the stiffness of the parallel elastic component and uncouple smooth muscle from the load provided by lung recoil, allowing exaggerated smooth muscle shortening. Increase in muscle mass may be associated with an increase, a decrease or no change in smooth muscle contractility. If an increased muscle mass was not associated with any other phenotypic changes it would be expected to contribute to exaggerated airway narrowing.

Animal models of allergic airway remodelling

The description of the structural changes in the airways of asthmatics who have chronic allergic inflammation is dependent on the post-mortem examination of airways from subjects who die of asthma or asthmatics who die of other causes, and on the examination of small samples of the superficial layers of the airway wall obtained by bronchoscopic biopsy. Although these sources have provided important qualitative and quantitative data, they do not allow a systematic study of the time course of the changes or of the cellular and molecular mechanisms involved in remodelling. In addition, it is difficult to obtain pathological material to assess potential interventions that might attenuate or reverse the structural changes. These problems have stimulated a search for animal models that demonstrate the airway damage and repair which characterize the structural remodelling observed in chronic allergic asthma. Structural changes reminiscent of those seen in chronic allergic asthma have recently been reported following repeated allergen challenge in rats (Sapienza et al 1991), mice (Blyth et al 1996), cats (Padrid et al 1995) and guinea pigs (Wang et al 1995). In the brown Norway rat, a strain which shows many similarities with atopic subjects, including a propensity to generate an exaggerated IgE response to inhaled aero-allergens, Sapienza et al (1991) showed that airway smooth muscle area can increase two- to threefold after as few as three ovalbumin challenges. Although they did not attempt to measure individual airway smooth muscle cell volume as an indicator of hypertrophy, they did show a 35-fold and a ninefold increase in the number of airway smooth muscle cell nuclei that took up bromodeoxyuridine in large and small airways, respectively. Bromodeoxyuridine is a thymidine analogue that is incorporated into dividing cells and can be detected using immunohistochemistry. These results suggest that airway smooth muscle cell proliferation (hyperplasia) occurs during chronic allergic inflammation.

Padrid et al (1995) have shown similar changes in the airways of mongrel cats sensitized and challenged with *A scaris suum* antigen. Twice-a-week challenges with antigen for four to six weeks led to marked eosinophilic inflammation, a 1.5 log leftward shift in the airway response to acetylcholine and approximately a 30% increase in smooth muscle layer thickness. There was also hypertrophy and hyperplasia of epithelial goblet cells and submucosal glands: all features of chronic allergic inflammation in asthmatics. In mice Blyth et al (1996) found marked epithelial changes in the airways of ovalbumin-sensitized BALB/c mice challenged by inhalation six times, with three days between challenges. In addition to peribronchial and epithelial inflammatory cell infiltration they observed a marked increase in goblet cell number, increased epithelial layer thickness and deposition of type III collagen beneath the basement membrane and within the thickened peribronchial space.

TABLE 1 Summary of morphological and morphometric changes following chronic antigen challenge in the guinea pig (from Wang et al 1995)

Challenge	Proliferation index (%)		Wall area (%)[a]		Eosinophils (area fraction, %)		Bromodeoxyuridine-positive eosinophils (proliferation index, %)	
	Smooth muscle	Epithelial	Inner	Outer	In epithelium	In adventitia	In epithelium	In adventitia
Control	2.7±1.1 (10, 27)	4.8±0.8 (10, 27)	17.3±0.8 (10, 32)	7.2±1.1 (10, 32)	0.7±0.2 (10, 27)	9.3±1.3 (10, 27)	30.3±9.1 (10, 27)	2.9±2.9 (10, 27)
Chronic antigen	23.0±3.7* (9, 29)	16.0±3.7 (9, 29)	16.1±0.8 (10, 47)	13.5±2.1* (10, 47)	6.4±1.2* (9, 29)	6.2±1.7 (9, 29)	58.5±11.9 (9, 29)	66.6±24.5* (9, 29)

[a]The wall areas are expressed as a per cent of the total area within the outer perimeter, assuming the luminal area conformed to a perfect circle (i.e. Ao, outer airway area).

Values given are per cent ± S.D. (number of guinea pigs, number of airways).

*$P < 0.05$.

Wang et al (1995) have developed a similar chronic model in the guinea pig. They challenged the ovalbumin-sensitized guinea pigs twice-a-week for six weeks, and by injecting bromodeoxyuridine intraperitoneally prior to each antigen challenge they were able to examine which of the resident and inflammatory cells in the airway wall had divided during the exposure protocol. In addition, they made precise measurements of airway wall compartments using the epithelial basement membrane perimeter as a marker of airway size as described earlier in this chapter. They quantified the hyperplasia of airway smooth muscle and epithelial cells by calculating a proliferation index as the number of bromodeoxyuridine-stained nuclei/total nuclei. Table 1 summarizes the results of these studies. There was a significant increase in the proliferation index in airway smooth muscle cells and epithelial cells, but no significant increase in the area occupied by smooth muscle. The outer or adventitial area was significantly increased but the inner wall area was not despite the proliferation of epithelial cells. These structural changes were associated with *in vivo* and *in vitro* functional changes. *In vivo* dose–response curves to inhaled acetylcholine were shifted about 0.5 log units to the left and the maximal pulmonary resistance achieved at the highest concentration of acetylcholine was doubled. *In vitro*, the trachealis smooth muscle stress generation in response to acetylcholine was also increased by 100%.

The results of these studies suggest that the structural changes seen in chronic allergic asthma can be reproduced in animals by chronic allergen exposure. We anticipate that the dissection of the cellular and molecular mechanisms involved in the development of airway remodelling in these models will provide new insights into the human disease and open the way for novel preventative and therapeutic strategies.

Acknowledgements

Our work is supported by the Medical Research Council of Canada and the British Columbia Lung Association.

References

Aubert J-D, Dalal BI, Bai TR, Roberts CR, Hayashi S, Hogg JC 1994a Transforming growth factor-β1 gene expression in human airways. Thorax 49:225–232

Aubert J-D, Hayashi S, Hards J, Bai TR, Paré PD, Hogg JC 1994b Platelet-derived growth factor and its receptor in lungs from patients with asthma and chronic airflow obstruction. Am J Physiol 266:655L–663L

Bai A, Eidelman DH, Hogg JC et al 1994 Proposed nomenclature for quantifying subdivisions of the bronchial wall. J Appl Physiol 77:1011–1014

Bai TR, Prasad FW 1990 Abnormalities in airway smooth muscle in fatal asthma. Am Rev Respir Dis 141:552–557

Blackwood RA, Cantor JO, Moret J, Mandl I, Turino GM 1983 Glycosaminoglycan synthesis in endotoxin-induced lung injury. Proc Soc Exp Biol Med 174:343–349

Blyth DI, Pedrick MS, Savage TJ, Hessel EM, Fattah D 1996 Lung inflammation and epithelial changes in a murine model of atopic asthma. Am J Respir Cell Mol Biol 14:425–438

Bosken CH, Wiggs BR, Paré PD, Hogg JC 1990 Small airway dimensions in smokers with obstruction to airflow. Am Rev Respir Dis 142:563–570

Boulet LP, Boulet M, Laviolette M et al 1994 Airway inflammation after removal from the causal agent in occupational asthma due to high and low molecular weight agents. Eur Respir J 7:1567–1575

Bousquet J, Chanez P, Lacoste JY et al 1992 Asthma: a disease remodelling the airways. Allergy 47:3–11

Bramley AM, Thomson RJ, Roberts CR, Schellenberg RR 1994 Hypothesis: excessive bronchoconstriction in asthma is due to decreased airway elastance. Eur Respir J 7:337–341

Bramley AM, Roberts CR, Schellenberg RR 1995 Collagenase increases shortening of human bronchial smooth muscle in vitro. Am J Respir Crit Care Med 152:1513–1517

Brewster CEP, Howarth PH, Djukanović R, Wilson J, Holgate ST, Roche WR 1990 Myofibroblasts and subepithelial fibrosis in bronchial asthma. Am J Respir Cell Mol Biol 3:507–511

Buttle DJ, Abrahamson M, Burnett D et al 1991 Human sputum cathepsin B degrades proteoglycan, is inhibited by α_2-macroglobulin and is modulated by neutrophil elastase cleavage of cathepsin B precursor and cystatin C. Biochem J 276:325–331

Cambrey AD, Kwon OJ, Gray AJ et al 1995 Insulin-like growth factor 1 is a major fibroblast mitogen produced by primary cultures of human airway epithelial cells. Clin Sci 89:611–617

Carroll N, Elliot J, Morton A, James A 1993 The structure of large and small airways in nonfatal and fatal asthma. Am Rev Respir Dis 147:405–410

Coflesky JT, Jones RC, Reid LM, Evans JN 1987 Mechanical properties and structure of isolated pulmonary arteries remodeled by chronic hyperoxia. Am Rev Respir Dis 136:388–394

Colebatch HJH, Greaves IA, Ng CKY 1979 Pulmonary mechanics in diagnosis. In: deKock MA, Nadel JA, Lewis CM (eds) Mechanics of airway obstruction in human respiratory disease. Balkema, Cape Town, p 25–47

de Jongste JC, Mons H, Bonata IL, Kerrebijn KF 1987 In vitro responses of airways from an asthmatic patient. Eur J Resp Dis 71:23–29

Deguchi Y 1992 Spontaneous increase of transforming growth factor beta production by bronchoalveolar mononuclear cells of patients with systemic autoimmune diseases affecting the lung. Ann Rheum Dis 51:362–365

Dunnill MS, Massarella GR, Anderson JA 1969 A comparison of the quantitative anatomy of the bronchi in normal subjects, in status asthmaticus, in chronic bronchitis, and in emphysema. Thorax 24:176–179

Ebina M, Yaegashi H, Chiba R, Takahashi T, Motomiya M, Tanemura M 1990 Hyperreactive site in the airway tree of asthmatic patients revealed by thickening of bronchial muscles. Am Rev Respir Dis 141:1327–1332

Ebina M, Takahashi T, Chiba T, Motomiya M 1993 Cellular hypertrophy and hyperplasia of airway smooth muscles underlying bronchial asthma. A 3-D morphometric study. Am Rev Respir Dis 48:720–726

Ghahary A, Shen Y, Nedelec B, Scott P, Tredget E 1995 Enhanced expression of mRNA for insulin-like growth factor 1 in post-burn hypertrophic scar tissue and its fibrogenic role in dermal fibroblasts. Mol Cell Biochem 148:25–32

Halayko AJ, Salari H, Ma H, Stephens NL 1996 Markers of airway smooth muscle cell phenotype. Am J Physiol 270:1040–1051

Hamalainen L, Oikarinen J, Kivirikko KI 1985 Synthesis and degradation of type I procollagen in cultured human skin fibroblasts and the effect of cortisol. J Biol Chem 260:720–725

Harkonen E, Virtanen I, Linnala A, Laitinen LL, Kinnula VL 1995 Modulation of fibronectin and tenascin production in human bronchial epithelial cells by inflammatory cytokines in vitro. Am J Respir Cell Mol Biol 13:109–115

Heard BE, Hossain S 1973 Hyperplasia of bronchial muscle in asthma. J Pathol 110:319–331

Houston JC, de Nevasquez S, Trounce JR 1953 A clinical and pathological study of fatal cases of status asthmaticus. Thorax 8:207–213

Huber HL, Koessler KK 1922 The pathology of bronchial asthma. Arch Intern Med 30:689–760

James AL, Hogg JC, Dunn LA, Paré PD 1988a The use of internal perimeter to compare airway size and to calculate smooth muscle shortening. Am Rev Respir Dis 138:136–139

James AL, Paré PD, Hogg JC 1988b Effects of lung volume, bronchoconstriction, and cigarette smoke on morphometric airways dimensions. J Appl Physiol 64:913–919

James AL, Paré PD, Hogg JC 1989 The mechanics of airway narrowing in asthma. Am Rev Respir Dis 139:242–246

Karnovsky MJ, Edelman ER 1994 Heparin/heparan sulphate regulation of vascular smooth muscle cell behaviour. In: Page C, Black J (eds) Airways and vascular remodelling. Academic Press, Cambridge, p 45–69

Khalil N, Whitman C, Zuo L, Danielpour D, Greenberg A 1993 Regulation of alveolar macrophage transforming growth factor beta secretion by corticosteroids in bleomycin-induced pulmonary inflammation in the rat. J Clin Invest 92:1812–1818

Koller ME, Woie K, Reed RK 1993 Increased negativity of interstitial fluid pressure in rat trachea after mast cell degranulation. J Appl Physiol 74:2135–2139

Kuwano K, Bosken CH, Paré PD, Bai TR, Wiggs BR, Hogg JC 1993 Small airways dimensions in asthma and in chronic obstructive pulmonary disease. Am Rev Respir Dis 148:1220–1225

Laitinen LA, Laitinen A 1994 Modulation of bronchial inflammation: corticosteroids and other therapeutic agents. Am Rev Respir Crit Care Med 10:87S–90S

Macklem PT 1995 Theoretical basis of airway instability. Roger S. Mitchell lecture. Chest 107:87S–88S

Ohno I, Nitta Y, Yamaguchi K et al 1995 Eosinophils as a potential source of platelet-derived-growth-factor B-chain (PDGF-β) in nasal polyps and bronchial asthma. Am J Respir Cell Mol Biol 13:639–647

Padrid P, Snook S, Finucane T et al 1995 Persistent airway hyperresponsiveness and histologic alterations after chronic antigen challenge in cats. Am J Repir Crit Care Med 151:184–193

Roberts CR, Burke A 1995 Is asthma a fibrosis disease? Chest 107:111S–117S

Robinson P Okazawa M, Bai T, Paré PD 1992 In vivo loads on airway smooth muscle: the role of noncontractile airway structures. Cdn J Physiol Pharmacol 70:602–606

Roche WR, Beasley R, Williams JH, Holgate ST 1989 Subepithelial fibrosis in the bronchi of asthmatics. Lancet I:520–524

Romberger DJ, Beckmann JD, Claasen L, Ertl RF, Rennard SI 1992 Modulation of fibronectin production of bovine bronchial epithelial cells by transforming growth factor-beta. Am J Respir Cell Mol Biol 7:149–155

Saetta M, Maestrelli P, Turato G et al 1995 Airway wall remodelling after cessation of exposure to isocyanates in sensitized asthmatic subjects. Am J Respir Crit Care Med 151:489–494

Saklatvala J, Sarsfield SJ 1988 How do interleukin 1 and tumour necrosis factor induce degradation of proteoglycan in cartilage? In: Glauert AM (ed) The control of tissue damage. Elsevier, New York, p 97–108

Sapienza S, Du T, Eidelman DH, Wang NS, Martin JG 1991 Structural changes in the airways of sensitized brown Norway rats after antigen challenge. Am Rev Respir Dis 144:423–427

Schellenberg RR 1992 Evidence of smooth muscle dysfunction in asthma. In: Busse WW, Holgate SL (eds) Asthma and rhinitis. Blackwell Scientific Publications, Oxford, p 1150–1158

Thomson RJ, Bramley AM, Schellenberg RR 1997 Airway muscle stereology-implications for increased shortening in asthma. Am J Respir Crit Care Med, in press

Tiddens HA, Paré PD, Hogg JC, Hop WC, Lambert R, de Jongste JC 1995 Cartilaginous airway dimensions and airflow obstruction in human lungs. Am J Respir Crit Care Med 152:260–266

Toole BP 1981 Proteoglycans and hyaluronan in morphogenesis and differentiation. In: Hay ED (ed) Cell biology of extracellular matrix, 2nd edn. Plenum, New York, p 305–341

Wang ZL, Bramely AM, McNamara A, Paré PD, Bai TR 1995 Chronic fenoterol exposure
    increases *in vivo* and *in vitro* airway responses in guinea pigs. Am Rev Respir Dis 149:960–965
Wiggs BR, Bosken C, Paré PD, James A, Hogg JC 1992 A model of airway narrowing in asthma
    and in chronic obstructive pulmonary disease. Am Rev Respir Dis 145:1251–1258
Wilson JW, Li X, Pain MC 1993 The lack of distensibility of asthmatic airways. Am Rev Respir
    Dis 148:806–809

DISCUSSION

Pauwels: It has been shown that increased intravascular pressure can lead to remodelling of the blood vessel walls (Mulvany 1993). Is there any evidence that broncho-constriction can cause a similar remodelling of the airway?

Paré: Your question is a good one. Could one produce smooth muscle hypertrophy and remodelling by introducing a repetitive stimulus for smooth muscle contraction that didn't have concomitant inflammatory effects? I don't know the answer. Most stimuli that cause smooth muscle contraction also have pro-inflammatory roles. One possible approach would be to give repeated cholinergic stimulation with methylcholine, for example, over many weeks or months, and as far as I know no one has done this.

Bleecker: Is there an intrinsic defect in the cartilage that causes it to change its character or is this due to a mechanical effect?

Paré: I don't know. There could have been a steroid-induced change in the cartilage of those fatal asthmatics or the damage may have been due to severe inflammatory airway disease. Cartilage is relatively resistant to digestion, but sufficient protease release could cause cartilage destruction. The changes could be secondary to the treatment or to mechanical events. I don't want to put too much emphasis on these cartilage changes. It may be a reflection of the severity of some of the proteolytic events that are going on in the airways.

Holgate: We have measured the levels of glycososaminoglycans in the urine during acute episodes of spontaneous asthma and have observed up to 10-fold increases in the excretion of these proteoglycan-derived metabolites. We have separated these by FPLC and found that about 75–80% are chondroitin sulfate and the remainder are highly sulfated products of heparin and heparan. Since these elevated levels do not occur in patients with exacerbations of cystic fibrosis we believe that they reflect matrix turnover as a result of the acute inflammatory response (Shute et al 1997).

Holt: Is there any real evidence that there are structural changes in the parenchyma of the lung in chronic asthma rather than just around the airways?

Paré: No, there is no evidence. However, the evidence is difficult to obtain because only a small amount of parenchyma, if any, is obtained from biopsies.

Holt: Could you look at asthma fatalities?

Paré: We could but we have not systematically examined the parenchyma in those subjects. Kinsella et al (1988) have performed high resolution computed tomography on asthmatics who had hyperinflation, but there was no evidence of emphysema or parenchymal destruction.

Busse: Are some of these airway changes specific to allergen sensitization or are they observed in other circumstances? For example, are similar changes observed in rhinovirus-infected animal models?

Paré: Rick Hegele in our laboratory has looked at respiratory syncytial virus infections in guinea pigs. He has observed chronic inflammation associated with persistence of viral genome but he hasn't yet quantitated whether that inflammation is associated with thickening of the airway wall (Hegele et al 1994).

Magnussen: Is it more useful to study the constriction of airways or the relaxation of constricted airways?

Paré: In my opinion it is more useful to study airway constriction because there first has to be some degree of airway smooth muscle constriction to enable one to study relaxation. Therefore, you're not necessarily looking at an intrinsic property of an individual's airway smooth muscle when you look at bronchdilation — it's influenced by whether or not they initially had smooth muscle contraction. Asthmatic airway smooth muscle does show impaired relaxation *in vitro*, however.

Boushey: I have two observations that support your line of reasoning. First, Cerrina et al (1986) obtained airway smooth muscle from lung tissue and found that the difference in the samples from asthmatics and non-asthmatics *in vitro* was in the relaxation response to β-agonists rather than the contractile response to different agonists. My second point, which is implied in your model, is that thickening of the adventitia around the airways will diminish the bronchodilatory effects of a deep inhalation. The loss of mechanisms of reversing smooth muscle contraction may contribute to airway hyper-responsiveness.

Corris: There are many different types of collagen. Is there anything specific about the collagen that is involved in the remodelling process in the asthmatic airway compared to other diseases?

Holgate: The epithelium is attached to a basement membrane via hemidesmosomes. The lamina reticularis of the basement membrane contains type IV and type VII collagen, as well as laminin. In asthma these collagen subtypes are replaced by interstitial collagens types I, III and V, which are secreted by myofibroblasts. Until recently, asthma was considered a disease of smooth muscle, then one of inflammation. It is our view that it is also a disease of repair in which the epithelium plays a central role.

Burney: I would like to mention some of the epidemiological studies. I'm struck by the divergence between your results, which suggest that there is a large effect of remodelling on the development of long-term obstruction, and the paucity of epidemiological evidence that this actually occurs. Ann Woolcock's data suggest that asthmatics on average have a worse prognosis in terms of lung function (Peat et al 1987), but there are other studies that seem not to show this (Ulrik & Lange 1994). Could you put what you're saying in the context of what happens in unselected populations, rather than in fatal asthmatics or those who are selected for special study?

Paré: I didn't mean to imply that the irreversible structural changes cause sufficient obstruction to result in CO_2 retention and respiratory failure. We are suggesting that the structural changes which do occur will change the airway behaviour irreversibly, i.e. to produce hyper-responsiveness. Occupational asthma is a good model: exposure to certain occupational agents results in the development of airway hyper-responsiveness. However, when the individuals are removed from their occupational environment they're often left with airway hyper-responsiveness, which can result in persistent symptoms in response to a wide variety of non-specific stimuli. I believe that the reason for this is the structural changes which have occurred in the airway; these changes may be irreversible.

Burney: So they don't actually have any airway obstruction as measured by spirometry.

Paré: They get some degree of fixed obstruction, but the structural changes predominantly result in hyper-responsiveness rather than a decrease in FEV_1 (forced expiratory volume in one second), although there is evidence for accelerated and fixed decline in FEV_1 in some asthmatics.

Woolcock: A decline in FEV_1 depends on the kind of asthma. In our study the group of asthmatics who had a decline in lung function were those who we defined as having persistent asthma, airway hyper-responsiveness and symptoms. However, in large populations of asthmatics the majority of them will have mild asthma and only minor changes in their FEV_1 with time.

Holgate: This highlights the paucity of knowledge on the natural history of asthma.

Weiss: There are now four or five studies which show that airway responsiveness in the absence of asthma *per se* predicts an accelerated decline in lung function (Frew et al 1992, Rijcken et al 1995, Villar et al 1995, O'Connor et al 1995). Airway responsiveness, even in the absence of an asthmatic state, predicts an accelerated decline in lung function. It's a mistake to think of asthma only as a disease of the airways. Peter Paré has described a phenomenon that is relevant early on, but I don't believe that chronic eosinophilic inflammation, which persists for years, won't influence the development of chronic obstructive pulmonary disease (COPD). The site of the airway inflammation is the small airways, which are exactly the same airways that are involved in cigarette smoking-induced inflammation and COPD. Although there are no data to support this, a conceivable scenario is that lung function is maximal early in adult life and stays stable for a period of time before declining. If one looks at IgE levels to determine when the eosinophilic inflammation is likely to occur, one finds that it's likely to occur between the ages of 15 to 40 when peoples' lung functions are maximal. Therefore, it will be difficult for the clinician to observe any decrease in lung function and any damage to the parenchyma. One could postulate that if a substantial amount of damage occurred in an individual they would be prone to severe disease later on in life as a result of the silent inflammation that's occurring. It's possible that there is a parenchymal component of this disease which we have not yet recognized.

Woolcock: There's some evidence which backs this up. If one measures vital capacity rather than FEV_1 one finds further changes in a subgroup of asthmatics. They have a progressive decline in vital capacity, which is greater than the decline in FEV_1. They lose lung volume and some airways appear to close off permanently.

The increased smooth muscle bulk down the airways was not linear. Judy Black studied a collection of asthmatic lungs in Peter Jeffery's laboratory, and she found that the increase of the bronchial smooth muscle was uneven and that the most substantial increases occurred in the middle-sized airways, which were 2–4 mm in diameter, rather than the smaller or larger airways.

Paré: We have not studied that carefully, but I agree that the most important changes are in intermediate-sized airways. Ebina et al (1990, 1993) have characterized groups of asthmatics based on whether or not they showed smooth muscle hypertrophy or hyperplasia and whether it occurred mainly in the central or the peripheral airways. They defined two patterns of smooth muscle change, which I described in my presentation.

References

Cerrina J, Ladurie ML, Labat C, Raffestin B, Bayol A, Brink C 1986 Comparison of human bronchial muscle response to histamine *in vivo* with histamine and isoproterenol agonists *in vitro*. Am Rev Respir Dis 134:57–61

Ebina M, Yaegashi H, Chiba R, Takahashi T, Motomiya M, Tanemura M 1990 Hyperreactive site in the airway tree of asthmatic patients revealed by thickening of bronchial muscles. Am Rev Respir Dis 141:1327–1332

Ebina M, Takahashi T, Chiba T, Motomiya M 1993 Cellular hypertrophy and hyperplasia of airway smooth muscles underlying bronchial asthma. A 3-D morphometric study. Am Rev Respir Dis 48:720–726

Frew AF, Kennedy SM, Chan-Yeung M 1992 Methacholine responsiveness, smoking, and atopy as risk factors for accelerated FEV_1 decline in male working populations. Am Rev Respir Dis 146:878–883

Hegele RG, Hayashi S, Bramley AM, Hogg JC 1994 Persistence of respiratory syncytial virus genome and protein after acute bronchiolitis in guinea pigs. Chest 105:1848–1854

Kinsella M, Muller NL, Staples C, Vedal S, Chan-Yeung M 1988 Hyperinflation in asthma and emphysema. Assessment by pulmonary function testing and computed tomography. Chest 94:186–189

Mulvany MJ 1993 Resistance vessel structure and the pathogenesis of hypertension. J Hypertens (suppl 5) 11:7S–12S

O'Connor GT, Sparrow D, Weiss ST 1995 A prospective study of methacholine airway responsiveness as a predicator of pulmonary function decline: the Normative Aging Study. Am J Respir Crit Care Med 152:87–92

Peat JK, Woolcock AJ, Cullen K 1987 Rate of decline in lung function in subjects with asthma. Eur J Respir Dis 70:171–179

Rijcken B, Schouten JP, Xu X, Rosner B, Weiss ST 1995 Bronchial hyperresponsiveness to histamine is associated with accelerated decline of FEV_1. Am J Respir Crit Care Med 151:1377–1382

Shute JK, Parmar J, Holgate PH 1997 Urinary GAG levels are increased in acute severe asthma — a role for eosinophil-derived gelatinase B? Int Arch Allergy Immunol, in press

Ulrik CS, Lange P 1994 Decline of lung function in adults with bronchial asthma 150:629–634

Villar MT, Dow L, Coggon D, Lampe FC, Holgate ST 1995 The influence of increased bronchial responsiveness, atopy, and serum IgE on decline in FEV_1: a longitudinal study in the elderly. Am J Respir Crit Care Med 151:656–662

Genetic susceptibility to asthma in a changing environment

Eugene R. Bleecker, Dirkje S. Postma* and Deborah A. Meyers†

*University of Maryland School of Medicine, Division of Pulmonary and Critical Care Medicine, 10 South Pine Street, Suite 800, Baltimore, MD 21201, USA, *University Hospital Groningen, The Netherlands and † Johns Hopkins University, Baltimore, MD, USA*

Abstract. There is a major interest in investigating the genetic components of allergy and asthma. Four different areas are involved in the study of complex genetic diseases: family studies, assessment of phenotype, segregation analysis and gene mapping. Initial assessment of phenotype must be practical, reproducible and relatively independent of compounding variables. Phenotypes important in allergy and asthma include atopic parameters such as total serum IgE, bronchial hyper-responsiveness and the presence/absence of clinical asthma. Numerous family and twin studies have suggested the presence of a heritable component for allergy, bronchial hyper-responsiveness and asthma. The number of genes involved in these complex genetic disorders and their mode of inheritance have not been fully determined. Our group has been involved in a collaborative US–Dutch study in which 92 families with over 500 individuals have been phenotyped and DNA has been obtained for genotyping. Initial results of the classification of family members show that approximately 26% of the offspring of families ascertained through a parent with asthma have an asthmatic phenotype. A large number of these offspring with clinical evidence of asthma do not have a prior physician diagnosis of asthma, suggesting that there is a spectrum which ranges from preclinical to symptomatic asthma. The familial aggregation of asthma and other obstructive airway diseases in these families is consistent with a significant genetic component. Initial linkage studies have been performed on two characteristics of the allergic and asthmatic phenotype. Total serum IgE was analysed because this measure correlates with the clinical expression of allergy, bronchial hyper-responsiveness and asthma. Segregation analysis of total serum IgE provided evidence for a recessive mode of inheritance. Sib pair analyses and maximum likelihood scores suggest that a gene regulating IgE production maps to chromosome 5q. Bronchial hyper-responsivenss and total serum IgE are related to asthma in population-based studies. Sib pair analyses for bronchial responsiveness showed significant linkage to markers on chromosome 5q.

1997 The rising trends in asthma. Wiley, Chichester (Ciba Foundation Symposium 206) p 90–105

Asthma is a respiratory disease that is characterized by variable airways obstruction, airways inflammation and bronchial hyper-responsiveness (BHR) (Sheffer 1991). There has been a recent increase in morbidity associated with asthma (Gergen & Weiss 1992), and epidemiological studies have provided strong evidence that asthma and allergic disorders are increasing both in prevalence and severity (Ninan & Russell 1992, Peat et al 1994). While the precise reasons for these changes are unknown, there is some evidence to indicate that these rising trends are associated with increased levels of sensitization to common environmental allergens and early life exposure to adjuvant factors including air pollutants and viral respiratory infections in susceptible individuals (Burr 1993).

Understanding the genetic mechanisms responsible for allergy and asthma has widespread public health consequences because it may lead to a better understanding of the pathogenesis of asthma. Briefly, the potential benefits are:

(1) an understanding of the heritable component(s) of the trait or disease;
(2) presymptomatic and early disease diagnosis;
(3) the elucidation of pathogenic mechanisms;
(4) the determination of the importance of gene–environment interactions; and
(5) the development of interventions, i.e. disease prevention (environmental control), specific pharmacological treatments and gene therapy.

Asthma is a complex genetic disease whose development is determined by the interaction between host susceptibility and environmental exposures (Fig. 1). It is possible that gene–environment interactions initially cause presymptomatic conditions before they cause symptomatic disease. The presence of atopy or BHR may characterize this presymptomatic state (Boushey et al 1980, Weiss et al 1984, Holgate et al 1987). The understanding of these gene–environment interactions may lead to therapeutic interventions for asthma that prevent disease progression and the development of irreversible changes in airway function.

It is clear that multiple genes as well as environmental factors are important in determining susceptibility to asthma. To investigate the complex genetic components found in asthma, we need to adopt the following logical stepwise experimental approach (Liggett & Meyers 1996, Panhuysen et al 1995):

(1) define the phenotype;
(2) identify a genetic component to the trait or disorder;
(3) select families or population samples;
(4) determine the mode of inheritance by segregation analysis;
(5) perform linkage analysis, i.e. genome screening to identify regions of interest;
(6) characterize the regions of interest;
(7) do fine mapping and gene localization studies; and
(8) determine gene–gene, genotype–phenotype and gene–environment interactions.

Genetic studies require the combined skills of experts in several disciplines including asthma, genetic analysis (epidemiology), molecular genetics, biology and physiology (Fig. 2). Because of the complex nature of these interactions, collaborative approaches are required to provide the statistical power to obtain linkage and map genes in allergy

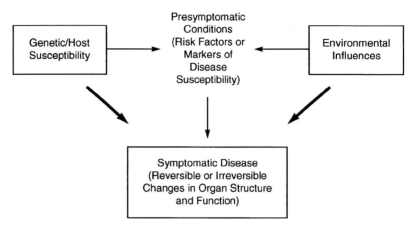

FIG. 1.   Schematic showing gene–environment interactions of complex genetic diseases.

and asthma. Careful clinical evaluation is necessary to characterize the families for linkage analysis, and physical mapping of appropriate susceptibility genes is then required (Fig. 2). Even at the initial stages of this integrated plan, biological studies employing relevant animal models and manipulated genetic mouse strains will compliment molecular mapping studies. Thus, multidisciplinary studies are necessary to determine the role of susceptibility genes and specific environmental exposures in the development and progression of asthma.

Phenotype definition

Defining the asthma phenotype is a central issue in dissecting the genetic components and their relationship to environmental influences. While current definitions of asthma now emphasize the importance of inflammatory mechanisms in addition to physiological changes associated with asthma (Global Initiative for Asthma 1995), often they are not helpful for the early identification of asthma or for its differentiation from other closely related conditions. Since one uniform phenotype defining asthma does not exist, investigators have used different, subjective or more concrete definitions for asthma: a reported prior doctor diagnosis of asthma, questionnaire data, the presence of BHR or combinations of the above (Wiesch et al 1996). In the past, many studies on the genetics of asthma have relied on only historical data to document the presence or absence of asthma (Wiesch et al 1996). Use of subjective clinical data alone without corroborative objective studies and testing of asymptomatic individuals can lead to misclassification. Overdiagnosis or underdiagnosis in family members may incorrectly classify individuals as showing recombination and add critical errors during fine mapping and gene localization (Xu & Meyers 1996). For example, in a study of 92 Dutch families, an algorithm was

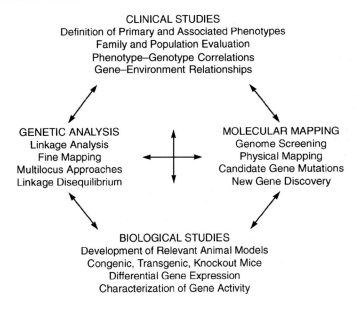

CLINICAL STUDIES
Definition of Primary and Associated Phenotypes
Family and Population Evaluation
Phenotype–Genotype Correlations
Gene–Environment Relationships

GENETIC ANALYSIS
Linkage Analysis
Fine Mapping
Multilocus Approaches
Linkage Disequilibrium

MOLECULAR MAPPING
Genome Screening
Physical Mapping
Candidate Gene Mutations
New Gene Discovery

BIOLOGICAL STUDIES
Development of Relevant Animal Models
Congenic, Transgenic, Knockout Mice
Differential Gene Expression
Characterization of Gene Activity

FIG. 2.   Schematic showing an integrated approach for mapping genes in complex diseases.

derived incorporating both subjective and objective measures of asthma (Panhuysen et al 1994). Family members in class 1 'definite asthma' had to be symptomatic, non-smokers with BHR. Using this scheme, 26% of 320 offspring were classified as having definite asthma. However, only 60% of these offspring had a prior physician's diagnosis, demonstrating the presence of preclinical asthma and probable underdiagnosis in these asthma families.

Most patients with asthma have clinical and serological evidence of atopy. Even in children who are asymptomatic, BHR appears to be closely linked to an allergic diathesis, as reflected by the association of serum IgE level with BHR and asthma (Sears et al 1991). Despite the close relationship between asthma, high total serum IgE and atopy, these traits cannot be simply interchanged. The same is true for asthma and BHR: though virtually all asthmatics show BHR, not all subjects with BHR have asthma. BHR may precede the expression of asthma and indeed constitute a risk factor (Hopp et al 1990) or it may be present in association with chronic obstructive pulmonary disease (Tashkin et al 1992). However, both total serum IgE levels and BHR are useful measurements that can be analysed in genetic family studies as quantitative traits. In addition, skin test responses, which have been shown to be closely related to BHR and asthmatic symptoms, can be studied (Burrows et al 1995). The value of studying these associated phenotypes, and especially quantitative traits, is that a larger percentage of the family members provide useful information for genetic analysis (Lander & Kruglyak 1995, Xu et al 1995, Kruglyak et al 1996).

Familial aggregation and segregation analysis

Significant familial aggregation of asthma and phenotypes associated with asthma have been described in numerous studies (Longo et al 1987, Sibbald et al 1980), probably due to an interaction of environmental and genetic factors that influence susceptibility to the development of asthma. The results from numerous twin studies, including the one from the Australian twin register (Duffy et al 1990) and those reported by Hopp et al (1988), showed significant differences between monozygotic and dizygotic twin-pairs, providing evidence for a genetic component. The latter group also found evidence for heritability of phenotypes associated with asthma such as BHR, skin test responses and total serum IgE levels, as well as clinical allergy (Hopp et al 1984, 1988, 1990). However, segregation analysis of the asthma phenotype did not show evidence for a single major gene (Holberg et al 1996) but that multiple genes are probably important in determining susceptibility.

There have been numerous segregation studies of the associated phenotype, i.e. total serum IgE levels demonstrating the presence of at least one major gene (Blumenthal et al 1974, 1981, 1992, Marsh et al 1981,1992, Friedhoff et al 1981, Meyers et al 1983, 1987, 1994, Martinez et al 1994). In an analysis of the Dutch family data by our group, evidence for two unlinked major loci was observed (Xu et al 1995). Martinez et al (1994) reported evidence for co-dominant inheritance in a large sample of families. Therefore, IgE levels represent an important associated phenotype for linkage studies.

Mapping studies

Previous evidence for susceptibility genes for asthma and/or allergy (Table 1) mapping to chromosomes 5, 6, 11, 12 and 14 have suggested that multiple genes are important in determining genetic susceptibility (Cookson et al 1989, 1992, Shirakawa et al 1994, Young et al 1994, Marsh et al 1994, Meyers et al 1994, Postma et al 1995, Doull et al 1996, Moffatt et al 1994, Barnes et al 1996). In addition, several genome screens are underway, which have reported additional areas of proposed linkage in different population and racial groups (Daniels et al 1996, Meyers et al 1996).

One candidate region that has been studied is chromosome 5q, where there are multiple candidate genes, including a number of proinflammatory cytokines — such as interleukin (IL)-3, IL-4, IL-5, IL-9, IL-13 and granulocyte macrophage colony-stimulating factor — and the $\beta 2$-adrenergic receptor. Results of these linkage studies illustrate the approaches required to study complex disorders such as allergy and asthma. Evidence for linkage of a locus regulating total serum IgE levels to chromosome 5q in the isolated Amish population was observed by Marsh et al (1994). In our studies in Dutch families, we found evidence for recessive inheritance of high IgE levels and linkage to chromosome 5q in families ascertained through a parent with asthma originally studied 25 years ago (Meyers et al 1994). Using a two-locus segregation analysis model, Xu et al (1995) reported evidence that approximately

TABLE 1   **Proposed chromosomal locations for asthma and allergy susceptibility genes**

Chromosomal location	Characteristics
5q	A region with multiple candidate genes
	Total serum IgE and bronchial hyper-responsiveness map here
6q	Association with responses to specific allergens and HLA haplotypes
11q	Maternal inheritance of atopy
	Proposed mutation in high affinity IgE receptor ($Fc_\varepsilon R1_\beta$)
12q	Linkage of asthma phenotype to a region of candidate genes including γ-interferon
14q	Linkage to the T cell receptor α and β

50% of the variability in total serum IgE levels was regulated on chromosome 5q. He also reported findings of a second locus on another unidentified chromosome that was involved in the regulation of serum IgE levels. Using the two-locus model the LOD score (maximum likelihood analysis) improved from 3.0 to 4.6 (odds for linkage > 10 000 : 1). By sib-pair analysis, evidence for linkage for both BHR and the asthma phenotype was also observed in this region (Postma et al 1995, Bleecker et al 1995). Additional evidence for linkage to this region has been observed in a study of randomly ascertained families in Southampton, UK (Doull et al 1996). These linkage findings support efforts at fine mapping this region to identify susceptibility genes for asthma and allergy.

Heterogeneity studies show that 60% of the Dutch families are linked to this region with a multipoint LOD score of 7.6 at 6 cM from the marker D5S1480 (Bleecker et al 1996). The cytokine cluster of genes fall within the confidence interval for this linkage. An association with specific IL-9 alleles and IgE levels was observed in a set of randomly ascertained families (Doull et al 1996). Further studies of IL-9 as a candidate gene were performed in the Dutch families. A novel polymorphism in exon 5, a C→T nucleotide substitution at position 4130 that results in the amino acid change Thr to Met, was found by direct DNA sequencing of probands. Probands and spouses (non-asthmatic) were evaluated in the 26 families that show the strongest evidence for linkage to chromosome 5q. The frequency of this polymorphism is similar in probands (21.7% are CT, freq(T) = 10.9%) and in spouses (19.5% are CT, freq(T) = 9.8%). Geometric mean IgE levels were low in both groups (< 100 IU) and not significantly different, 47 IU in CC individuals vs. 38 i.u. in CT individuals. Thus, this IL-9 polymorphism does not appear to be related to the regulation of elevated IgE levels in these asthmatic Dutch families.

Another example is the linkage that has been reported for atopy to chromosome 11q (Cookson 1989, 1992). While other investigators have not been able to replicate this linkage in their populations (Lympany 1992 et al, Hizawa et al 1992, Amelung 1992, Rich et al 1992), Shirakawa et al (1994) have reported evidence for a polymorphism in the β subunit of the high affinity IgE receptor. Additional studies are required to determine the presence of this association in other populations and if there is maternal inheritance of atopy in families who demonstrate the reported polymorphism.

These analyses raise several important issues. In view of the genetic complexity of asthma susceptibility, it is possible that one or two important major genes may not be found but that multiple genes are important. Polymorphisms in these multiple genes may be relatively frequent but may interact with environment influences for their expression. Besides the genetic components of asthma, there are multiple environmental factors that are important in the pathogenesis of this disease, such as breast-feeding, diet, viral respiratory infections in early childhood, exposure to allergens and parental smoking, especially maternal smoking during pregnancy (Burr et al 1989, Schwartz et al 1990, Arshad & Hide 1992). Therefore, it will be very important to evaluate gene–environment interactions in order to delineate genetic susceptibility to asthma. This can accomplished using the statistically powerful technique of transmission disequilibrium with logistic regression (Speilman et al 1993). In studies using linkage disequilibrium analytical techniques, a large number of patients with clinical asthma should be studied with blood samples obtained from the parents. It would then be possible to detect associations between polymorphisms in candidate genes and measures of the disease phenotype and environmental influences. The alleles present in the parents that were not transmitted to the child would serve as control alleles, avoiding the requirement to evaluate a large sample of control subjects. Different environmental exposures can be used as parameters in the regression analysis.

Summary

Studies of gene–environment interactions are emerging in the field of asthma. Genetic susceptibility to the development of asthma may require specific environmental exposures dependent on the genotype of the patient. Since the human genome is being rapidly mapped, it is becoming increasingly easier to characterize candidate loci. As suggested by Risch & Merikangas (1996), future studies should be focused on studying large samples of patients, rather than families, to determine the interactions between genes and the environment. Since several genome screens for candidate regions have now been completed (Daniels et al 1996, Meyers et al 1996), the candidate genes in these regions need to studied in patient populations to determine their relevancy and the relationship between their expression and environmental exposures.

Acknowledgements

This study was supported by the National Institutes of Health R01-HL48341, the National Institutes of Health U01-HL49602, the Dutch Asthma Fonds grant no. 90.39, and the Foundations CARA bestrijding and de Kock.

References

Amelung PJ, Panhuysen CIM, Postma DS et al 1992 Atopy and bronchial hyperresponsiveness: exclusion of linkage to candidate loci on chromosome 11q and 6p. Clin Exp Allergy 22:1077–1084

Arshad SH, Hide DW 1992 Effect of environmental factors on the development of allergic disorders in infancy. J Allergy Clin Immunol 90:235–241

Barnes KC, Neely JD, Duffy DL et al 1996 Linkage of asthma and total serum IgE concentration to markers on chromosome 12q: evidence from Afro-Carribean and Caucasian populations. Genomics 37:41–50

Bleecker ER, Amelung PJ, Levitt RC, Postma DS, Meyers DA 1995 Evidence for linkage of total serum IgE and bronchial hyperresponsiveness to chromosome 5q: a major regulatory locus important in asthma. Clin Exp Allergy 25:84–88

Bleecker ER, Scott AF, Xu J, Panhuysen CIM, Postma DS, Meyers DA 1996 Fine mapping of asthma susceptibility locus to 5q31–33. Am J Hum Genet 59:213A

Blumenthal MN, Amos DB, Noreen H, Mendell NR, Yunis EJ 1974 Genetic mapping of Ir locus in man: linkage to second locus of HLA. Science 184:1301–1303

Blumenthal MN, Namboodiri K, Mendell N, Gleich G, Elston RC, Yunis E 1981 Genetic transmission of serum IgE levels. Am J Med Genet 10:219–228

Blumenthal MN, Marcus-Bagley D, Awdeh Z, Johnson B, Yunis EJ, Alper CA 1992 Extended major HLA-DR2, [HLA-B7, SC31, DR2], and [HLA-B8, SC01, DR3] haplotypes distinguish subjects with asthma from those with only rhinitis in ragweed pollen allergy. J Immunol 148:411–416

Boushey HA, Holtzman MJ, Sheller JR, Nadel JA 1980 Bronchial hyperresponsiveness. Am Rev Respir Dis 121:389–413

Burr ML 1993 Epidemiology of clinical allergy. Karger, Basel (Monographs Allergy Series 31) p 1–8

Burr ML, Miskelly FG, Butland BK, Merrett TG, Vaughan-Williams E 1989 Environmental factors and symptoms in infants at high risk of allergy. J Epidemiol Community Health 43:125–132

Burrows B, Sears MR, Flannery EM, Herbison GP, Holdaway MD 1995 Relationship of bronchial responsiveness to allergy skin test reactivity, lung function, respiratory symptoms, and diagnosis in 13-year-old New Zealand children. J Allergy Clin Immunol 95:548–556

Cookson WOCM, Sharp PA, Faux JA, Hopkin JM 1989 Linkage between immunoglobulin E responses underlying asthma and rhinitis and chromosome 11q. Lancet I:1292–1295

Cookson WO, Young RP, Sandford AJ et al 1992 Maternal inheritance of atopic IgE responsiveness on chromosome 11q. Lancet 340:381–384

Daniels SE, Bhattacharrya S, James A et al 1996 A genome-wide search for quantitative trait loci underlying asthma. Nature 383:247–250

Doull IJM, Lawrence S, Watson M et al 1996 Allelic association of gene markers on chromosomes 5q and 11q with atopy and bronchial hyperresponsiveness. Am J Resp Crit Care Med 153:1280–1284

Duffy DL, Martin NG, Battistuta D, Hopper JL, Mathews JD 1990 Genetics of asthma and hay fever in Australian twins. Am Rev Respir Dis 142:1351–1358

Freidhoff LR, Meyers DA, Bias WB, Chase GA, Hussain R, Marsh DG 1981 A genetic–epidemiologic study of human immune responsiveness to allergens in an industrial population. I. Epidemiology of reported allergy and skin-test positivity. Am J Med Genet 9:323–340

Gergen PJ, Weiss KB 1992 The increasing problem of asthma in the United States. Am Rev Respir Dis 146:823–824

Global Initiative for Asthma 1995 Global strategy for asthma management and prevention (National Institutes of Health, National Heart, Lung and Blood Institute and World Health Organisation Workshop Report). NIH publication no. 95-3659

Hizawa N, Yamaguchi E, Ohe M et al 1992 Lack of linkage between atopy and locus 11q13. Clin Exp Allergy 22:1065–1069

Holberg CJ, Elston RC, Halonen M et al 1996 Segregation analysis of physician-diagnosed asthma in hispanic and non-hispanic white families. A recessive component? Am J Respir Crit Care Med 154:144–150

Holgate ST, Beasley R, Twentyman OP 1987 The pathogenesis and significance of bronchial hyperresponsiveness in airway disease. Clin Sci 73:561–572

Hopp RJ, Bewtra AK, Watt GD, Nair NM, Townley RG 1984 Genetic analysis of allergic disease in twins. J Allergy Clin Immunol 73:265–270

Hopp RJ, Bewtra AK, Biven R, Nair NM, Townley RG 1988 Bronchial reactivity pattern in nonasthmatic parents of asthmatics. Ann Allergy 61:184–186

Hopp RJ, Townley RG, Biven R, Bewtra AK, Nair NM 1990 The presence of airway reactivity before the development of asthma. Am Rev Respir Dis 141:2–8

Kruglyak L, Daly MJ, Reeve-Daly MP, Lander ES 1996 Parametric and nonparametric linkage analysis: a unified multipoint approach. Am J Hum Genet 58:1347–1363

Lander E, Kruglyak L 1995 Genetic dissection of complex traits: guidelines for interpreting and reporting linkage results. Nat Genet 11:241–247

Liggett S, Meyers DA (eds) 1996 The genetics of asthma. Marcel Dekker, New York (Lung Biology in Health and Diseases Series 96)

Longo G, Strinati R, Poli F, Fumi F 1987 Genetic factors in nonspecific bronchial hyperreactivity. An epidemiologic study. Am J Dis Child 141:331–334

Lympany P, Welsh KI, Cochrane GM, Kemeny DM, Lee TH 1992 Genetic analysis of the linkage between chromosome 11q and atopy. Clin Exp Allergy 22:1085–1092

Marsh DG, Meyers DA, Bias WB 1981 The epidemiology and genetics of atopic allergy. N Engl J Med 305:1551–1559

Marsh DG, Meyers DA, Freidhoff LR et al 1992 HLA-Dw2: a genetic marker for human immune response to short ragweed pollen allergen Ra5.II. Response after ragweed immunotherapy. J Exp Med 155:1452–1463

Marsh DG, Neely JD, Breazeale DR et al 1994 Linkage analysis of IL-4 and other chromosome 5q31.1 markers and total serum IgE concentrations. Science 264:1152–1156

Martinez FD, Holberg CJ, Halonen M, Morgan WJ, Wright AL, Taussig LM 1994 Evidence for Mendelian inheritance of serum IgE levels in Hispanic and non-Hispanic white families. Am J Hum Genet 55:555–565

Meyers DA, Hasstedt SJ, Marsh DG et al 1983 The inheritance of immunoglobulin E: genetic linkage analysis. Am J Med Genet 16:575–581

Meyers DA, Beaty TH, Freidhoff LR, Marsh DG 1987 Inheritance of total serum IgE (basal levels) in man. Am J Hum Genet 41:51–62

Meyers DA, Postma DS, Panhuysen CIM, Amelung PJ, Levitt RC, Bleecker ER 1994 Evidence for a locus regulating total serum IgE levels mapping to chromosome 5. Genomics 23:464–470

Meyers DA, Banks-Schlegel S, Bleecker ER et al 1996 A genome-wide search for asthma susceptibility loci in ethnically diverse populations. Am J Hum Genet 59:228A

Moffatt MF, Hill MR, Cornelis F et al 1994 Genetic linkage of T-cell receptor alpha/delta complex to specific IgE responses. Lancet 343:1597–1600

Ninan TK, Russell G 1992 Respiratory symptoms and atopy in Aberdeen schoolchildren: evidence from two surveys 25 years apart. Br Med J 304:873–875

Panhuysen CIM, Bleecker ER, van Altena R, Meyers DA, Koeter GH, Postma DS 1994 Results of an algorithm to characterize obstructive airways disease in families of probands with asthma. Am J Respir Crit Care Med 149:910A

Panhuysen CIM, Meyers DA, Postma DS, Levitt RC, Bleecker ER 1995 The genetics of asthma and atopy. Allergy 50:863–864

Peat JK, van den Berg RH, Green WF, Mellis CM, Leeder SR, Woolcock AJ 1994 Changing prevalence of asthma in Australian children. Br Med J 308:1591–1596

Postma DS, Bleecker ER, Amelung PJ et al 1995 Genetic susceptibility to asthma: bronchial hyperresponsiveness coinherited with a major gene for atopy. New Engl J Med 333:894–900

Rich SS, Roitman-Johnson B, Greenberg B, Roberts S, Blumenthal MN 1992 Genetic analysis of atopy in three large inbreds: no evidence for linkage to D11S97. Clin Exp Allergy 22:1070–1076

Risch N, Merikangas K 1996 The future of genetic studies of complex human diseases. Science 273:1516–1517

Schwartz J, Gold D, Dockery DW, Weiss ST, Speizer FE 1990 Predictors of asthma and persistent wheeze in a national sample of children in the United States. Association with social class, perinatal events, and race. Am Rev Respir Dis 142:555–562

Sears MR, Burrows B, Flannery EM, Herbison GP, Hewitt CJ, Holdaway MD 1991 Relation between airway responsiveness and serum IgE in children with asthma and in apparently normal children. N Engl J Med 325:1067–1071

Sheffer AL 1991 Guidelines for the diagnosis and management of asthma. J Allergy Clin Immunol 88:425–534

Shirakawa T, Li A, Dubowitz M et al 1994 Association between atopy and variants of the subunit of the high-affinity immunoglobulin E receptor. Nat Genet 7:125–130

Sibbald B, Horn MEC, Brain EA, Gregg I 1980 Genetic factors in childhood asthma. Thorax 35:671–674

Speilman RS, McGinnis RE, Ewens WJ 1993 Transmission test for linkage disequilibrium: the insulin gene region and insulin-dependent diabetes mellitus (IDDM). Am J Hum Genet 52:506–516

Tashkin DP, Altose MD, Bleecker ER et al 1992 The Lung Health Study. Airway responsiveness to inhaled methacholine in smokers with mild to moderate airflow limitation. Am Rev Respir Dis 145:301–310

Weiss ST, Tager IB, Weiss JW, Munoz A, Speizer FE, Ingram RH 1984 Airway responsiveness in a population sample of adults and children. Am Rev Respir Dis 129:898–902

Wiesch DG, Meyers DA, Samet JM, Bleecker ER 1996 Classification of the asthma phenotype in genetic studies. In: The genetics of asthma. Marcel Dekker, New York (Lung Biology in Health and Diseases Series 96) p 421–422

Xu J, Meyers DA 1996 Linkage analysis in complex disorders. In: The genetics of asthma. Marcel Dekker, New York (Lung Biology in Health and Diseases Series 96) p 351–366

Xu J, Levitt RC, Panhuysen CI et al 1995 Evidence for two unlinked loci regulating total serum IgE levels. Am J Hum Genet 57:425–430

Young RP, Dekker JW, Wordsworth BP et al 1994 HLA-DR and HLA-DP genotypes and immunoglobulin E responses to common major allergens. Clin Exp Allergy 24:431–439

DISCUSSION

Magnussen: Is it possible to use any of these techniques to diagnose asthma at a pre-symptomatic level?

Bleecker: One could probably begin to predict disease by combining genotyping with clinical data. If a gene, or linkage in a specific chromosomal region, in a given population group is closely related to the disease and one child in a family is affected, it may be possible to determine whether that child shares an identified chromosomal region with other siblings. There are methods of predicting whether this child will be affected soon or at some point in the future. This may be an interesting approach for early interventions, which may be pharmacological or preventive environmental control. These approaches may prevent some of the irreversible findings associated with chronic asthma. In the future we may be able to design diagnostic tests, such as those available for the early-onset breast cancer genes to use in specific early intervention studies or even in clinical medicine.

Holgate: One of the major difficulties is in describing the phenotype of asthma. Our colleagues who work on diabetes are in a better position because they can make a single measurement, i.e. blood sugar, whereas we have to deal with multiple combinations of measurements.

Bleecker: Some of these problems concerning approaches to defining asthma phenotype and making a diagnosis of asthma work both ways. In asthma there are intermediate phenotypes, some of which are quantitative traits (IgE levels and bronchial hyper-responsiveness [BHR]), which can provide information on all family members. Another approach, in terms of asthmatic and allergic combinations, is that if one only looks in families in the Dutch sample in which the proband is allergic and there is no smoking history in the proband, one can exclude about 30% of the families. In these cases we can observe a linkage to IgE and BHR: the LOD scores almost double. This is another way of looking at the asthma phenotype in family studies.

Paré: I have a comment regarding phenotypic heterogeneity in asthma and diabetes. The people who work on diabetes have found 13 linked loci! They would have to have some phenotypic heterogeneity so that they could look for patterns. In some ways the phenotypic heterogeneity of asthma might be an advantage.

Holgate: Heritability calculations indicated that 30–50% of the disease phenotype can be accounted for by genetic factors (Lawrence et al 1994).

Paré: If one calculates heritability using the prevalence of asthma in first degree relatives compared to the prevalence in the general population one finds a strong influence of heredity despite the low value for lambda. Lambda is low because the population prevalence is high. Unfortunately, the high prevalence is probably linked to a lot of genetic heterogeneity.

Holgate: I'm just saying that the difficulties of estimating these heritability values arise from methodological problems rather than from mathematical difficulties, judging from the wide range and lack of repeatability in the various techniques used to measure disease phenotypic markers by the various groups. This is an area of tremendous controversy and cause for uncertainty. Another is that groups interested in asthma genetics are entering into industrial contracts that greatly limit the amount of information they can share with others in the field. Finally, on account of the multiple statistical tests that we made, many of the apparent 'significant' linkages reported eventually turn out to have occurred by chance.

Bleecker: Even setting the levels of interest statistically when one analyses a genome screen is difficult because one does not want too many or too few areas to light up as significant. The ideal situation is to have something that allows one to identify a somewhat larger number of areas, so that minor genes are not missed.

Strachan: I have two points. The first refers to the data from the twin studies, which in my opinion are much more informative than data on heritability estimates. In monozygotic pairs only about half of the twins of probands have any form of asthma, which must be telling us something informative about the relative contributions of genes and the environment. Having said that, however, there is some utility in trying to identify genetic risk factors. My concern on the phenotypic characterization is that for much of the time we are dealing with a disease of children, and if we start to try and make comparisons across generations we have to think not only about the problems of ascertaining childhood asthma in the parental generation, but also what the parents were exposed to as children. Therefore, there are some techniques in the list that you have described which have more intrinsic validity for studies of asthma. For example, although the analysis of sib pairs is, from the laboratory angle, much more labour intensive, it is methodologically much more attractive.

Holgate: And of course it also does not make assumptions about the mode of inheritance.

Kay: Several groups are engaged on genome searches and there are many candidate genes. What is the heterogeneity of linkages in a single individual?

Bleecker: I can use diabetes as an example. At a meeting in Oxford last year, data were presented on different populations showing the relative importance of five or six different candidate genomic areas that may be important in modulating diabetes (Wellcome Trust meeting. Oxford, UK, Oct 29–Nov 1 1995). In one population group one particular genetic region accounted for about 60% of the variability, whereas that same region in another country only accounted for about 30% of the disease variability. This suggests that there are population differences and, in the case of asthma, there are also probably phenotype differences. I agree with David Strachan that there may be many differences between childhood and adult asthma. One of the nice things about the Dutch data set is that there are some retrospective data on at least one of the parents during childhood or early adulthood. The other part of your question is how to select these regions in individuals. We're beginning to examine that area, although at the moment the genome screening data are overwhelming. There were clear population and racial differences apparent in the collaborative studies on the genetics of asthma (National Heart, Lung and Blood Institute) performed at four universities (University of Chicago, Johns Hopkin's University, University of Minnesota and University of Maryland). In a uniform population clear linkages can be established. Indeed, one could propose that the chromosome 5 area in the Dutch population is an important determinant of atopy and possibly also hyper-responsiveness. Our calculations, which may be biased because of how the population was selected, e.g. an asthma proband, suggest that about 50% of the variability serum IgE levels can be explained by the linkage to chromosome 5q. This suggests that this is probably a major locus and further investigation is indicated. I also predict that a locus on chromosome 12q may be important, and there may even be an interaction between the two loci.

Boushey: Perhaps if they want to recover their investment they should start looking at the phenotype of airway inflammation, because that has been left off the genetic characterization list. Measuring eosinophils in induced sputum probably separates asthmatic and non-asthmatic populations as well as does measuring IgE levels in blood. Airway inflammation has been incorporated into the working definition of asthma so it should be added to the list of genetic characterizations.

Bleecker: I agree, but there is a small problem of logistics, i.e. there are enormous numbers involved in these approaches. We need practical methods to characterize bronchial inflammation.

Boushey: But that's the great advantage of sputum induction as opposed to other means of assessing bronchial mucosal inflammation, such as bronchial lavage or biopsy. It may be difficult, but it is much more feasible than the alternatives.

Bleecker: When you're trying to persuade entire families to be tested, the timing becomes important. On the other hand, if BHR is linked to 40% of the family, for example, one may want to go back to those families and perform a more detailed characterization of the affected individuals to determine clinical heterogeneity. Sputum analysis for inflammatory markers is an excellent idea.

Holgate: One marker that we have been using to follow disease activity in longitudinal studies is adenosine 5'-monophosphate (AMP) (Holgate et al 1991). This stimulus activates 'primed' mast cells in the asthmatic airway and therefore reflects more closely an index of inflammation rather than either histamine or methacholine, which contract airway smooth muscle directly and are, therefore, involved in more downstream events. Induced sputum would be another useful marker of airway inflammation.

Kay: Have you looked at nitric oxide?

Holgate: Nitric oxide is another possibility but one problem is that the apparatus required to measure the levels of nitric oxide at the moment isn't portable or easily handled. Hopefully, something more portable and robust will be developed soon.

Brostoff: It seemed to me that Eugene Bleecker manipulated his Dutch data somewhat by removing the smokers, which resulted in an increased LOD score. Could this not be turned the other way around by suggesting that there is a positive advantage in smoking in that it suppresses the levels of IgE and that this effect has confused your data?

Bleecker: It is possible, but all I was trying to show was that in secondary analyses novel approaches to understanding the asthma phenotype may be useful.

Holgate: I would like to bring up the subject of markers of disease severity as opposed to markers of disease origin because there have recently been numerous publications on this: for example, on genetic polymorphisms of the $\beta2$-adrenoceptors that either relate to an increased disease severity or greater chance of receptor down-regulation occurring (Green et al 1995a).

Britton: We've been involved with some of this work. We have looked for cross-sectional associations but not in any family or linkage studies. We haven't been able to find any association with the $\beta2$-adrenoceptor (I. Hall & J. Britton, unpublished observations 1995).

Potter: We've looked at restriction fragment length polymorphisms of the $\beta2$-adrenoceptor using the *Ban*I restriction enzyme and found no difference between asthmatics and non-asthmatics, or between asthmatics with or without rhinitis (Potter et al 1993). Reishaus et al (1993) have sequenced the $\beta2$-adrenoceptor gene in 51 patients and have found several mutations: arginine 16 to glycine and glutamine 27 to glutamic acid. In asthmatics, the former mutation identified a subset of patients who were more likely to be steroid dependent. In a multifactorial disease such as asthma it is likely that there will be some genetic markers which will select out particularly high risk patients or patients with particular types of asthma.

Bleecker: We've looked at two polymorphisms of the $\beta2$-adrenoreceptor, which lie in the chromosome 5q region, where there is linkage. We have no evidence that they are linked with asthma, hyper-responsiveness or IgE levels. There is some degree of linkage throughout the whole region but it is not confined to these polymorphisms. We are going to look at other parameters in collaboration with Steve Liggett, who first described the association with $\beta2$-adrenoreceptor polymorphisms (Liggett 1995), including asthma and other markers of severity that seem to have been important in their analyses.

Beasley: In our studies we have observed that the Gly16 allele is found at a higher frequency in asthmatics with very severe asthma compared to a group with mild to moderate asthma and a non-asthmatic control group. These findings are consistent with the previous work of Liggett, who reported that the Gly16 allele is strongly associated with nocturnal asthma (Turki et al 1995).

Holgate: Am I correct in saying that site-directed mutagenesis producing a Gly16 mutant results in increased desensitization of the $\beta2$-adrenoceptor?

Beasley: Yes, the Gly 16 polymorphism is associated with enhanced down-regulation following prolonged exposure to isoprenaline *in vitro* (Green et al 1995b). This suggests that this genotype might predispose individuals to more severe asthma.

Paré: Wouldn't a useful group to study be the asthmatics in New Zealand who died presumably in association with excessive use of fenoterol.

Beasley: Yes, and that is what we are now working on. Another approach we are taking is to determine the clinical phenotype of the different $\beta2$-adrenoreceptor polymorphisms in asthmatics and non-asthmatic controls *in vivo*. These studies need to be done because it has not yet been determined whether the Gly167 allele is associated with resistance to the bronchodilator effects of long-term β-agonist therapy in asthma.

Holgate: One could extract DNA from post-mortem tissue directly.

Beasley: Yes, that is one of the approaches we are taking.

Woolcock: I would like to ask a completely different question for clarification. In the Finnish population, 0.18% of those eligible to go into the army in 1961 had asthma, but this increased to 1.8% 28 years later. How can one study the associations of particular genetic polymorphisms with asthma when there have been such large increases in the the prevalence of asthma over time? One would obtain different results depending on when the analyses were performed.

Martinez: Changes in the prevalence of disease between cohorts have been occurring over time. This is why it is always better to work with subjects who are approximately the same age. You have raised an important point, because Eugene Bleecker showed us some LOD scores that were calculated using data from two generations, and the prevalence of asthma has globally increased during this time interval. Working with sib pairs is preferable because these 'epochal' changes will not influence the results.

Bleecker: In those families where the spouses of the primary proband were unaffected, the data were obtained when they were aged 15–35 years and again 25 years later. Therefore, there is some degree of longitudinal assurance. It doesn't solve the issue, and I am aware that it is a problem with all of these studies. I look at this from the opposite point of view — to be able to identify some sort of genetic signal amongst so much noise is fairly impressive, and it is possible that if we can control for some of this clinical variability the genetic linkage might be stronger.

Paré: I agree with you. Despite all of these problems, a growing number of linkages have been identified.

Sears: Couldn't the explanation be that the genetic basis hasn't changed over 20 years but the environmental component has. The genetics presumably haven't changed but the prevalence of asthma has, so how does one sort out whether there is indeed a genetic basis?

Bleecker: Even if genetic susceptibility has not changed, that is one of the advantages of longitudinal approaches, i.e. that you can determine whether environmental influences are greater than genetic influences. However, there will always be interactions between the environment and genetics. Studies on gene–environment interactions will be important. A major finding in the studies is that there is fairly significant susceptibility to asthma in these population groups. We have found, both in our Dutch and American studies, that there are some children who at some point in time have an asthma phenotype but who do not two or three years later. In contrast, if a 25-year old, for example, has a history of asthma they always have some symptoms of asthma. Therefore, there is a transition in the disease profile of asthma from childhood asthma, where it can be intermittent, to the asthma in adolescents and adults, where it is usually persistent and not reversible.

References

Green SA, Turki J, Hall IP, Liggett SB 1995a Implications of genetic variability of human β2-adrenergic receptor structure. Pulm Pharmacol 8:1–10

Green SA, Turki J, Bejarano P, Hall IP, Liggett SB 1995b Influence of beta 2-adrenergic receptor genotypes on signal transduction in human airway smooth muscle cells. Am J Resp Cell Mol Biol 13:25–33

Holgate ST, Church MK, Polosa R 1991 Adenosine: a positive modulator of airway inflammation in asthma. Ann N Y Acad Sci 629:227–237

Lawrence S, Beasley R, Doull I et al 1994 Genetic analysis of atopy and asthma as quantitative traits and ordered polychotomies. Ann Hum Genet 58:359–368

Liggett SB 1995 Genetics of β2-adrenergic receptor variants in asthma. Clin Exp Allergy 25:89S–94S

Potter PC, van Wyk L, Martin M, Lentes KU, Dowdle EB 1993 Genetic polymorphism of the β-2 adrenergic receptor in atopic and nonatopic subjects. Clin Exp Allergy 23:874–877

Reishaus E, Innis M, MacIntyre N, Ligget SB 1993 Mutations in the same gene encoding the β2-adrenergic receptor in normal and asthmatic subjects. Am J Resp Cell Mol Biol 8:334–339

Turki J, Pak, J, Green SA, Martin RJ, Liggett SB 1995 Genetic polymorphisms of the beta 2-adrenergic receptor in nocturnal and non-nocturnal asthma. Evidence that Gly16 correlates with the nocturnal phenotype. J Clin Invest 95:1635–1641

General discussion I

Holgate: I would like to bring up the antigen specificity side of human genetics. The data on the associations between the HLA haplotypes and some of the common antigens, such as cats and house dust mites, as opposed to some of the rare antigens, are rather disappointing. David Marsh's studies on *Amb b* 1 are the ones that are always quoted, probably because they are the tightest results that exist (Marsh et al 1989).

Platts-Mills: When David Marsh first started sorting out the ragweed data, he realized that *Amb a* 5 was a molecule with sufficiently restricted T cell epitopes so that an HLA association could be observed. This is not the case for *Der p* 1 because there are too many ways that it can be presented to a T cell.

Busse: Why are some aeroantigens more likely to be uniquely associated with the pathogenesis of asthma?

Platts-Mills: You say 'uniquely' but one of the things that has become apparent in the last 10 years is that cats, dogs, cockroaches, house dust mites and *Alternaria* can all trigger the disease, yet these allergens are biologically very diverse. The observation that many of these proteins are enzymes may be relevant, but *Fel d* 1 and *Der p* 2, which are powerful allergens, have no apparent enzymic activity. Therefore, there is no simple pattern.

Weiss: This situation may also be influenced by observer bias. We have looked only at the proteins we know and many other proteins that we have not yet looked at, such as endotoxins, may be influential.

Platts-Mills: I'm not denying that there could be other important allergens, but sufficient absorption studies have now been done which can explain a reasonable portion of the total IgE levels. I'm sure there are more, but it's unlikely that we are missing the major ones.

Busse: Is the manner of antigen presentation involved in determining the response? And by that, I don't just mean immunological presentation but rather the pattern of exposure. For example, house dust mites and *Alternaria* are not always delivered to the environment like ragweed, but rather appear to be present on a more constant basis. Is there something different about how these antigens are deposited in or cleared from the airway?

Platts-Mills: In the mouse repeated low dose (Levine & Faz 1972) immunization is a good way of inducing IgE antibody responses. Presumably, the switching on of IL-12 is avoided by this regime. Whether the chronicity is also important for symptoms or sensitization is an important issue.

Holgate: I agree. One of the great frustrations about working with animal models is that if one does keep presenting antigen in the way you have described then tolerance occurs, which is different from the situation in human asthma. In essence, we really do not have an adequate animal model for studying the chronicity of allergen sensitization. Patrick Holt, with your knowledge of immunology could you extrapolate what might be missing in our animal models?

Holt: Now that we're starting to obtain information on the natural history of IgE responses to environmental allergens in humans, we can say that in most cases they are biphasic, i.e. they start up soon after initial exposure, but if exposure persists they almost always shut down, which is precisely what we see in the relevant animal models. On this basis it is reasonable to propose that allergic disease represents a failure of a set of T helper (Th) cell selection processes which are identical to those documented in animals. Why these processes which are so efficient in the animal models should have such a high failure rate in humans is unknown. The chronicity of the disease process is likely to be the major missing factor in the animal models. There's no way in a murine experimental system that we can reproduce the effects of repeated allergen stimulation over a number of years, as occurs in humans.

Platts-Mills: It is unlikely that an increase in failure rate can explain why the prevalence of asthma has increased. There are studies from the Brown University, USA in 1965 which show that 25% of the incoming classes had symptomatic ragweed hay fever. As early as 1960, the American population had a high rate of symptomatic atopy, which was predominantly hay fever, but then switched over to a different set of antigens that were predominantly associated with asthma.

Holgate: This observation of a switch in antigen specificity over time is likely to be important. Is there any other evidence for such a switch occurring?

Burney: I know of two studies that have looked at IgE levels in children over time: one from Switzerland (Gassner 1992) and one from Japan (Nagagomi et al 1994). Both of those show an increased sensitivity to a batch of allergen rather than being restricted to a particular allergen. The historical data which relate to an increase in atopy as measured by radioallergosorbent tests seem to indicate that people are responding to a wide range of potential allergens that they encounter in the environment.

Holgate: This argues against a shift in the proportions of allergens against which children are sensitive.

Sears: There are three studies in the UK (Taylor et al 1984, Burr et al 1989, Ninan & Russell 1992) which show that the proportion of children with eczema over a 10–20 year period has more than doubled, suggesting that eczema is another disease associated with atopy which has increased substantially over time. This contrasts with the proportion of adults who suffer from hay fever, which probably hasn't changed that much over 20 years, although childhood hay fever has increased (Ninan & Russell 1992).

Strachan: Hagy & Settipane (1969) compiled a series of prevalence studies of allergic rhinitis in American college students from the 1920s through to the 1970s. In the later series the prevalence was relatively high, 20% reporting asthma or allergic rhinitis. What seemed to be clear from that series was that the prevalence of asthma or allergic rhinitis had increased during that time period, but with the proviso that there has been increased labelling and increased awareness. The question is what is the prevalence of allergic rhinitis amongst American college students nowadays? We have looked at the prevalence of hay fever in two British birth cohorts and we have found that it is increasing alongside other markers of allergy. There is also some interesting anecdotal evidence that in the 1920s a large-scale population survey of 77 000 Swiss came up with a remarkably low prevalence of 0.8% (Rehsteiner 1926).

Britton: We tried to explain the changes in the prevalence of asthma between two British birth cohorts: the 1958 National Child Development Study (NCDS) and the 1970 British Cohort Study (BCS70). We looked at several potential risk factors, such as low maternal age, maternal smoking, social class, birth weight and breast feeding, but none of these factors explained more than a few per cent of the increase (Lewis et al 1996).

Strachan: We need to identify the nature of the underlying trends in children and in adolescents. Most studies indicate that the trends are rising, suggesting a general increase in allergic disease, although there are a few exceptions to the rule. However, most of our discussions so far have been about chronic adult asthma, which is probably a different condition, and we shouldn't leap too easily from one to the other.

Woolcock: It is often thought that rhinitis is a modern disease. In populations in Africa, Papua New Guinea and Indonesia rhinitis is very rare in both adults and children.

Holgate: Do they have the 'right sort' of pollen in this part of the world, i.e. pollens from wind-pollinated plants?

Woolcock: Yes.

Weiss: Hay fever is almost unheard of in rural China, but migrants of these areas living in the USA can develop hay fever.

Brostoff: The increase in asthma, which began in the 1960s, is undoubted. This occurred simultaneously with numerous changes in social habits; for example, the rising popularity of double glazing and the television. It has been estimated that children spend at least 30 h a week watching television. Such changes in social habits may underlie the changes in allergen exposure.

Nelson: Ragweed pollen is abundant in the North Central United States. Maternowski & Mathews (1962) showed that in the student population at that time the prevalence of allergic rhinitis was about 17%, of asthma 5.7%, and of one or the other or both about 19%. Chinese students who came to study in Michigan took only two or three seasons to develop the same prevalences, demonstrating the importance of the availability of potent allergens (Maternowski & Mathews 1962).

Woolcock: Asthma is not a new illness, but its prevalence has recently been increasing. In contrast, allergic rhinitis may have arisen more recently, but it is also increasing. It is possible that populations are being exposed to new antigens. Alternatively, we may always have been at risk of developing allergic rhinitis but have been protected by inhibitory factors, which we are now gradually losing.

Beasley: Another way of looking at the time course of the development of allergic diseases is to study communities that have adopted a western lifestyle. This approach has been undertaken by Hsieh's group. They looked at the prevalence of asthma, rhinitis and eczema in Taiwan since the 1970s (Hsieh & Tsai 1991). They found that the increase in asthma occurred first, and that was followed five to 10 years later by increases in eczema and rhinitis, suggesting that the development of these diseases follows a different time course.

Potter: I have a similar comment. In the rural Transkei region of South Africa 20 years ago there were very few cases of hay fever. One of my graduate students, H. Steinman, has gone back to that region recently and studied a similar group of people, who still live in a rural community but have adopted a more western lifestyle. He found that the prevalence of hay fever is now greater than 20%.

I have another anecdote relating to the allergens: rural Africans don't experience hay fever due to Kikuyu grass because the Kikuyu grass doesn't produce pollen in the rural environment. This grass species propagates by rhizomatous propagation in the wild. However, if Kikuyu grass is cultivated, it readily produces anthers and pollen is released. The pollen is highly allergenic and people in inner cities become sensitive to Kikuyu grass. This species of grass is not a problem in the rural areas because pollen is not produced there. Thus, the effects of urbanization and cultivation can alter the biological and reproductive characteristics of a plant species and in this way influence its allergenicity.

Bleecker: Many studies that rely on the histories of these allergic diseases may suffer from misclassification, either because of over- or under-diagnosis of the phenotype. Under-diagnosis may miss people who are susceptible. If susceptible individuals move into a new exposure situation, for example if they adopt a more western lifestyle, they may become symptomatic and seek health care. They will then have a diagnosis of asthma or allergic disease. However, when one is studying these families or populations, one will see many people who don't have that diagnostic label. Thus, we have adapted an approach that employs objective testing as well as historical information (clinical data) when performing genetic epidemiological studies

References

Burr ML, Butland BK, King S, Vaughan-Williams E 1989 Changes in asthma prevalence: two surveys 15 years apart. Arch Dis Child 64:1452–1456

Gassner M 1992 Immunologische: allergologische Reactionen unter veranderten Umweltbedungingen. Schweitz Rundsch Med Prax 81:426–430

Hagy GW, Settipane GA 1969 Bronchial asthma, allergic rhinitis, and allergy skin tests among college students. J Allergy 44:333–332

Hsieh K-H, Tsai Y-T 1991 Increasing prevalence of childhood allergic disease in Taipei, Taiwan, and the outcome. Proceedings of 14th ICACI Meeting, Kyoto, p 223–225

Levine BB, Vaz NM 1970 Effect of combinations of inbred strain, antigen, and antigen dose on immune responsiveness and reagin production in the mouse. A potential mouse model for immune aspects of human atopic allergy. Int Archs Allergy Appl Immunol 39:156–171

Lewis S, Butland B, Strachan D et al 1996 Study of the aetiology of wheezing illness at age 16 in two national British cohorts. Thorax 51:670–676

Marsh DG, Zwollo P, Ansari AA 1989 Genetic and immunological studies of human responsiveness: the allergy model. In: Pickler W J, Stadler BM, Dakindenn CA et al (eds) Progress in allergy and clinical immunology. Hogrefe & Huber, Berne, p 117–124

Maternowski C J, Mathews KP 1962 The prevalence of ragweed pollinosis in foreign and native students at a midwestern university and its implications concerning methods of determining the inheritance of atopy. J Allergy 33:130–140

Nagagomi T, Itaya H, Tominaga T, Yamaki M, Hisamatsu S-I, Nakagomi O 1994 Is atopy increasing? Lancet 343:121–122

Ninan TK, Russell G 1992 Respiratory symptoms and atopy in Aberdeen schoolchildren: evidence from two surveys 15 years apart. Br Med J 304:873–875

Rehsteiner R 1926 Beiträge zur Kenntris der Verbreitung des Henfiebers. Schweiz Zeitung Gesundheitspflege 1:3–34

Taylor B, Wadsworth J, Wadsworth M, Peckham C 1984 Changes in the reported prevalence of childhood eczema since the 1939–45 war. Lancet II:1255–1257

Interpretation of epidemiological surveys of asthma

Peter Burney

Department of Public Health Medicine, UMDS, Block 8, South Wing, St Thomas' Hospital, Lambeth Palace Road, London SE1 7EH, UK

Abstract. Two particular issues make the interpretation of epidemiological studies in asthma problematic. The first is the lack of any clear definition of asthma. This is a perennial area of controversy. Thirty-eight years ago a Ciba Foundation guest symposium addressed this issue and suggested a solution. However, as J. G. Scadding, one of the participants of that symposium, pointed out after further consideration of the problem, what they had proposed was a description, not a definition. Since then, further attempts have been made but with little progress. They remain descriptive rather than definitive and have become, if anything, vaguer. The second problem has been the widespread failure to be precise about hypotheses or to define more precisely the hypothetical influences on asthma. Examples of this are the notions of 'inflammation' and 'atopy'. Standardization of methods for epidemiological studies of asthma is likely to provide a more rigorous framework for the comparison of results and the testing of hypotheses. Nevertheless, the development of such protocols should itself be seen as a hermeneutic device rather than an assertion of established knowledge.

1997 The rising trends in asthma. Wiley, Chichester (Ciba Foundation Symposium 206) p 111–121

The very broad nature of the title that has been given to me, though generous, leaves me with a problem in selecting which particular issues to raise without covering issues that will be dealt with more thoroughly by later speakers. After much thought, I have decided to raise some issues that featured centrally in an earlier Ciba Foundation symposium (Ciba Foundation guest symposium 1959), and which I still think remain of great importance. I refer to the definitions that are used and some of the confusion that surrounds these. In doing this I recognize that some of what I have to say will be controversial and will be at variance with the views of other people. But, then, that seems to me to be to make the subject all the more suitable for a Ciba Foundation symposium.

The Ciba Foundation guest symposium of 1958 and the definition of asthma

The Ciba Foundation symposiasts of 1958 defined asthma, with a few qualifications, as

'... the condition of subjects with widespread narrowing of the bronchial airways which changes its severity over short periods of time either spontaneously or under treatment.'

It is notable that the definition is a clinical and physiological definition. This had not been inevitable. The same group defined emphysema in strictly pathological terms. Nevertheless, the definition of 1958 has had a strong and lasting influence and has been difficult to improve. The American Thoracic Society were the first to try and they reinforced the physiological nature of the definition by introducing the concept of bronchial hyper-responsiveness to the definition. This additional assumption has seen variable fortunes over the succeeding 35 years.

In spite of its success, the principal weakness of this part of the work of the Ciba Foundation symposium of 1958 was soon identified by one of its principal contributors. Scadding (1963) pointed out that what had been provided was not a definition at all, but a description of asthma. A true definition should, he argued, provide unambiguous criteria by which an individual could be judged to have asthma or not. However, despite a further attempt to improve on the first definition at a Ciba Foundation study group in 1971, the contributors gave up and concluded that under current knowledge no further progress could be made towards a better definition of the condition (Ciba Foundation study group 1971).

An epidemiological approach

Part of the difficulties encountered in defining asthma have arisen from the clinical perspective of the main contributors to this debate. The practice of clinical medicine demands above all a division of the world into clear groups: generally, those who should be given specific treatments, and those who should not. There has also been a desire to define these groups in terms of characteristics that are observable and verifiable in the clinic. So Scadding (1963) objected to the inclusion of 'allergy' in the definition of asthma, although his argument now seems somewhat circular, on the grounds that the term was vague ('I have a better idea of what asthma is than I have of what an allergic condition is') and that in his view there were many cases of 'asthma' that were not allergic in origin.

The view that clear-cut syndromes could ever be defined in terms of clinical findings seems optimistic. A consideration of clearly dichotomous biological states, such as the presence or absence of an abnormal gene, suggests that clinical expression will be highly variable depending on gene–gene and gene–environment interactions. Moreover, most measured characteristics show unimodal distributions even where extreme values pose evident risks to life or health.

What we are able to define are physiological states and subjective states described in terms of perceived symptoms. Our assessment of each of these can be characterized by the reliability of the measurements and their ability to predict other characteristics that are of interest, including future health status or other disease states.

Epidemiological studies are observational and comparative and therefore dependent on the equivalence of the measurements made, although the measurements do not need to relate directly to standard diagnoses. In talking about the interpretation of epidemiological studies of asthma, the first point to make is that these are often far more dependent on the standardization of measurement than on the 'validity' of measurement. If measurements are not well standardized then the results may be highly misleading. As the epidemiology of asthma is painted on a wider and wider canvas both across time, as will be discussed by Richard Beasley and Ann Woolcock (this volume: Beasley et al 1997, Woolcock & Peat 1997), and across geographical areas as in the European Community Respiratory Health Survey (Burney et al 1994) and the ISAAC study (Pearce et al 1993), the need for standardization becomes paramount, while that of validity, even if the concept was clear in this context, takes a secondary place.

Studies of 'asthma' have relied on a number of different strategies for the identification of asthma. It is difficult to suggest that any one of them is correct or incorrect but the limitations of each need to be recognized. Questionnaires are now available for use in such studies and provide standardized questions to elicit a diagnosis of asthma or the presence of symptoms suggestive of asthma (Burney et al 1989a, 1994, Pearce et al 1993).

Questions relating to the diagnosis of asthma

Questions relating to the diagnosis of asthma are commonly used to identify patients with asthma. They give highly repeatable responses which are reckoned to be highly specific to the condition. Few people who do not have clinical asthma claim to have the condition. The corollary of this is that such questions are not very sensitive and that many people who would have been diagnosed as having asthma will deny that they have the condition, and this appears to be true even in health care settings (Burney et al 1989b). The most problematic issue here is that the responses are likely to be biased by the local health care providers. Those receiving adequate care for their asthma are more likely to say that they have asthma (Speight et al 1983). This makes such questions unhelpful and misleading in any context in which the health services are themselves being evaluated as they will always overestimate the proportion of the population with 'asthma' that is being treated. It might make comparisons between areas or countries unreliable.

Questions relating to symptoms

Questions on symptoms are generally less repeatable, although improvements in repeatability have been achieved by administering them with a video (Shaw et al 1995). Symptoms are also less specific to particular conditions. Nevertheless, several symptoms are regarded as being typical of patients with asthma. They are generally the symptoms of airway obstruction or airway responsiveness and are therefore also associated with other pathological states not generally associated with a diagnosis of asthma (Burney et al 1987). However, they are less influenced by the local health services and should be independent of diagnostic fashion. In the comparison of results between communities, particularly communities speaking different languages, there is little knowledge so far about the equivalence of questions. The decision on which of a list of standardized questions should be taken to be equivalent to clinical asthma is arbitrary and some have taken combinations of questions, where others have used single questions, such as that on the admission of waking at night with breathlessness.

The European Community Respiratory Health Survey (1996) has produced comparative results which suggest that the concept of asthma may be quite similar between centres. In comparing those who say that they have had an attack of asthma in the previous 12 months or are currently taking medication for asthma with those who claim to have been woken with an attack of shortness of breath in the previous 12 months, we find a relatively good relationship between the prevalence of the two. This is encouraging, though there appear to be some differences between countries and these will need to be examined in greater detail.

Measures of airway responsiveness

Measures of airway responsiveness are increasingly used in epidemiological studies and their short-term reliability is generally good (Dehaut et al 1983). They provide objective measures of physiological function but the term is vague and poorly defined. On these grounds alone the validity of the claim that these measure 'asthma' has rightly been challenged.

Measures of hyper-responsiveness include: challenge with direct smooth muscle agonists, such as histamine and methacholine, and agents that release mediators from inflammatory cells, such as adenosine and hypertonic saline; changes in bronchial tone after exercise; spontaneous variability in peak expiratory flow rate; and responses to bronchodilators. Different methods of assessing hyper-responsiveness give different results when applied to the same individuals (Higgins et al 1992). Using common methods of challenge, such as histamine challenge, tests give abnormal results in subjects who have airway disease that would not be conventionally regarded as asthma (Burney et al 1987). Although there are contested claims that challenge with an indirect agonist is more specific for asthma (Avital et al 1995, Wilson et al 1995), these have not been widely used and the choice of methods for use in a survey also depends on other considerations. These include reliability, standardization and practicability. Paradoxically, it is also true that measures of hyper-responsiveness which correlate poorly with each other are associated with similar risk factors (Higgins et al 1993).

Standardization of challenge tests remains a problem. Major advances have been made in this field, particularly in the development by Ann Woolcock's group of simple methods of challenge suitable for epidemiological studies (Yan et al 1983).

Nevertheless, for comparative surveys standardization remains problematic because of the technical difficulties in reliable aerosol generation. Similar methods of nebulization using similar equipment can produce very different 'effective' doses and care has to be exercised in comparing figures that superficially seem similar (Dennis et al 1992). Alternative methods of challenge such as exercise challenge are even more difficult to standardize, although some progress has been made in this area (Haby et al 1995).

The assessment of atopy

The assessment of atopy is an important part of any study of asthma. Here again, however, the terminology has been used very loosely and the methods of assessment have not been standardized. Apart from questions about the 'atopic diseases' asthma, eczema and hay fever, the principal measures used have been the results of skin tests and the measurement of total and specific serum IgE. It seems that these are often regarded as interchangeable. In surveys undertaken in narrowly defined populations this may indeed be the case, but it is not likely to be true otherwise. In comparing the East and West German populations (Behrendt et al 1993) it has become apparent that the levels of total IgE are very much higher in East Germany, although the prevalence of atopic disease is higher in West Germany. This discrepancy may be important and it raises questions at least about the relevance of total IgE to the aetiology of asthma. This again is important, considering that much of the research on the genetics of asthma has defined the phenotype in terms of total IgE levels.

Skin tests can be more convenient and cheaper than tests of serum IgE, but the best methods for assessing skin sensitivity are still unclear. In clinical practice it is widely believed that small skin weals are not clinically relevant, because they are not generally associated with disease, and should be ignored. However, the evidence from the European Community Respiratory Health Survey is that the measurement of skin weal diameter is exceedingly difficult to standardize with current methods, even when training is standardized (Chinn et al 1996). The better standardized measure is therefore the presence or absence of a weal, and additional criteria, for instance the presence of a weal greater than 3 mm in diameter, introduce poorly controlled variation between observers into the assessment. Others have suggested the comparison of the skin weal produced by allergen to the skin weal produced by histamine. Again, it can be shown that the skin response to histamine is the least reliable of all the measurements and introduces further error into the assessment of atopy if used in this way.

Progress since 1958

In many ways it is difficult to see very much progress in the definition of asthma since the symposium of 1958. The International Consensus Report on the Diagnosis and Treatment of Asthma (1992) provided as their operational definition of asthma:

'. . . a chronic inflammatory disorder of the airway in which many cells play a role, including mast cells and eosinophils. In susceptible individuals this inflammation causes symptoms which are usually associated with widespread but variable airflow obstruction that is often reversible either spontaneously or with treatment, and causes an associated increase in airway responsiveness to a variety of stimuli.'

This definition represents a radical departure from J. G. Scadding's plea for clear unambiguous and observable criteria without the intrusion of tendentious hypothesis.

It is tempting to suggest in the face of this that we should retreat from studies of 'asthma' and concentrate on studying those things that we can define clearly, even if these are not exactly what we mean by asthma. Studying the epidemiology of wheeze, or of waking at night with breathlessness, or the bronchial response to methacholine may not be the same as studying asthma but they may, treated with caution, tell us a great deal about the epidemiology of asthma all the same. In doing this, however, we will need to bear in mind the heterogeneity of some of the measures that we are using. It is no more reasonable to assume that airway responsiveness is aetiologically or pathologically homogeneous than it is to assume that height or blood pressure are. It is no more necessary to think that waking at night with breathlessness represents a single process than it is to assume this for jaundice or chest pain. The additional difficulties that this introduces, however, should be clearly stated. It can be predicted that different authors will report different results depending on the populations and the mixture of diseases represented within the study. The consistency that epidemiologists generally seek in establishing causal associations may need to wait for more precise definitions. At the same time the inconsistencies are themselves clues that may reveal more about these individual processes.

A difficulty still arises from the desire to be relevant to the work of clinicians and the health services. It is for this reason, rather than for any scientific reason, that we will continue to try to define asthma. And perhaps it is, after all, part of our responsibility to say to what extent findings are likely to relate to what clinicians call asthma. For this reason, some rule of thumb that allows us to make such a translation is to be welcomed. Ann Woolcock's group has made a proposal of how to do this, suggesting that airway responsiveness with symptoms should be taken to be the equivalent of asthma (Toelle et al 1992). The rationale for this is that symptomatic children who are not hyper-responsive are very similar in other respects to asymptomatic children, and this proposal has been taken up in a number of quarters. As a rule of thumb for translating epidemiological studies back into some kind of common currency, this definition has the advantages of being based on observable criteria and of making the measurement more specific, a useful characteristic in many settings. However, it also raises the question of why diseases are not diseases if they are not symptomatic, an unusual assumption, particularly in asthma where differences between people in their ability to perceive physiological changes has been documented. In effect, the definition amounts to removing those from the definition of disease who have only mild symptoms or making the definition of hyper-responsive more stringent, and there may be a simpler way of achieving the same ends. Even this, however, leaves unresolved the issue of what defines asthma, it simply asserts that asthma is not a trivial condition.

References

Avital A, Springer C, Bar-Yishay E, Godfrey S 1995 Adenosine, methacholine, and exercise challenges in children with asthma or pediatric chronic obstructive pulmonary disease. Thorax 50:511–516

Beasley R, Pearce N, Crane J 1997 International trends in asthma mortality. In: The rising trends in asthma. Wiley, Chichester (Ciba Found Symp 206) p 140–156

Behrendt H, Krämer U, Dolgner R et al 1993 Elevated levels of total IgE in East German children: atopy, parasites or pollutants? Allergol J 2:31–40

Burney PGJ, Britton JR, Chinn S et al 1987 Descriptive epidemiology of bronchial reactivity in an adult population: results from a community study. Thorax 42:38–44

Burney PGJ, Chinn S, Britton JR, Tattersfield AE, Papacosta AO 1989a What symptoms predict the bronchial response to histamine? Int J Epidemiol 18:165–173

Burney PGJ, Laitinen LA, Perdrizet S et al 1989b Validity and repeatability of the IUATLD (1984) bronchial symptoms questionnaire: an international comparison. Eur Respir J 2:940–945

Burney PGJ, Luczynska C, Chinn S et al 1994 The European Community Respiratory Health Survey. Eur Respir J 7:954–960

Chinn S, Jarvis D, Luczynska CM, Lai E, Burney PGJ 1996 Measuring atopy in a multi-centre epidemiological study. Eur J Epidemiol 12:155–162

Ciba Foundation guest symposium 1959 Terminology, definitions and classification of chronic pulmonary emphysema and related conditions (a report of the conclusions of a Ciba guest symposium). Thorax 14:286–299

Ciba Foundation study group 1971 Identification of asthma. Churchill Livingstone, Edinburgh (Ciba Found study group 38)

Dehaut P, Rachiell A, Martin RR, Malo JL 1983 Histamine dose–response curves in asthma: reproducibility and sensitivity to different indices to assess response. Thorax 38:516–522

Dennis JH, Avery AJ, Walters EH, Hendrick DJ 1992 Calibration of aerosol output from the Mefar dosimeter: implications for epidemiological studies. Eur Respir J 5:1279–1282

European Community Respiratory Health Survey 1996 Variations in the prevalence of respiratory symptoms, self-reported asthma attacks, and use of asthma medication in the European Community Respiratory Health Survey (ECRHS). Eur Respir J 9:687–695

Haby MM, Peast JK, Mellis CM, Anderson SD, Woolcock AJ 1995 An exercise challenge for epidemiological studies of childhood asthma: validity and repeatability. Eur Respir J 8:729–736

Higgins BT, Britton JR, Chinn S, Cooper S, Burney PGJ, Tattersfield AE 1992 Comparison of bronchial reactivity and peak expiratory flow variability measurements for epidemiologic studies. Am Rev Respir Dis 145:588–593

Higgins BT, Britton JR, Chinn S, Lai KK, Burney PGJ, Tattersfield AE 1993 Factors affecting peak expiratory flow variability and bronchial reactivity in a random population sample. Thorax 48:899–905

International Consensus Report on the Diagnosis and Treatment of Asthma 1992 Eur Respir J 5:601–641

Pearce N, Weiland S, Keil U et al 1993 Self-reported prevalence of asthma symptoms in children in Australia, England, Germany and New Zealand: an international comparison using the ISAAC protocol. Eur Respir J 6:1455–1461

Scadding JG 1963 Meaning of diagnostic terms in broncho-pulmonary disease. Br Med J 2:1425–1430

Shaw R, Woodman K, Ayson M et al 1995 Measuring the prevalence of bronchial hyper-responsiveness in children. Int J Epidemiol 24:597–602

Speight ANP, Lee DA, Hey EN 1983 Underdiagnosis and undertreatment of asthma in childhood. Br Med J 286:1253–1256

Toelle BG, Peat JK, Salome CM, Melis CM, Woolcock AJ 1992 Toward a definition of asthma for epidemiology. Am Rev Respir Dis 146:633–637

Wilson MN, Bridge P, Silverman M 1995 Bronchial responsiveness and symptoms in 5–6 year old children: a comparison of a direct and indirect challenge. Thorax 50:339–345

Woolcock AJ, Peat JK 1997 Evidence for the increase in asthma worldwide. In: The rising trends in asthma. Wiley, Chichester (Ciba Found Symp 206) p 122–139

Yan K, Salome C, Woolcock AJ 1983 Rapid method for measurement of bronchial responsiveness. Thorax 38:760–765

DISCUSSION

Bleecker: A number of practical approaches are evident. One is evaluating asthma, which is a somewhat dichotomous variable, versus looking at associated phenotypes, such as IgE levels, which can be used as quantitative traits. The latter are often more informative. Hyper-responsiveness is another associated phenotype that may be possible to use as a quantitative trait across the population. We conducted a survey on the classification of asthma in which we sent 50 offspring to two clinicians, two epidemiologists and two paediatricians, and we found that there was total agreement in only six of the 50 cases (Bleecker et al 1997, this volume). Also, in our classification scheme atopy and allergy were noted as being present or absent, but we found that they were not useful in determining cases of asthma. Therefore, many of the points you brought up are relevant, but it is important to have operational definitions rather than descriptive ones.

Burney: I agree. One of the things that we are always asked to do is to relate our findings to clinical and health service issues. For instance, determining whether asthma is under-diagnosed and under-treated in a particular country becomes difficult unless one has an idea of what ought to be treated. Therefore, in that sense, asthma can be redefined as a condition that would benefit from being treated for asthma. However, at what point do you treat people? Different clinicians will use different cut-off points when they are diagnosing someone as asthmatic. The fashion now is away from saying that asthma is a stigmatizing condition and is better left alone towards saying that everyone who wheezes should have early steroid treatment just in case things get worse later. At the moment, we haven't made a final judgement on the criteria to be used in the next European Community study, and we need to do many more detailed studies before we can come up with any kind of consensus as to where that point might be. Even then, it is debatable whether it should be taken as normative, rather than being a standard. Saying that it is normative and that everybody ought to be treated at this particular level is not the job of epidemiologists.

Britton: I would like to endorse your scepticism about some of the methods used to define or measure asthma. There is a need to define the phenotype both for the geneticists and the epidemiologists; however, there is no clear answer. I am not convinced that hyper-reactivity is a better phenotype than any of the others because it is so heavily dependent on atopy and the baseline level of lung function. If one allows for lung function much of the effect of smoking disappears, so that hyper-reactive people tend to be those with either positive skin tests or low lung function. Therefore, why measure hyper-reactivity at all?

Burney: Presumably, one would want some sort of measure of the lung component. It's true that there are few people who haven't had a long history of smoking, who are not allergic and who are hyper-responsive, but that's not the same as saying that all hyper-responsiveness is explained by those two variables.

Weiss: I would like to make a point about lung function and its relationship to airway responsiveness because it's critical in the context of a specific study design. In a cross-sectional study it's impossible to determine whether low lung function is causing the responsiveness or responsiveness is causing the low lung function. These sorts of questions can be answered by longitudinal studies in which one can control for baseline lung function and look at the effect of both responsiveness on declining lung function and responsiveness as a predictor of declining lung function. This suggests, at least in a directional sense, that responsiveness is associated with a decline regardless of the initial level. Responsiveness is not just low lung function. It's important to distinguish between the two.

Burney: Neil Pride's data probably argue against that. He has shown that if people with hyper-responsiveness stop smoking their lung function stops declining and their reactivity doesn't get worse (Taylor et al 1985). If they continue smoking their lung function continues to decline and their reactivity does get worse. This doesn't explain your data, but I suspect an alternative explanation of your data is that some of the early changes in the morphology of the lung, which are not picked up simply by looking at FEV_1 (forced expiratory volume in one second), may affect bronchial hyper-responsiveness. The problem is that these changes may not be picked up sufficiently early by spirometry so that the changes in hyper-responsiveness are picked up before the changes in FEV_1. In this case it is not possible to determine which develops first.

Platts-Mills: John Britton said that hyper-reactive people either have positive skin tests or have low lung function. However, this statement depends on being in the UK, where there are many experienced people who can give advice on which skin test to do. It also has a homogeneous climate and a homogeneous population. If you extend that argument to the rest of the world then you may become lost because you don't know which skin tests to do.

Britton: I take your point. I was just concerned about the practicality of those measures. We are substituting asthma and allergy, neither of which we can define, with hyper-responsiveness, which we can measure but can't define. It is important to look at the components of that, but it is extremely difficult.

H. R. Anderson: I would like to raise the issue of questionnaires. We're talking about trends in asthma but most data are confined to trends in questionnaire measures. In the 1960s, at least in the UK, there was a preoccupation with bronchitis. Mothers who were hearing their children cough may not have noticed a wheeze because that was something which wasn't emphasized. In contrast, the emphasis is now on wheezing rather than on coughing. This may be a serious problem in trying to determine whether asthma is increasing.

My second point is related to using questionnaires for determining severity. One way to make sure that we are not observing an increased prevalence that is being driven by an increased reporting of mild symptoms is to develop better questionnaire measures of severity. Asthma, at least in children, is a remitting disease; therefore, questionnaires that measure the situation at a particular point in time are much less useful than questionnaires that give some sort of summary assessment over a period of time. Is there anything we can do now in terms of designing questionnaires so that we will not be in this position when we're trying to assess the trends in asthma in the future?

Burney: We know that there are problems with the asthma questionnaires because the reported prevalence of asthma has increased at a faster rate than the reported prevalence of symptoms. The increased reporting of asthma is probably tied in with the encouragement of general practitioners to treat almost all cases of wheezing as asthma.

The data on trends over time should be taken together with other information. I take your point, but when all the evidence is taken together it is difficult to conclude anything else except that asthma trends are rising. Furthermore, because there are large geographic variations in the prevalences of asthma, which we believe are environmentally induced, it is not implausible that there are equally large changes over time. The best approach for obtaining good standardized measures is to do cross-sectional studies where one can plan and control the measures that are being made. This is one of the rationales for doing the European study.

On the question of whether we could improve the questionnaires, I suspect that the answer is yes for studies of severity, but I'm not sure that this is a logical solution to the real problem that you have identified because perceptions of severity may also change over time as may the readiness to report specific symptoms. However, the more specific the diagnosis, the less likely it will be open to various interpretations by respondents. Nevertheless, even this is not a complete answer to the problem. For example, the question 'have you woken at night with breathlessness?' is more specific, but we suspect that people who wake up with nightmares may interpret this as breathlessness. Indeed, there are many reasons why people might wake up or interpret things differently.

Warner: What are your comments on whether or not asthmatic children who cough are being missed in the questionnaires? These are generally the patients who don't recognize that they have asthma, even though the doctor might diagnose them as being asthmatic.

Burney: Cough in children is probably different from that in adults. In our questionnaire we ask whether the patients wake at night with cough, and we find that this is a common symptom affecting 30% of the population. It is also more prevalent in women than in men. I'm not sure, however, whether this can be regarded as pathological.

Holgate: We have a paper in *Thorax* which reports the results of a survey on cough versus wheezing in children of school age (Doull et al 1996). These results are very much in agreement with what you are saying.

Strachan: I would like to try to draw the distinction between defining in a population who has asthma and with what degree of severity, and the question of comparing the burden of asthma in whole populations between areas or over time. Peter Burney has concentrated on the problems of standardizing the measure of population burden, because that bears on the time trends and we can use geographical examples to illustrate this. Defining phenotypes in studies within populations demands a different type of definition. It may be appropriate in some of these studies to define the case group on the basis of relatively specific but insensitive criteria that ignore a lot of the data on the burden of illness but do draw clear black-and-white distinctions between a group of affected and unaffected individuals.

Burney: This sacrifice of sensitivity for specificity would also be true for a number of other epidemiological studies.

References

Bleecker ER, Postma DS, Meyers DA 1997 Genetic susceptibility to asthma in a changing environment. In: The rising trends in asthma. Wiley, Chichester (Ciba Found Symp 206) p 90–105

Doull IJM, Williams AA, Freezer NJ, Holgate ST 1996 Descriptive study of cough, wheeze and school absence in childhood. Thorax 51:630–631

Taylor RG, Joyce H, Gross E, Holland F, Pride NB 1985 Bronchial reactivity to inhaled histamine and annual rate of decline in FEV_1 in male smokers and ex-smokers. Thorax 40:9–16

Evidence for the increase in asthma worldwide

Ann J. Woolcock and Jennifer K. Peat

Institute of Respiratory Medicine, Royal Prince Alfred Hospital, Camperdown, Sydney, NSW 2050, Australia

Abstract. This chapter reviews the evidence that asthma is increasing and that changes in exposure to environmental risk factors may explain the increase. Although asthma is difficult to define for epidemiological studies, the prevalence of asthma as measured by the questionnaire definitions 'asthma ever diagnosed' and 'wheeze ever' is large and increasing. In all countries where serial studies using the same methods have been undertaken over the last 20 years, an increase in wheezing illness in children and adolescents has been recorded but there are insufficient data to determine whether the disease is increasing in adults. Despite the recorded increases, there remains a large difference in the prevalence of asthma between populations, with high rates of wheezing illness in Australasia and low rates in villages in poor countries. The male to female ratio for the occurrence of asthma remains at about 1.5 in children, 1.0 in late adolescence and less than 1.0 in adults, when more females than males have symptoms. The risk factors for childhood asthma are atopy (positive skin tests), parental asthma, allergen load, respiratory infections, some aspects of diet and an 'affluence' factor. There is some evidence for an increase in the prevalence of atopy in children but this may be due to earlier acquisition of atopy. Changes in the other risk factors have not been documented. The evidence for changes in indoor allergen loads, in diet, in the severity and nature of respiratory infections, and in 'affluence' is indirect and comes from a number of small studies rather than from serial epidemiological studies. It seems unlikely that a single, environmental risk factor has changed dramatically worldwide. Rather, a number of lifestyle changes may have combined to cause the disease to be expressed in children who, in previous times, were immunologically protected from developing asthma, perhaps by their T helper cell phenotype, or were not exposed to high allergen levels.

1997 The rising trends in asthma. Wiley, Chichester (Ciba Foundation Symposium 206) p 122–139

The theme of this symposium is the increase in asthma — is it real and if so what are the causes? The aim of this chapter is to review the literature relating to the prevalence of asthma worldwide, with emphasis on children, and then to review the known and putative risk factors for the disease that have been obtained from epidemiological studies. The risk factors for attacks of asthma (acute asthma) are not reviewed.

Childhood asthma

There seems little doubt that asthma and wheezing illness are increasing in children and young adults. Data for 'asthma ever diagnosed' or 'current asthma' are shown in Table 1, which lists studies that have used the same methods in the same populations on at least two occasions. The data clearly show an increase worldwide, in both affluent and non-affluent countries. Figure 1 shows the increase in current asthma in Taiwan (Hsieh & Tsai 1992) and in diagnosed asthma in Scotland (Ninan & Russell 1992, Omran & Russell 1996) as examples of two different populations in which asthma is increasing. Furthermore, Bauman (1993) has collected the data for Australia from different studies

TABLE 1   Changes in prevalence of asthma in children and young adults from questionnaire studies

Country	Study year	Number	Age	Current asthma (%)	Asthma ever diagnosed (%)	References
Australia	1982	769	8–11		12.9	Britton et al 1986
	1992	795	8–11		29.7	Peat et al 1994
New Zealand	1975	715	12–18		26.2	Shaw et al 1990
	1989	435	12–18		34	Shaw et al 1990
Wales	1973	818	12		6	Burr et al 1989
	1988	965	12		12	Barry et al 1991
Scotland	1964	2743	8–13		4.1	Ninan & Russell 1992
	1989	3942	8–13		10.2	Ninan & Russell 1992
	1994	4034	8–13		19.6	Omran & Russell 1996
USA	1971–1974	4941	6–11		4.8	Gergen et al 1988
	1976–1980	7399	3–17		7.6	Gergen et al 1988
Finland	1961	38 000	19	0.1		Haahtela et al 1990
	1989	38 000	19	0.8		Haahtela et al 1990
France	1968	8140	21		3.3	Perdrizet et al 1987
	1982	10 559	21		5.4	Perdrizet et al 1987
Japan	1982	55 388	5–11	3.17		Nishima 1993
	1992	45 674	5–11	4.6		Nishima 1993
Taiwan	1974	23 678	7–15	1.3		Hsieh & Tsai 1992
	1991	92 471	7–15	5.8		Hsieh & Tsai 1992
	1994	NK	7–15	10.8		Hsieh & Tsai 1992
Norway	1981	1772		2.2	3.4	Skjonsberg et al 1995
	1993	4521		4.2	8	Skjonsberg et al 1995

NK, not known.

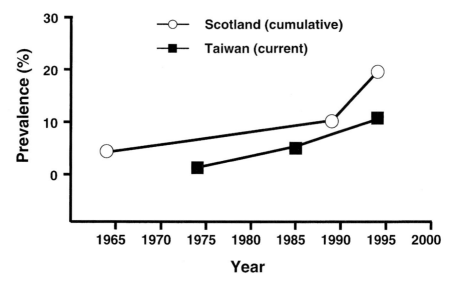

FIG. 1.   Changes in the prevalence of asthma in two populations studied on three occasions using the same questionnaires. The Scottish data are for 'diagnosed asthma', a cumulative prevalence, while those for Taiwan are for 'current asthma'. Asthma has increased in these widely different populations in the last 25 years. References for these studies are given in the text.

and shown that the trend has continued into the early part of this decade. This increase has attracted much attention leading to a number of review articles (Woolcock et al 1995, Peat 1996a, Gergen & Weiss 1995).

It is not possible to list all of the studies on the prevalence of childhood asthma in the world during the last 30 years, but a review by Gregg (1983) showed that the prevalence of childhood asthma in most affluent countries was 2–5%, with higher values in New Zealand, Australia and Tristan da Cunha. In addition, he showed that the prevalence of asthma was higher in boys than in girls but that this excess disappears during teenage years.

An analysis of all the published data suggests that the increase in prevalence began in the 1970s. Initially, there was debate about whether the increases were real or due to diagnostic transfer and increased awareness of the population with widespread publicity. However, authors who have looked carefully at the data agree that both wheezing illness and asthma have increased (Peat et al 1994, Bauman 1993, Burney et al 1990). In addition, there is evidence that asthma was rare in children in Africa up to the late 1970s. Recent studies suggest that asthma is emerging in Kenya (Odhiambo et al 1994) and Zimbabwe (Keeley et al 1991) and that there is a gradient in prevalence from low in rural to high in urban populations (Fig. 2).

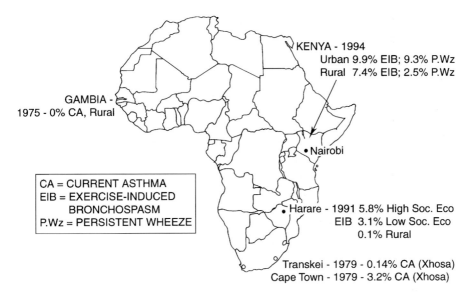

FIG. 2.   Prevalence of asthma in children in several African countries. The studies in 1975 and 1979 are reported by Gregg (1983). The studies documented either 'current' asthma or exercise-induced bronchospasm. The prevalence has increased from low levels in 1975 to levels similar to those found in affluent countries in 1994.

Adults

There are fewer data for adults and it is not known if asthma is increasing in adult populations. In Busselton we found increased symptoms and diagnosed asthma, especially in young adults, but no change in the prevalence of bronchial hyper-responsiveness (Peat et al 1992a). There have been few other studies that have compared the same population of adults with time. Early data from the second study of the inhabitants of Tristan da Cunha suggest that current asthma has increased from 11% in 1974 (Mantle & Pepys 1974) to a value of over 20% (Zamel 1995).

Other allergic diseases

There is evidence that other allergic diseases are increasing in children, but not in all populations. Hay fever has greatly increased in Australia (Peat et al 1994), New Zealand (Barry et al 1991, Sears et al 1993), Scotland (Ninan & Russell 1992) and Sweden (Aberg 1989), but not in Norway (Skjonsberg et al 1995). The questionnaire definitions of rhinitis are less precise than those for asthma, so the magnitude of the change may not be precise. It is suggested that hay fever is, in fact, a 'new' disease. It appears to be a disease associated with good hygiene and is rarely seen in village populations of developing countries.

Risk factors

Until recently, there were few studies that used logistic regression analysis to identify, in terms of odds ratios, the magnitudes of different putative risk factors. In Australia (Peat 1994), Germany (von Mutius & Nicolai 1996), the USA (Sporik et al 1995) and New Zealand (Sears et al 1989) being atopic has been shown to be the greatest risk for asthma. The allergens, identified by skin prick tests, shown to be significant risk factors are house dust mites, cat, *Alternaria* and pollens, depending on the environment. After atopy, the next most important risk factor is parental asthma. Having a parent with asthma approximately doubles the risk of airway hyper-responsiveness and asthma in childhood (von Mutius & Nicolai 1996, Peat et al 1992b, Jenkins et al 1994). It is not yet possible to determine how much of this association is due to genetic factor(s) and how much to shared environmental exposures.

Other risks include the amount of allergen in the home, environmental tobacco smoke (in young children), early respiratory illness, length of breast feeding and diet (particularly in relation to salt intake and oily fish). These risk factors have recently been reviewed in the context of preventive strategies (Peat 1996b). Factors that do not appear to be involved in the development of asthma are air pollution, being allergic to pollens only, and being allergic to foods and cigarette smoking, although these factors have not been studied in large populations.

Environmental factors

If asthma is increasing which of the risk factors are changing to cause the increase?

Atopy

Table 2 outlines the studies of skin prick tests undertaken in random populations of children and young adults during the last 12 years. These were undertaken in random samples except for the last one in the USA, which was a group of asthmatic children plus a control population (Sporik et al 1995). Several populations of children and adults have been studied twice and the data from the USA (Barbee et al 1987), Australia (Peat et al 1995), Italy (Forastiere et al 1996), France (Oryszczcn et al 1995) and Switzerland (Wuthrich et al 1995) are shown in Fig. 3. In all studies an increase was shown but these increases were smaller than the increases that are shown in Table 1 for asthma. The data are of interest in spite of the fact that different methods, different allergens and different weal size cut-off values were used in the studies and in some early studies mite allergen was not included. The range of prevalence in skin tests is extremely high and it is not explained by differences in methods. The relationship between the prevalence of atopy and the prevalence of 'diagnosed asthma' in the same population is poor. In populations living traditional lifestyles, such as in Indonesia, Papua New Guinea and the Australian Aborigines, both atopy and asthma are uncommon, and this also applies to the parts of Eastern Europe for which there are data. Within the populations with 25–45% of the population atopic, Australia and New Zealand have much higher levels of diagnosed asthma than countries in Europe. In populations where 50% or more are atopic, the prevalence of asthma

TABLE 2 **Prevalence of atopy (as measured by skin prick tests) and diagnosed asthma (as measured by questionnaire in children and young adults)**

Country	Atopy (%)	Diagnosed asthma (%)	n	Age	Comments[a]	References
Indonesia (rural)	24	2.0	597	7–17	3 mm	Woolcock et al 1982
Papua New Guinea (rural)	14	0.5	197	6–20	2 mm	Turner et al 1986
Australia, Aborigines (rural)	20.9	1.0	263	8–12	3 mm	Veale et al 1996
Estonia (rural)	8.1	2.5	774	10–12	3 mm	Riikjarv et al 1995
Estonia (urban)	14.3	3.2	806	10–12	10–12 mm	Riikjarv et al 1995
Poland (urban)	13.7	2.9	358	10–12	3 mm	Braback et al 1994
Italy (Rome)	29.1	5.9	892	14–15	3 mm	Forastiere et al 1996
England (Southampton)	32.0	9.5	311	7–11	3 mm	Clifford et al 1989
Denmark (Copenhagen)	30	5.3	524	7–16	NK M>F	Backer et al 1992
Sweden (urban)	35.3	9.5	351	10–12	3 mm	Braback et al 1994
Sweden (urban, north)	43.2	6.8	1112	14	3 mm M=F	Norrman et al 1994
Germany (Munich)	36.7	5.9	5030	9–11	3 mm	von Mutius et al 1994a
Germany (Leipzig)	18.2	3.9	2623	9–11	3 mm	von Mutius et al 1994a
Australia (rural)	34.8	29.7	873	8–11	3 mm	Peat et al 1995
Australia (Sydney)	42.4	23.5	1339	8–11	3 mm	Peat et al 1995
New Zealand (Dunedin)	43.8	35.5	662	13	2 mm M>F	Sears et al 1993
Hong Kong	57.7	11.6	471	13–17	3 mm	Leung & Ho 1994
Malaysia (urban/ rural)	63.9	8.2	321	13–17	3 mm	Leung & Ho 1994
China (urban/rural)	49.0	1.9	737	14–18	3 mm	Leung & Ho 1994
USA (Los Almos)	69	17.4	120	12–14	3 mm	Sporik et al 1995

[a]Weal size and gender distribution if known.
F, females; M, males; NK, not known.

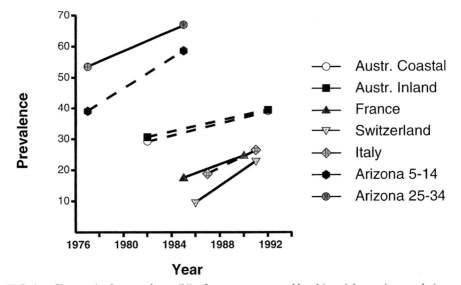

FIG. 3.   Changes in the prevalence (%) of atopy as measured by skin prick tests in populations
where the same methods and allergens have been used at different times. The French study in
adults used only two groups of allergens (mites and pollens) and the Italian study is in the same
cohort at an older age. Small increases have occurred. The figure shows the wide range of
prevalence from Switzerland (low) to Arizona, USA (high). Some of the differences are
probably due to different methods and allergens tested. References for these studies are given
in the text.

varies greatly from extremely low in China to high in the USA. Thus, it appears that the
factors which determine atopy are not the same as those which determine asthma.

In New Zealand skin prick tests were repeated in the Dunedin cohort (at age 21)
studied by Sears and the prevalence had increased to 66% (Sears 1995). These high
values for atopy, together with those found in some Chinese populations and in the
USA, suggest that, given the appropriate environment, the majority of populations
can become sensitized to aero-allergens. It seems unlikely that a genetic factor is
predisposing to the atopic status as such, although it may predispose to the severity
of atopy present. The relationship between the prevalence of asthma and the severity
of atopy, as defined by the radioallergosorbent test or by the size and number of
positive skin prick tests, has not been reported.

There are data which indicate that atopy acquired early in life may be important.
Atopy acquired after the age of seven is not a risk factor for the later development of
asthma (Peat & Woolcock 1991) and the first three years of life may be important for
the acquisition of atopy (Van Asperen et al 1990). More precise studies will be needed
to determine if populations are becoming more atopic or acquiring atopy at a younger
age. However, it seems unlikely that the increase in asthma can be explained simply by
an increase in atopic sensitization.

Allergen load

Allergen load may well be increasing but the evidence for this is circumstantial. There are some data that show increases in mite allergen levels (Green et al 1993) and most people agree that indoor environments have changed in the last 20 years in climates where some household heating is required in the winter. Evidence that allergen load may be important comes from two of our studies. In a study of children in Sydney, those born in Australia were more likely to have asthma than those born in South-East Asia (Peat et al 1992) and children who are skin test positive to house dust mites are more likely to have asthma if they live in towns with high mite levels than in towns with low mite levels (Peat et al 1996).

Family history

Logistic regression analysis shows that parental history of asthma is an important risk factor for asthma after adjusting for atopy (Peat et al 1992). Even in non-atopic children with asthma, a family history of asthma was a risk factor (von Mutius & Nicolai 1996). The risk ratio for family history appears to be about two to three. Although the data from certain populations such as Tristan da Cunha (Mantle & Pepys 1974, Zamel 1995) suggest that there is a genetic component in asthma which is independent of atopy, the relative roles of genes and of shared environments still have to be defined.

Early respiratory infection

Respiratory infections before the age of two years have been found to be a risk factor when this question has been asked in studies in affluent societies (Peat et al 1992). In addition, viral respiratory tract infections appear to cause attacks of asthma. However, there is circumstantial evidence, based on the lack of asthma in children living in traditional lifestyles (Veale et al 1996, Woolcock et al 1981), that early respiratory infections may be protective and this would make sense if some infections stimulate T helper (Th) 1 rather than Th2 lymphocytes.

Diet

As Seaton et al (1994) pointed out, a change in diet may be a factor responsible for the increasing prevalence of childhood asthma. Peat (1996) has recently reviewed the literature from epidemiological studies of asthma and the role of diet is also discussed by Weiss (1997, this volume). It seems likely that the change in diet with the higher intakes of some nutrients and the decrease in others will be shown to be a factor in the increasing prevalence of asthma. Dietary habits are changing rapidly in many countries and, if the resulting effects interact with exposure at an early age to allergens and to environmental tobacco smoke, the overall effect in terms of numbers of wheezy children in communities may be large.

Environmental tobacco smoke

This has been studied extensively and has been shown to be a small but consistent risk factor for early wheezing illness (Peat 1994). In many affluent countries, where all the other risk factors mentioned above are present, young adult women of child-bearing age are continuing to smoke, and this may be another factor adding to the burden of illness. There is enough evidence to suggest that this is a definite risk and that programmes to stop smoking throughout pregnancy and in the environment of the newborn child are definite public health measures that can be introduced.

Other 'lifestyle' factors

Taken together, the world data suggest that asthma is increasing in societies that no longer live in traditional lifestyles and that the 'cleaner' the living conditions of populations, the more likely it is that asthma will be present. What additional factors associated with modern (and perhaps clean) lifestyles, and not yet identified in epidemiological studies, could account for the increase of asthma symptoms amongst atopic children? Perhaps having fewer serious infections in early childhood (due to fewer worms, fewer children per household, fewer shared bedrooms, more immunization and increased use of antibiotics) is a one of the factors responsible for the increase in asthma prevalence. Theoretically, a protective factor related to Th1 pathways may be being lost. It is not known if all atopic children have eosinophilic inflammation of the airways but it is conceivable that, even in the presence of atopy, the airways can be protected from severe inflammation by Th1 cells.

Another potential risk factor relates to lack of exercise. Since asthma is a disease in which the airways are prone to narrow too much, there seems little doubt that the bronchial smooth muscle is behaving abnormally. It has been postulated that bronchial smooth muscle, when at short fibre length, can easily shorten to a point where the cross-bridges between actin and myosin increase so that the muscle fibres act as though they are in a 'latch' state and it becomes more difficult for them to relax (Fredberg 1997). In severe asthma the inflammation extends to the adventitial layer, which is thickened, and it is thought to prevent the stretching effects of big breaths on the muscle fibres. Without this stretch, muscle may more easily go into the 'latch' state (Wiggs et al 1990). In atopic children without asthma, airway inflammation due to ongoing reactions to allergens may result in the development of asthma if these children have a low level of exercise (e.g. if they watch many hours of television) (Heath et al 1994) because these children do not stretch their lungs, thus allowing some airways to narrow or close. The combination of a low level of inflammation with release of mediators and muscle that is insufficiently stretched causes the muscle to behave in an asthmatic way. In addition, there is evidence that children are exercising less in societies where television is freely available (Heath et al 1994).

Summary

There seems little doubt that asthma and wheezing illnesses are increasing worldwide in children. The increase appears to have started in the early 1970s and data up to 1994 show a continuing increase. The increases have been greatest in affluent populations and large differences in prevalences remain between different parts of the world, with high values in affluent populations of the southern hemisphere followed by the UK and the USA. Non-affluent societies have the lowest rates of asthma but there is evidence for an increase in Asia and in some African countries.

The risk factors for asthma are beginning to be defined. The risks include: being allergic to mites, to the mould *Alternaria* or to cats; the allergen load and the time at which exposure occurs; parental asthma; diet; environmental tobacco smoke; and perhaps excessive levels of hygiene. The role of respiratory infections as being protective or as a risk factor is unclear. Information about changes in these environmental factors is sparse. There is some evidence for an increased prevalence of atopy but this increase is not large enough to explain the large increase in wheezing illness. The data concerning allergen load, changes in diet, changes in environmental tobacco smoke and respiratory infections are all circumstantial since, until recently, these risk factors were not measured in epidemiological studies.

Overall one can conclude from the literature that affluent populations with good hygiene who are exposed to consistently high levels of aero-allergen, who have a diet relatively low in fresh fruit, vegetables and fish, and who experience low levels of exercise have an increased risk of asthma. These environmental changes are perhaps lessening the effect of factors that previously protected against asthma. Undoubtedly, there are genetic factors that predispose to asthma and that are independent of atopy, and in some families asthma may occur in the absence of the defined risk factors but the nature of these genetic factors awaits further research.

References

Aberg N 1989 Asthma and allergic rhinitis in Swedish conscripts. Clin Exp Allergy 19:59–63

Backer V, Ulrik CS, Hansen KK, Laursen EM, Dirksen A, Bach-Mortensen N 1992 Atopy and bronchial responsiveness in a random population sample of 527 children and adolescents. Ann Allergy 69:116–122

Barbee RA, Kaltenborn W, Lebowitz MD, Burrows B 1987 Longitudinal changes in allergen skin test reactivity in a community population sample. J Allergy Clin Immunol 79:16–24

Barry DMJ, Burr ML, Limb ES 1991 Prevalence of asthma among 12-year-old children in New Zealand and South Wales: a comparative survey. Thorax 46:405–409

Bauman A 1993 Has the prevalence of asthma symptoms increased in Australian children? J Paediatr Child Health 29:424–428

Braback L, Breborowicz A, Dreborg S, Knutsson A, Pieklik H, Bjorksten B 1994 Atopic sensitization and respiratory symptoms among Polish and Swedish school children. Clin Exp Allergy 24:826–835

Britton WJ, Woolcock AJ, Peat JK, Sedgwick CJ, Lloyd DM, Leeder SR 1986 Prevalence of bronchial hyperresponsiveness in children: the relationship between asthma and skin reactivity to allergens in two communities. Int J Epidemiol 15:202–209

Burney PGJ, Chinn S, Rona RJ 1990 Has the prevalence of asthma increased in children? Evidence from the national study of health and growth 1973–86. Br Med J 300:1306–1310

Burr ML, Butland BK, King S, Vaughan-Williams E 1989 Changes in asthma prevalence: two surveys 15 years apart. Arch Dis Child 64:1452–1456

Clifford RD, Radford M, Howell JB, Holgate ST 1989 Prevalence of atopy and range of bronchial response to methacholine in 7- and 11-year-old schoolchildren. Arch Dis Child 64:1126–1132

Forastiere F, Corbo GM, Dell'Orco V, Pistelli R, Agabiti N, Kriebel D 1996 A longitudinal evaluation of bronchial responsiveness to methacholine in children: role of baseline lung function, gender, and change in atopic status. Am J Respir Crit Care Med 153:1098–1104

Fredberg JJ 1997 Friction in airway smooth muscle: mechanism, latch and implications in asthma. J Appl Physiol, in press

Gergen PJ, Weiss KB 1995 Epidemiology of asthma. In: Busse WW, Holgate ST (eds) Asthma and rhinitis. Blackwell Scientific, Oxford, p 15–31

Gergen PJ, Mullally DI, Evans R 1988 National survey of prevalence of asthma among children in the United States, 1976 to 1980. Pediatrics 81:1–7

Green W, Toelle B, Woolcock AJ 1993 House dust mite increase in Wagga Wagga houses. Aust NZ J Med 23:23

Gregg I 1983 Epidemiological aspects. In: Clark TJH, Godfrey S (eds) Asthma. Chapman Hall, London, p 242–284

Gregg I 1986 Epidemiological research in asthma: the need for a broad perspective. Clin Allergy 16:17–23

Haahtela T, Lindohlm H, Björkstén F, Koskenvuo K, Laitinen LA 1990 Prevalence of asthma in Finnish young men. Br Med J 301:266–268

Heath GW, Pratt M, Warren CW, Kann L 1994 Physical activity patterns in American high school students. Results from the 1990 Youth Risk Behavior Survey. Arch Pediatr Adolesc Med 148:1131–1136

Hsieh K-H, Tsai Y-T 1992 Increasing prevalence of childhood allergic disease allergic disease in Taipei, Taiwan, and the outcome. In: Miyamoto T, Okuda M (eds) Progress in allergy and clinical immunology, vol 2: Proceedings of the 14th International Congress of Allergology and Clinical Immunology. Hogrefe & Huber, Gottingen, p 223–225

Jenkins MA, Hopper JL, Bowes G, Carlin JB, Flander LB, Giles GG 1994 Factors in childhood as predictors of asthma in adult life. Br Med J 309:90–93

Keeley DJ, Neill P, Gallivan S 1991 Comparison of the prevalence of reversible airways obstruction in rural and urban Zimbabwean children. Thorax 46:549–553

Leung R, Ho P 1994 Asthma, allergy, and atopy in three south-east Asian populations. Thorax 49:1205–1210

Mantle J, Pepys J 1974 Asthma amongst Tristan da Cunha islanders. Clin Allergy 4:161–170

Ninan TK, Russell G 1992 Respiratory symptoms and atopy in Aberdeen schoolchildren: evidence from two surveys 25 years apart. Br Med J 304:873–875

Nishima S 1993 A study on the prevalence of bronchial asthma in school children in western districts of Japan: comparison between the studies in 1982 and in 1992 with the same methods and same districts. The Study Group of the Prevalence of Bronchial Asthma, the West Japan Study Group of Bronchial Asthma (translated from Japanese). Arerugi-Jpn J Allerg 42:192–204

Norrman E, Rosenhall L, Nystrom L, Jonsson E, Stjernberg N 1994 Prevalence of positive skin prick tests, allergic asthma, and rhinoconjunctivitis in teenagers in northern Sweden. Allergy 49:808–815

Odhiambo J, Ng'ang'a L, Mungai M et al 1994 Rural and urban respiratory health. Surveys in Kenya schoolchildren: participation rates and prevalence of markers of asthma. Am J Resp Crit Care Med 149:385A

Omran M, Russell G 1996 Continuing increase in respiratory symptoms and atopy in Aberdeen schoolchildren. Br Med J 312:34

Oryszczyn M-P, Annesi I, Neukirch F, Dore M-F, Kauffmann F 1995 Longitudinal observations of serum IgE and skin prick test response. Am J Respir Crit Care Med 151:663–668

Peat JK 1994 The rising trend in allergic illness: which environmental factors are important? Clin Exp Allergy 24:797–800

Peat JK 1996a The epidemiology of asthma. Curr Opin Pul Med 2:7–15

Peat JK 1996b Prevention of asthma. Eur Respir J 9:1545–1555

Peat JK, Woolcock AJ 1991 Sensitivity to common allergens: relation to respiratory symptoms and bronchial hyperresponsiveness in children from three different climatic areas of Australia. Clin Exp Allergy 21:573–581

Peat JK, Haby M, Spijker J, Berry G, Woolcock AJ 1992a Prevalence of asthma in adults in Busselton, Western Australia. Br Med J 305:1326–1329

Peat JK, Salome CM, Woolcock AJ 1992b Factors associated with bronchial hyperresponsiveness in Australian adults and children. Eur Respir J 5:921–929

Peat JK, van den Berg RH, Green WF, Mellis CM, Leeder SR, Woolcock AJ 1994 Changing prevalence of asthma in Australian children. Br Med J 308:1591–1596

Peat JK, Toelle B, Gray L et al 1995 Prevalence and severity of childhood asthma and allergic sensitisation in seven climatic regions of New South Wales. Med J Aust 163:22–26

Peat JK, Tovey E, Toelle BG et al 1996 House-dust mite allergens: a major cause of childhood asthma in Australia. Am J Resp Crit Care Med 152:141–146

Perdrizet S, Neukirch F, Cooreman J, Liard R 1987 Prevalence of asthma in adolescents in various parts of France and its relationship to respiratory allergic manifestations. Chest 91:104S–106S

Riikjarv MA, Julge K, Vasar M, Braback L, Knutsson A, Bjorksten B 1995 The prevalence of atopic sensitization and respiratory symptoms among Estonian schoolchildren. Clin Exp Allergy 25:1198–1204

Sears MR 1995 Natural history of asthma from childhood to young adulthood: a longitudinal study. Am J Resp Crit Care Med 152:24

Sears MR, Herbison GP, Holdaway MD, Hewitt CJ, Flannery EM, Silva PA 1989 The relative risks of sensitivity to grass pollen, house dust mite and cat dander in the development of childhood asthma. Clin Exp Allergy 19:419–424

Sears MR, Burrows B, Flannery EM, Herbison GP, Holdaway MD 1993 Atopy in childhood. I. Gender- and allergen-related risks for development of hay fever and asthma. Clin Exp Allergy 23:941–948

Seaton A, Godden DJ, Brown K 1994 Increase in asthma: a more toxic environment or a more susceptible population? Thorax 49:171–174

Shaw RA, Crane J, O'Donnell TV, Porteous LE, Coleman ED 1990 Increasing asthma prevalence in a rural New Zealand adolescent population: 1975–1989. Arch Dis Childhood 65:1319–1323

Skjonsberg OH, Clenchaas J, Leehaard J et al 1995 Prevalence of bronchial asthma in schoolchildren in Oslo, Norway: comparison of data in 1993 and 1981. Allergy 50:806–810

Sporik R, Ingram JM, Price W, Sussman JH, Honsinger RW, Platts-Mills TAE 1995 Association of asthma with serum IgE and skin test reactivity to allergens among children living at high altitude. Tickling the dragon's breath. Am J Respir Crit Care Med 151:1388–1392

Turner KJ, Dowse GK, Stewart GA, Alpers MP 1986 Studies on bronchial hyperreactivity, allergic responsiveness, and asthma in rural and urban children of the highlands of Papua New Guinea. J Allergy Clin Immunol 77:558–566

Van Asperen PP, Kemp AS, Mukhi A 1990 Atopy in infancy predicts the severity of bronchial hyperresponsiveness in later childhood. J Allergy Clin Immunol 85:790–795

Veale A J, Peat JK, Tovey ER, Salome CM, Thompson JE, Woolcock AJ 1996 Asthma and atopy in four rural Australian Aboriginal communities. Med J Aust 165:192–196

von Mutius E, Nicolai T 1996 Familial aggregation of asthma in a South Bavarian population. Am J Respir Crit Care Med 153:1266–1272

von Mutius E, Martinez FD, Fritzsch C, Nicolai T, Roell G, Thiemann H-H 1994a Prevalence of asthma and atopy in two areas of West Germany and East Germany. Am J Respir Crit Care Med 149:358–364

von Mutius E, Martinez FD, Fritzsch C, Nicolai T, Reitmeir P, Thiemann HH 1994b Skin test reactivity and number of siblings. Br Med J 308:692–695

Weiss ST 1997 Diet as a risk factor for asthma. In: The rising trends in asthma. Wiley, Chichester (Ciba Found Symp 206) p 244–257

Wiggs BR, Moreno R, Hogg JC, Hilliam C, Paré PD 1990 A model of the mechanics of airway narrowing. J Appl Physiol 69:849–860

Woolcock A J, Green W, Alpers MP 1981 Asthma in a rural highland area of Papua New Guinea. Am Rev Respir Dis 123:565–567

Woolcock A J, Konthen PG, Sedgwick C 1982 Bronchial reactivity in the students of an Indonesian village (translated from French). Bull Int Union Tuberc 57:163–168

Woolcock A J, Peat JK, Trevillion LM 1995 Changing prevalence of allergies worldwide. In: Johansson SGO (ed) Progress in allergy and clinical immunology, vol 3: Proceedings of the 15th International Congress of Allergology and Clinical Immunology and the 1994 Annual Meeting of the European Academy of Allergology and Clinical Immunology, Stockholm, June 6–July 1 1994. Hogrefe & Huber, Gottingen, p 167–171

Wuthrich B, Schindler C, Leuenberger P et al 1995 Prevalence of atopy and pollinosis in the adult population of Switzerland (SAPALDIA Study). Int Arch Allergy Immunol 106:149–156

Zamel N 1995 In search of the genes of asthma on the island of Tristan da Cunha. Can Respir J 2:18–22

DISCUSSION

Busse: Have the instruments used to assess asthma changed over the last 10 years?

Woolcock: Each questionnaire is slightly different, so the instruments have changed slightly. However, if one looks at all the studies that have used exactly the same questionnaire and the ones that have used bronchial hyper-responsiveness, all the evidence is that asthma has been increasing. It is not yet known whether this trend is continuing in 1995/1996.

Busse: Your 'latch' hypothesis is intriguing. Am I correct in assuming that in the equation the latch doesn't change significantly but the changes in the risk factors which drive the latch or its susceptibility change so that it becomes more expressed?

Woolcock: Yes, that is my hypothesis. We believe that there is factor which affects bronchial smooth muscle formation independently of T helper 2 cells and inflammation. This is not yet well defined but would explain why bronchial hyper-responsiveness is independent of atopy in genetic studies.

Holgate: It could just be an ion channel, for example.

Woolcock: Yes, it could be one of a number of factors.

Busse: Can you explain the observation that when asthma lungs are transplanted into normal recipients they develop asthma? Because presumably normal recipients do not have the ability to go into latch.

Woolcock: Anyone can go into latch. Latch appears to depend on the initial length of the smooth muscle. However, there may also be an inherited abnormality that makes individuals more likely to go into latch.

Brostoff: I attended the Ciba Foundation study group in 1971, where the term atopy was debated over coffee and dinner with vigour. The first description of atopy by Coca & Cooke (1923) was that of a state of hypersensitivity to include asthma, eczema, hay fever and food allergy. The description that we're seeing here is that atopy equals a positive skin test. I suspect that many of us would feel rather uncomfortable with this change in definition because a positive skin test is not a clinical definition.

Woolcock: I used the two terms interchangeably. Instead of writing 'prevalence of atopy' I could have written 'prevalence of positive skin tests'.

Brostoff: But the definitions are quite different. To a clinician, someone who has atopy has asthma, eczema, hay fever or food allergy. I regret the definition of atopy as equivalent to the presence of weal and flare skin reaction with an allergen for a number of reasons. For example, local mucosal production of IgE, which I showed over 20 years ago (Huggins & Brostoff 1975), can predict atopy in terms of hay fever only by nasal provocation with the patient having negative skin and negative radioallergosorbent test (RAST) results. These subjects by your definition are not atopic but clearly have true allergic rhinitis. Many people who had hay fever 15 years ago, for example, and who have now grown out of it still have positive RAST and skin test results — they are no longer allergic.

Holgate: It may be better if we used specific IgE hyper-responsiveness or bronchial hyper-responsiveness with methacholine or histamine, which are laboratory measures.

Platts-Mills: At the time these experiments were performed, there was little information about house dust mites, which are the key allergens. At least today we can define what we mean by a skin test. Skin tests or serum IgE levels are standardizable phenomena that we can measure. I'm in favour of the transfer from atopy as a disease state to atopy as a measurement.

Brostoff: In that case you should re-define what you mean by atopy.

Paré: Are there any good data on changes in the levels of total IgE within the same populations?

Woolcock: No. There are very few data for total IgE levels measured in exactly the same way in the same populations at the same time and in which the parasite status was also known.

Holt: There's another missing link we should discuss because the data suggest that atopy is necessary but not sufficient for the development of asthma. The challenge is to find the link between skin test reactivity and bronchial hyper-reactivity. One possibility is that allergen-specific T cells have to develop tissue-specific homing receptors before they can take up residence in the airways. We do not yet know if this is correct, but recent work on the expression of the CLA antigen on skin-homing

T cells points in this direction. Antigen-presenting cells in airway tissues could also be involved, by promoting excessive local T cell activation. This is a new area and one that is technically extremely demanding.

Holgate: Some gene-manipulated mouse models could help by deleting one molecule in the cascade at a time.

Holt: There is also room for some new epidemiology. The questions would have to be re-cast but at least we now have the insight to be able to ask the relevant questions.

Platts-Mills: Is it possible to combine epidemiology with T cell studies? It's been a general rule in the past that T cell technology was not at a level of consistency where it could be studied epidemiologically.

Holt: We have now reached the stage where this is just about possible. We're currently involved in these sorts of studies with collaborators in Sweden and Estonia. These involve cryopreservation of T cells such that they can be transferred between labs around the world, and we've now managed to solve the logistical problems involved.

Britton: On the point of which questions need to be asked, if I understood Patrick Holt correctly, he implied that we treat atopy as a component but not an absolute cause for asthma. However, there has been a rise in the prevalence of positive skin tests in many studies, and most notably in the East and West European studies. Therefore, we have to ask not only why is the proportion of atopics, as defined by positive skin tests, becoming asthmatic, but also why is the prevalence of positive skin tests increasing?

Nelson: In drier areas, such as Broken Hill, where there are fewer house dust mites, there is an increased sensitivity towards *Alternaria*. Is this because there is more *Alternaria* in these regions or is *Alternaria* just an antigen of convenience in the absence of house dust mites?

Woolcock: No one has measured the levels of *Alternaria* anywhere in Australia because it's extremely difficult. However, from the few studies that we have done using pollen traps, there does appear to be more *Alternaria* in rural areas than there is in Sydney.

Holgate: If one attaches primacy to certain allergens in the environment, such as house dust mites, cats, *Alternaria* or birch pollen, I have never been able to understand why that if the primary allergen is removed another soon takes its place.

Woolcock: This situation has not occurred in Broken Hill. *Alternaria* has probably always been there.

Holgate: But in Calgary, for example, there are almost no house dust mites on account of the cold and dry climate, and there the asthma cases are explained by exposure to cat allergens. As far as I can tell, the cat population in Calgary is similar to that in Southampton, for example.

Woolcock: The cat allergen, however, is extremely allergenic. The logistic regression analyses on allergens suggest that there are only four major allergens: house dust mites, *Alternaria*, cats and cockroaches. Rye grass and birch are only minor allergens.

Holgate: If these are the four important sources of allergens that seem to be driving the disease across the world we have to look carefully at why they have taken primacy.

Weiss: It is interesting that the Chinese have a high prevalence of atopy and a low prevalence of asthma. We obtained the same results in our genetic studies in China, i.e. a high degree of skin test positivity, high IgE levels and a low prevalence of asthma compared to western countries. We are also looking at parasites, which are clearly part of the equation and may also be part of the reason for the uncoupling of the atopic and asthmatic responses.

Holgate: Is it possible to inherit allergen-specific responses? On the island of Tristan da Cunha there have not been any cats since the early 1960s and yet children born on the island after that time who have never seen a cat are skin test positive to cats despite extremely low, if not negligible, concentrations of *Fel d* 1 in homes (Zamel et al 1996).

Platts-Mills: In general it is not possible to inherit IgE or allergen-specific responses.

Strachan: I have a point on attribution and causality, and their relationship with allergen sensitization and asthma. You showed that a sizeable proportion of the recently wheezy children were non-atopic according to your definition, although they may have been classified as atopic if the definition was based on a smaller weal size. This suggests that there is a capacity for non-atopic wheezing, and one might presume that a proportion of those who are atopic are also suffering from non-atopic wheezing. Therefore, it's dangerous to assume that all atopic asthmatics are having allergic asthma attacks.

Also, on the topic of specific allergens, I wonder whether the problem is that when we find relationships between the more severe forms of wheezing and specific allergen sensitivities within a population we're simply picking up the more severely atopic individuals. In addition, the allergens being tested may be capable of discriminating between more and less severe atopy, and some may be more effective at doing that within a given environment than others. Therefore, I'm not surprised that different allergens are the major culprits in different environments, or that in a mite-free environment *Alternaria* is the discriminator. *Alternaria* may not necessarily be causing severe asthma.

Holgate: This is an important point because causality is being attached to this.

Martinez: I also feel strongly about this. The strongest risk factor for sensitization to *Alternaria* in Tucson, Arizona is not a positive skin test in the mother but asthma in the mother or the father. Therefore, people with genetic susceptibilities to asthma are easily sensitized to certain antigens. This is important but not necessarily a cause–effect relationship. Our latest data, which are not yet published, show that in many children who were sensitized at age six years to *Alternaria* if they are tested again with exactly the same techniques at age 11 years many lose their skin test reactivity to *Alternaria*, yet they're still asthmatic by our definition. They still have symptoms and they are becoming sensitized to other things. They may have inherited a certain peculiar way of reacting to the environment such that certain agents are associated causally to the condition and other agents are not. I caution against assuming that when there is an association between two factors, a cause–effect relationship is the only possible explanation for the association.

Sears: I would like to take the definition of atopy equals positive skin tests one step further and mention the problems of the definition of a positive skin test, which is a continuous variable. We encounter the same problems with airway responsiveness, i.e. that a PC_{20} of 8.0 mg/ml is deemed positive and 8.1 is negative. In most of the studies you presented the definition of a positive skin test was a weal size of 3 mm, so that by this definition someone with a weal size of 2.5 mm is classified as non-atopic, which is not appropriate. We and others have shown that even a 1 mm weal has meaning in predicting the development of asthma (Sears et al 1993a,b, Weirings et al 1995).

Nelson: It's also important to determine the background, non-specific reactivity for skin testing. Depending on the device that's used, below a certain weal size or flare reaction you start picking up reactions from the trauma of skin testing (Nelson et al 1993). Therefore, even though in theory there may be a continuum of allergic reactivity beginning with the first observable reaction, you have to define a size above which you can be fairly certain that there are no false positives.

Magnussen: You presented data on the comparisons between skin test reactivity and asthma in different countries. von Mutius et al (1994) and Nowak et al (1996) have observed in children and adults, respectively, that in those parts of the country with poor living standards skin test reactivity was less prevalent. This may have something to do with air pollution. Recently, von Mutius et al (1996) demonstrated that particles may be protective, and particles are the main component of air pollution in East Germany. On the other hand, Jörres et al (1996) have indicated that ozone promotes allergic airway responsiveness. You didn't mention these possibilities in your list of risk factors.

Woolcock: I agree. There are no epidemiological data to support the hypothesis that the oxidant air pollutants, such as ozone and nitrogen dioxide, are risk factors for the development of asthma. However, it is possible that particulate pollution is protective.

Potter: You showed that there has been an increase in house dust mites in Wagga Wagga. Is this not the most important risk factor for the development of asthma in this area?

Woolcock: It is unlikely. The main problem in Wagga Wagga is *Alternaria*. There has been an increase in childhood asthma throughout Australia, and not just in Wagga Wagga. Therefore, there has to have been a universal change in a particular factor. It is unlikely that the levels of allergens have increased dramatically in Australia, suggesting that factors other than allergen load are involved. The loss of a protective factor that is associated with poor hygiene and exposure to infectious agents appears to be more likely. The lifestyle changes are complex and finding a way to tease them out and test them in epidemiological studies represents a real challenge.

References

Coca AF, Cooke RA 1923 On the clarification of the phenomenon of hypersensitiveness. J Immunol 8:163

Huggins KG, Brostoff J 1975 Local production of specific IgE antibodies in allergic rhinitis patients with negative skin tests. Lancet II:148–152

Jörres R, Nowak D, Magnussen H 1996 The effect of ozone exposure on allergen responsiveness in subjects with asthma or rhinitis. Am J Respir Crit Care Med 153:56–64

Nelson HS, Rosloniec DM, McCall LI, Ikle, D 1993 Comparative performance of five commercial prick skin test devices. J Allergy Clin Immunol 92:750–756

Nowak D, Heinrich J, Jörres R et al 1996 Prevalence of respiratory symptoms, bronchial hyperresponsiveness and atopy among adults: West and East Germany. Eur Resp J 9:2541–2552

Sears MR, Burrows B, Flannery EM, Herbison GP, Holdaway MD 1993a Atopy in childhood. I. Gender and allergen-related risks for development of hay fever and asthma. Clin Exp Allergy 23:941–948

Sears MR, Burrows B, Herbison GP, Holdaway MD, Flannery EM 1993b Atopy in childhood. II. Relationship to airway responsiveness, hay fever and asthma. Clin Exp Allergy 23:949–956

von Mutius E, Martinez FD, Fritzsch C, Nicolai T, Roell G, Thiemann H-H 1994 Prevalence of asthma and atopy in two areas of West Germany and East Germany. Am J Respir Crit Care Med 149:358–364

von Mutius E, Illi S, Nicolai T, Martinez F 1996 Relation of indoor heating with asthma, allergic sensitisation and bronchial responsiveness: survey of children in South Bavaria. Br Med J 312:1448–1450

Weirings M, Weyler J, Vermiere P 1995 Definition of house dust mite allergy in epidemiological surveys: 1 mm versus 3 mm weal size. Eur Respir J Suppl 19:53S

Zamel N, McClean PA, Sandell PR, Siminovitch KA, Slutsky AS 1996 Asthma on Tristan da Cuhna: looking for the genetic link. Am J Respir Crit Care Med 153:1902–1906

International trends in asthma mortality

Richard Beasley, Neil Pearce and Julian Crane

Asthma Research Group, Department of Medicine, Wellington School of Medicine, PO Box 7343, Wellington South, New Zealand

Abstract. Throughout the 20th century many different patterns of asthma mortality have been observed. Following relatively stable asthma mortality rates during the first half of this century, there has been a gradual increase in asthma mortality in many countries over the last 50 years. Although a number of possible explanations have been proposed to explain this trend — including increases in asthma prevalence, increases in exposure to factors that trigger asthma attacks and changes in asthma management — their relative contribution in different countries is uncertain. Another pattern is that of sudden marked increases in asthma mortality occurring in at least seven countries in the 1960s and in New Zealand in the 1970s. Available evidence indicates that the cause of these 'epidemics' was the use of high dose preparations of two specific β-agonist drugs, namely isoprenaline forte and fenoterol. The most recent trend observed in a number of western countries during the last decade has been a gradual reduction in asthma mortality; this may relate to improvements in the management of asthma.

1997 The rising trends in asthma. Wiley, Chichester (Ciba Foundation Symposium 206) p 140–156

It was once held that 'the asthmatic pants into old age' and that asthmatics rarely died of their disease (Osler 1901). This is now known to be incorrect, but asthma deaths were certainly very rare in the first half of this century. Since then, the time trends of asthma mortality have become considerably more complex with a number of different patterns apparent. There were epidemics of asthma deaths in at least seven countries in the 1960s and again in New Zealand in the 1970s. In other countries, more gradual and less marked increases in asthma mortality have been observed. While this pattern has occurred in different countries at different periods during the last 50 years, it has been observed in many countries in the 1970s to 1980s. More recently, the asthma mortality rate has begun to decrease again in a number of western countries.

Interpretation of these international time trends in asthma mortality is inherently difficult due to the many different factors that have changed in different countries over such prolonged periods. As a result, they should be interpreted with caution and considered together with the findings from other epidemiological studies of asthma mortality. It is with these considerations in mind that the different patterns of

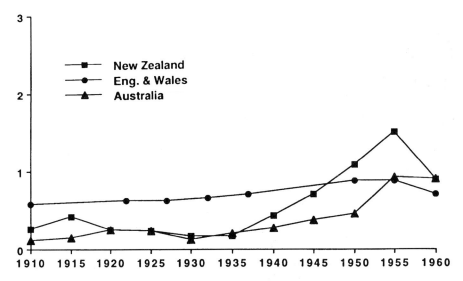

FIG. 1. Asthma mortality (deaths per 100 000 persons) in persons aged five to 34 years in New Zealand, Australia, England and Wales, 1910–1960. Adapted from Speizer & Doll (1968), Beasley et al (1990) and Baumann & Lee (1990).

asthma mortality which have been observed in different countries during this century are discussed. As in previous analyses of this type, attention has been confined to the group aged five to 34 years, since the diagnosis of asthma, as distinct from other obstructive respiratory diseases, is more firmly established in this age group (Speizer & Doll 1968, Jackson et al 1982).

1900 to 1960

Examination of the time trends in asthma mortality in the first half of the 20th century is limited by a paucity of data. Those western countries in which the relevant data have been published indicate that asthma mortality was uniformly low and relatively stable between 1900 and 1940 (Fig. 1) (Speizer & Doll 1968, Beasley et al 1990, Baumann & Lee 1990). The death rate began to increase gradually in the 1940s with the magnitude being greatest in New Zealand and Australia, in which a threefold increase over a 15-year period was observed. Mortality declined again in the late 1950s in New Zealand, England and Wales, but not in Australia. Although the interpretation of death rates over such an extended period is difficult, the historical data are likely to be of acceptable accuracy in this five- to 34-year age group. Examination of the time trends for deaths from other obstructive respiratory disorders does not suggest that changes in diagnostic fashion were responsible for the low death rate prior to 1940 or the increase in mortality during the 1940s and 1950s (Beasley et al 1990).

Epidemics in the 1960s

Following the relatively stable asthma death rates during the first half of this century, asthma mortality increased dramatically in at least seven western countries in the 1960s: England and Wales, Scotland, Ireland, New Zealand, Australia and Norway (Fig. 2) (Stolley 1972). In these countries, the mortality rates increased two- to 10-fold within a two- to five-year period. Other countries such as the USA, Denmark, Canada and Germany did not experience epidemics, although in some countries such as Japan, significant increases in asthma mortality were noted within more narrowly defined age groups (Mitsui 1986). The initial detailed examination of mortality trends in the five- to 34-year age group in England and Wales concluded that the epidemic was real and was not due to changes in death certification, disease classification or diagnostic practice (Speizer et al 1968). It was also considered that it was unlikely to be due to a sudden increase in asthma prevalence, with the most likely explanation being an increase in case fatality, possibly due to new methods of treatment.

Subsequent examination of international time-trend data suggested that the epidemics were related to the use of the high dose β-agonist aerosol isoprenaline forte (Stolley 1972). Epidemics occurred only in countries where the high dose preparation of isoprenaline was available, there was a close association between the sales of isoprenaline forte and asthma mortality, and case series identified that many

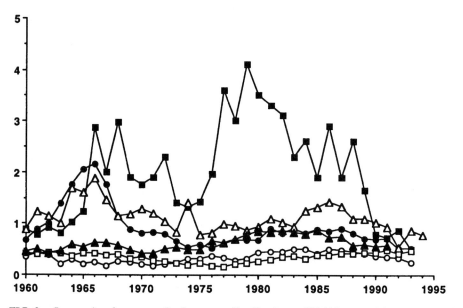

FIG. 2.   International patterns of asthma mortality (deaths per 100 000 persons) in persons aged 5–34 years, 1960–1994, showing the different trends. ■—■, New Zealand; ●—●, England and Wales; △—△, Australia; ▲—▲, West Germany; ○—○, Canada; □—□, United States. Adapted from Sears & Taylor (1994) and Jackson et al (1988).

of the patients who died from asthma had used excessive amounts of this drug in the situation of severe asthma (Fraser et al 1971). Unfortunately, formal analytical epidemiological studies were not undertaken because the epidemic declined before there was time to conduct them. Nevertheless, the weight of evidence suggested that the use of the isoprenaline forte inhaler was the major, although probably not the only, cause of the epidemics of asthma mortality. In some countries in which less marked (non-epidemic) increases in asthma mortality were noted, associations were observed with the sales of the general class of β-agonist drugs (Stolley 1972, Mitsui 1986); in other countries in which there were no significant changes in asthma mortality, marked increases in the sales of β-agonist drugs were observed (Stolley 1972).

Although the isoprenaline forte hypothesis was subsequently disputed in many texts and reviews, this reinterpretation was not based on any new substantial evidence (Pearce et al 1991), and in fact the further analyses that were undertaken strengthened the original conclusions (Stolley & Schinnar 1978). The mortality rate in countries experiencing epidemics declined following warnings from regulatory bodies, a marked reduction in the sales of isoprenaline forte and other changes in medical practice, such as increases in hospital admissions.

The second New Zealand epidemic

In the mid-1970s a second asthma mortality epidemic began in New Zealand, but not in other countries (Fig. 2). Formal investigation of this epidemic identified that it was real and could not be explained by changes in the classification of asthma deaths, inaccuracies in death certification or changes in diagnostic fashion (Jackson et al 1982). It was also concluded that it was unlikely that the epidemic could be due to changes in the incidence or prevalence of asthma in New Zealand, and that the most likely explanation, as for the 1960s epidemics, appeared to be an increased case fatality rate related to changes in the management of asthma in New Zealand.

These initial investigations led to the formal examination of prescribed drug therapy and asthma mortality in New Zealand. In a series of three case-control studies, which employed different methods and incorporated different data sources, at different time periods throughout the epidemic, an increased risk of asthma death was found in patients prescribed fenoterol but not other asthma medications (Table 1) (Crane et al 1989, Pearce et al 1990, Grainger et al 1991). The association between fenoterol and asthma deaths was particularly strong in subgroups with more severe asthma, a pattern which essentially rules out the possibility that the findings were due to confounding by severity (Beasley et al 1994). This interpretation was supported by more detailed analyses, which indicated that the association between fenoterol and asthma mortality could not be attributed to confounding by severity (Sackett et al 1990).

A subsequent case-control study from Saskatchewan, Canada undertaken specifically to address the 'fenoterol hypothesis' also found that the prescription of the high dose preparation of fenoterol was associated with an increased risk of death when compared with the more commonly prescribed β-agonist, salbutamol (Table 1)

TABLE 1   Prescribed inhaled β-agonist and the relative risk of dying from asthma: results from published case-control studies when analysed in an identical manner

Specific β-agonist [b]	Relative risk [a]			
	1st NZ study	2nd NZ study	3rd NZ study	Saskatchewan study
Salbutamol	0.7	0.7	0.6	0.9
Fenoterol	1.6	2.0	2.1	5.3

[a] Relative risk of death, unadjusted odds ratios.
[b] During the period of these studies, salbutamol and fenoterol were available in preparations dispensing 100 μg/puff and 200 μg/puff, respectively.

(Spitzer et al 1992). Although the authors raised the possibility of a general β-agonist class effect, their subsequent analyses indicated that these particular findings may largely be due to confounding by severity (Suissa 1995). More recently, a cohort study in Germany found that in patients with chronic obstructive respiratory disease, the prescription of fenoterol was associated with an increased risk of mortality when compared with either salbutamol or terbutaline (Criée et al 1993).

By their nature, epidemiological studies such as those discussed are unable to identify the underlying mechanisms by which the high dose preparations of fenoterol and isoprenaline forte led to an increased risk of death in the populations in which they were widely used. There are two potential groups of mechanisms that have been proposed: those relating to their regular use leading to worsening asthma control; and those relating to their over-use in the situation of a life-threatening attack of asthma, in which the cardiac side-effects are likely to be particularly harmful in the presence of severe hypoxia (Sears & Taylor 1994, Taylor & Sears 1994, Beasley et al 1991, Collins et al 1969). Fenoterol and isoprenaline are relatively non-selective potent full β-agonists, which have been shown to have both greater adverse chronic and acute side-effects when compared with other β-agonist drugs (Sears & Taylor 1994, Beasley et al 1991, Trembath et al 1979, Bremner et al 1996). It is likely that both these groups of mechanisms are relevant to the increased mortality associated with their use.

The relationship between the reduction in mortality at the end of the New Zealand epidemic and the withdrawal of fenoterol is also of interest (Pearce et al 1995). In mid-1989 the New Zealand Department of Health issued warnings about the safety of fenoterol and in 1990 fenoterol was withdrawn from the drug tariff, which effectively removed it from the market. This was associated with a decrease in the asthma death rate in the five- to 34-year age group from an average of 2.3/100 000 per year during the previous five years to a level of 0.8 in 1990. The mortality remained low in the following three years, with the 1993 figure of 0.5 representing the lowest death rate from asthma in New Zealand for 50 years. Consistent with the case-control studies, the time-trend data do not suggest a class effect of inhaled β-agonist drugs in the

TABLE 2   The epidemic of asthma deaths in New Zealand and fenoterol: examining the epidemiological evidence using a comparable approach to that used for the relationship between smoking and lung cancer

Criteria	Smoking and lung cancer	Fenoterol and NZ epidemic of asthma deaths
Type of studies	Cohort and case-control (many) No randomized control trials	Cohort (one) and case-control (four) studies No randomized control trials
Strength of association	Relative risk 15–64	Relative risk 1.5–13
Consistency	Worldwide	NZ, Canada and Germany
Biologically appropriate temporal relationships	Yes	Yes
Dose–response relationship	Yes	Possible
Biological plausibility	Carcinogens in cigarette smoke	Acute and/or chronic effects greater than other commonly used β-agonist drugs
Analogy	Carcinoma of the scrotum in chimney sweeps	1960s epidemic — isoprenaline forte
Ecological evidence	Worldwide sales of cigarettes vs. lung cancer occurrence	NZ sales of fenoterol vs. onset and end of the epidemic of deaths

Modified with permission from Hensley (1992).

epidemic: there was no association between β-agonist sales and the start of the epidemic, and total sales of inhaled β-agonists increased during the period 1989–1991, when the epidemic came to an end. Time-trend data were also inconsistent with the hypothesis that the epidemic may have occurred because of under-prescribing of inhaled corticosteroids; similarly, it does not support the hypotheses postulating a major role for socioeconomic factors such as unemployment (Pearce et al 1995). Thus, time-trend data, when considered together with other epidemiological evidence, are consistent with fenoterol being the major, but not the only, cause of the second New Zealand asthma mortality epidemic, which is similar to the role of isoprenaline forte in the first New Zealand asthma mortality epidemic (Table 2) (Hensley 1992).

The gradual increase in asthma mortality

Another feature of the international trends in asthma mortality has been the gradual increase that has occurred in many countries during the last 25 years. This background increase has occurred not only in countries which experienced the first epidemic of deaths in the 1960s, but also in other countries unaffected by previous increases in mortality.

It has been difficult to determine the causes of this trend because death from asthma is a complex phenomenon and many factors relevant to the causation of asthma mortality have changed to differing degrees in different countries during this period. These factors could potentially include the characteristics of the disease and its treatment, the characteristics of the asthmatic population and changes in the underlying level of asthma prevalence. Despite this complexity, there are a number of observations worthy of comment.

The first is that in a number of countries the magnitude of this 'gradual' increase has been substantial. For example, between the mid-1970s and mid-1980s, the mortality rate increased between 1.5- and twofold in many countries throughout the world (Table 3) (Sears & Taylor 1994, Jackson et al 1988, Sears 1991). Although these trends have not been considered to represent epidemics, an increase in mortality of this magnitude within a decade, in many cases on the background of relatively stable asthma mortality rates, would suggest that they possess some features of an epidemic.

The second observation is that there is a wide variation in the reported asthma mortality rates in countries with similar lifestyles and comparable approaches to the management of asthma. In general, the highest rates have been observed in those countries with the highest reported asthma prevalence, suggesting that the prevalence of asthma (and in particular the prevalence of severe asthma) is a major, but not the only, determinant of international mortality rates (Pearce et al 1993).

This issue leads on to the third observation: that the gradual increase in mortality rates has occurred during the same period in which the prevalence of asthma has also

TABLE 3   Asthma mortality (deaths per 100 000 persons) in 10 countries between the mid-1970s and mid-1980s in persons aged five to 34 years

Country	1975–1977	1985–1987	Per cent increase
Australia	0.86	1.42	65
Canada	0.33	0.47	42
England and Wales	0.57	0.90	58
France	0.24	0.51	113
Japan	0.44	0.59	34
Singapore	0.75	0.88	17
Sweden	0.37	0.54	46
Switzerland	0.31	0.45	45
USA	0.19	0.40	111
West Germany	0.59	0.78	32

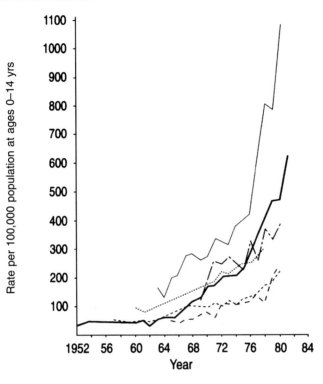

FIG. 3.   Admissions to hospital with asthma in 0–14 year olds in a number of different countries since the 1950s (reproduced with permission from Mitchell et al 1985). ———, Queensland, Australia; ····· Tasmania, Australia; —— New Zealand; .... , Canada; - - - - , England and Wales; – ———, USA.

increased. Asthma prevalence studies that have been repeated during this period using standardized methods in the same population group have demonstrated a consistent increase in the prevalence of asthma (National Institutes of Health 1995). This increase has been observed in a wide range of countries with differing lifestyles and in some countries it has been of considerable magnitude. For example, the prevalence of asthma in young adults in Finland has increased up to 20-fold since 1960 (Haahtela et al 1990). In addition, available data suggest a marked increase in the prevalence of severe asthma, as indicated by the international trends of increasing hospital admissions for asthma in children (Fig. 3) (Mitchell 1985). This would suggest that a significant part of the gradual increase in asthma mortality observed over recent decades may be due to the increased prevalence of severe asthma.

Another feature of the epidemiological studies of asthma mortality has been the observation that the increased mortality is concentrated in particular demographic groups. These studies have suggested that much of the increase is amongst the disadvantaged populations such as the Blacks and Hispanics in the USA (Weiss & Wagener 1990).

Finally, the possible relationship between β-agonist therapy and this gradual trend of increasing asthma mortality needs to be considered. Although it has been noted in several countries that a close association exists between increasing mortality and sales of β-agonist drugs, it is uncertain whether this represents a causal relationship, a response to changes in the prevalence of severe asthma or merely reflects changes in the approach to asthma management. Perhaps the two major issues which need to be considered are: (i) the extent to which fenoterol may have contributed to the more gradual increases in mortality observed in countries in which its use has been less widespread than in New Zealand; and (ii) the contribution of the more selective β-agonist drugs that have been marketed in lower dose preparations and that have not been incriminated in asthma mortality epidemics. Clearly, further studies will be needed to clarify these two important issues.

Most recent trends

Since the late 1980s there has been a significant gradual fall in asthma mortality in some but not all countries in which accurate mortality statistics are available (Fig. 2). This trend has been observed particularly in countries adopting modern approaches to asthma treatment. It is tempting to speculate that this reduction may relate to such changes in management, in particular the greater use of inhaled corticosteroid therapy. In support of this view are the studies that have shown improved clinical outcome with inhaled corticosteroid therapy (Toogood et al 1993) and their protective effects against mortality (Ernst et al 1992). However, the time-trend evidence is not conclusive in this regard, and other (unknown) factors may account for some or all of the recent mortality decline.

Summary

To date, the priority for epidemiological studies of asthma mortality has been to follow the time trends and to investigate the causes of the asthma mortality epidemics that were identified from the time-trend data. With the identification of the role of isoprenaline forte and fenoterol as the primary causes of the asthma mortality epidemics, and the resolution of the epidemics following regulatory action restricting their availability, attention has now shifted to the causes of the more gradual increases in mortality that have been observed in other countries at different times over the last 50 years. The relative contribution of different management and non-management factors in these time trends is less certain. There is a continuing need for further studies to monitor these trends, and to ascertain the causes. This will require assessment of the validity of time trends in asthma mortality (accuracy of death certificates, changes in disease classification and changes in diagnostic fashion), assessment of the contribution of changes in asthma prevalence, investigation of the possible explanations for an increase in case fatality (in particular pharmacological factors) and consideration of the reasons why the increased mortality disproportionately affects particular groups in the community.

Acknowledgements

The Wellington Asthma Research Group is supported by programmes grants from the New Zealand Health Research Council and the Guardian Trust. The authors thank Malcolm Sears for providing recent asthma mortality data.

References

Baumann A, Lee S 1990 Trends in asthma mortality in Australia, 1911–1986. Med J Aust 153:366

Beasley R, Smith K, Pearce N, Crane J, Burgess C, Culling C 1990 Trends in asthma mortality in New Zealand, 1908–1986. Med J Aust 152:570–573

Beasley R, Pearce N, Crane J, Windom H, Burgess C 1991 Asthma mortality and inhaled beta agonist therapy. Aust NZ J Med 21:753–763

Beasley R, Burgess C, Pearce N, Grainger J, Crane J 1994 Confounding by severity does not explain the association between fenoterol and asthma death. Clin Exp Allergy 24:660–668

Bremner P, Siebers R, Crane J, Pearce N, Beasley R, Burgess C 1996 Partial versus full beta receptor agonism — a clinical study of inhaled albuterol and fenoterol. Chest 109:957–962

Collins JM, McDevitt DG, Shanks RG et al 1969 The cardiotoxicity of isoprenaline during hypoxia. Br J Pharmacol 36:35–45

Crane J, Pearce N, Flatt A et al 1989 Prescribed fenoterol and death from asthma in New Zealand, 1981–83: case-control study. Lancet I:917–922

Criee C-P, Quast CH, Ludtke R, Laier-Groeneveld G, Huttemann U 1993 Use of beta agonists and mortality in patients with stable COPD. Eur Resp J 6:426S

Ernst P, Spitzer WO, Suissa S et al 1992 Risk of fatal and near-fatal asthma in relation to inhaled corticosteroid use. JAMA 268:3462–3464

Fraser PM, Speizer FE, Waters DM et al 1971 The circumstances preceding death from asthma in young people in 1968 to 1969. Br J Dis Chest 65:71–84

Grainger J, Woodman K, Pearce N et al 1991 Prescribed fenoterol and death from asthma in New Zealand, 1981–1987: a further case-control study. Thorax 46:105–111

Haahtela T, Lindholm H, Björkstén F, Koskenvuo K, Laitinen LA 1990 Prevalence of asthma in Finnish young men. Br Med J 301:266–268

Hensley MJ 1992 Fenoterol and death from asthma. Med J Aust 156:882

Jackson RT, Beaglehole P, Rea HH et al 1982 Mortality from asthma: a new epidemic in New Zealand. Br Med J 28:771S–774S

Jackson R, Sears MR, Beaglehole R et al 1988 International trends in asthma mortality: 1970 to 1985. Chest 94:914–918

Mitchell EA 1985 International trends in hospital admission rates for asthma. Arch Dis Child 60:376–378

Mitsui S 1986 Death from bronchial asthma in Japan. Sino-Jpn J Allergol Immunol Soshiran 3:249–257

National Institutes of Health 1995 Epidemiology. In: Global Initiative for Asthma: global strategy for asthma management and prevention (National Institutes of Health, National Heart, Lung and Blood Institute and World Health Organisation Workshop Report). NIH publication no. 95-3659, p 10–24

Osler W 1901 The principles and practice of medicine, 4th edn. Pentland, Edinburgh

Pearce N, Grainger J, Atkinson M et al 1990 Case-control study of prescribed fenoterol and death from asthma in New Zealand, 1977–1981. Thorax 45:170–175

Pearce NE, Crane J, Burgess C, Jackson R, Beasley R 1991 Beta agonists and asthma mortality: *déjà vu*. Clin Exp Allergy 21:401–410

Pearce N, Weiland S, Keil U et al 1993 Self-reported prevalence of asthma symptoms in children in Australia, England, Germany and New Zealand: an international comparison using the ISAAC protocol. Eur Resp J 6:1455–1461

Pearce N, Beasley R, Crane J, Burgess C, Jackson R 1995 End of the New Zealand asthma mortality epidemic. Lancet 345:41–44

Sackett DL, Shannon HS, Browman GW 1990 Fenoterol and fatal asthma. Lancet I:46

Sears MR 1991 Worldwide trends in asthma mortality. Bull Int Union Tuberc Lung Dis 66:79–83

Sears MR, Taylor DR 1994 The β_2-agonist controversy: observations, explanations and relationship to epidemiology. Drug Safety 11:259–283

Speizer FE, Doll R 1968 A century of asthma deaths in young people. Br Med J 3:245–246

Speizer FE, Doll R, Heaf P 1968 Observations on recent increases in mortality from asthma. Br Med J I:335–339

Spitzer WD, Suissa S, Ernst P et al 1992 The use of beta agonists and the risk of death and near death from asthma. New Engl J Med 326:501–506

Stolley PD 1972 Why the United States was spared an epidemic of deaths due to asthma. Am Rev Resp Dis 105:883–890

Stolley PD, Schinnar R 1978 Association between asthma mortality and isoproterenol aerosols: a review. Prev Med 7:319–338

Suissa S 1995 The case-time-control design. Epidemiology 6:248–253

Taylor DR, Sears MR 1994 Regular beta-adrenergic agonists: evidence, not reassurance, is what is needed. Chest 106:552–559

Toogood JH, Jennings BH, Baskerville JC, Lefcoe NM 1993 Aerosol corticosteroids. In: Weis ED, Stein M (eds) Bronchial asthma: mechanisms and therapeutics, 3rd edn. Little, Brown & Co, Boston, p 818–841

Trembath PW, Greenacre JK, Anderson M et al 1979 Comparison of four weeks treatment with fenoterol and terbutaline aerosols in adult asthmatics. J Allergy Clin Immunol 63:395–400

Weiss KB, Wagener DK 1990 Changing patterns of asthma mortality: identifying populations at high risk. JAMA 264:1683–1687

DISCUSSION

Busse: Could you expand on your studies of fenoterol by considering whether polymorphisms in the β-adrenergic receptor may play a role?

Beasley: One of the important unresolved issues is the mechanism by which fenoterol and isoprenaline, but not other β-agonists, markedly increase the risk of death. There are two major mechanisms that have been proposed: (1) that their regular use is more likely to lead to worsening asthma control; and (2) that the use of high doses of fenoterol or isoprenaline is more likely to cause cardiac toxicity in the situation of severe hypoxia (Crane et al 1993). The approach we have taken is to look at pharmacological properties of fenoterol and isoprenaline and determine how they are different from other β-agonists. The major differences are that they are more potent, less selective and have greater intrinsic activity than other β-agonist drugs. Another approach, rather than looking at the drug *per se*, is to determine whether it is possible to identify those individuals that may be at particular risk. In this respect, we're looking at polymorphisms in the $\beta2$-adrenergic receptor, particularly the Gly16 polymorphism, which in the New Zealand population appears to occur more frequently in the severe asthmatics compared to the mild asthmatics and non-asthmatic control groups. Although there are limited data on the phenotype, *in vitro* studies suggest that this particular allele is associated with enhanced down-regulation to prolonged exposure to isoprenaline. It is possible, therefore, that patients with this polymorphism are less responsive to β-agonist therapy. This could be relevant to the outcome of an acute attack of asthma, when these individuals would have to take a greater dose to obtain the maximum achievable bronchodilation and, as a result, experience greater cardiac effects that are predominantly $\beta1$-receptor mediated.

Potter: Polymorphisms generally tend to vary between populations. Are you sure that the Gly16 polymorphism is associated with steroid-dependent asthma in New Zealand? Because it's likely that the relevant mutations are quite different in different populations. Reishaus et al (1993) studied 51 patients and found nine different mutations, of which Gly16 was the commonest, but Green et al (1993) showed that the isoleucine/threonine polymorphism at residue 164 had a significant decreased affinity for epinephrine when expressed in the homozygous form in Chinese hamster CHWH-1102 fibroblasts, and it could be lethal if it occurred naturally.

Beasley: We have only studied the Gly16 and Glu27 polymorphisms at this stage. These studies are preliminary and there is much work to be done.

Busse: Are there any similarities in terms of any of the issues that have been raised with salmeterol?

Beasley: We have done a case-control study with Stephen Holgate looking at life-threatening attacks as a surrogate marker for asthma deaths. We found that salmeterol was not associated with an increased risk of life-threatening attacks, which contrasts with the similar case-control studies of fenoterol that showed an increased risk. These are preliminary results, and obviously looking at asthma deaths is preferable to looking at life-threatening attacks, but the study does suggest that salmeterol has a safety profile similar to salbutamol rather than fenoterol, which may be important from a mechanistic point of view.

Holgate: Is fenoterol a partial or full $\beta2$-adrenoceptor agonist?

G. Anderson: Fenoterol has a much higher efficacy at the $\beta2$-adrenoceptor than salmeterol. The best comparative studies that have been performed to date are those by Lemoine and of Barber in Texas, who have compared the coupling efficiency and efficacies of formoterol, salmeterol and other agents to the $\beta2$-adrenoceptor (Lemoine et al 1992, Lemoine & Overlack 1992, Clark et al 1996). The coupling efficiency of salmeterol to the $\beta2$-receptor is about 0.10, whereas for fenoterol this value is 0.85 (a full agonist has a coupling efficiency of 1.00), so there's a large difference in efficacy. Formoterol also has a high efficacy at the $\beta2$-adrenoceptor (0.9). However, a difference in efficacy doesn't necessarily translate into a difference in mortality risk because the follow-up data for formoterol suggested that it does not cause an increased mortality. It is possible that the duration of agonism at the β2-receptor is important. Some recent work on β2-adrenoceptor signal transduction suggests that pulsing the β2-adrenoceptors in order to cause large changes in the cAMP levels results in different effects on the CREB (cAMP response element binding) and CREM (cAMP response element modulator) proteins. These proteins may affect inflammatory responses by interfering with corticosteroid signal transduction. Stable levels of β2-adrenoceptor activation may not cause the same induction of CREB/CREM.

Sears: There are two alternative mechanisms by which the β-agonist may have led to these mortality epidemics: long-term worsening of the severity of asthma versus an acute cardiac or other toxic effect on the myocardium (Taylor & Sears 1994). Data that are important to add to this discussion are those concerning changes in morbidity at the time warnings were issued regarding fenoterol in 1989, followed by its effective withdrawal from sale in New Zealand in 1990. Richard Beasley has shown that the death rate decreased over the following two years down to levels reported before the two epidemics of asthma mortality. This could conceivably be explained by either a decrease in the severity of asthma or a decrease in adverse cardiac effects. However, hospital admissions over that two-year period also fell abruptly, i.e. by almost 50% (Sears 1997). Although numerous factors may affect some of the decrease, the majority of the decrease must represent a change in the severity of asthma. The decrease certainly cannot be explained by decreased cardiac effects because asthmatics are not hospitalized for arrhythmias. Therefore, potent β-agonists likely increase the severity of asthma, with effects on both morbidity and mortality.

Boushey: It is possible that you are referring to non-selective β-agonists because the sale of all β-agonists in New Zealand showed a rise through the period of the fall in mortality and hospitalizations. Perhaps the other agents were more truly selective β-agonists.

Sears: There are clear differences between the effects of different β-agonists. The epidemics of asthma mortality relate to marketing of the higher potency or higher dose full β-agonists, isoprenaline and fenoterol (Taylor & Sears 1994). However, Cockroft and colleagues have looked at the adverse effects of salbutamol, the standard β-agonist used internationally, and have shown deleterious effects of regular four-times daily dosing on the early asthmatic response (Cockroft et al 1993) and the late asthmatic response (Cockroft et al 1995). There are deleterious effects of probably all β-agonists if given frequently, and this also applies to partial agonists such as salbutamol.

Boushey: But the point I wished to emphasize was that Richard Beasley's data suggest that this is not necessarily a class effect, but one specific to fenoterol.

Beasley: Malcolm Sears is correct in his interpretation of the hospital admission data. However, one can put forward strong cases for both the long-term and the acute effects (Beasley et al 1991). It's probably going to be a combination of both mechanisms, and it will be necessary to determine the relative importance of each. With respect to Homer Boushey's point, the epidemiological data suggest that the first and second asthma mortality epidemics were not due to β-agonists as a class, but were due to two specific β-agonists — isoprenaline forte and fenoterol — which are both potent, less selective β-agonists with greater intrinsic activity than other β-agonist drugs, such as salbutamol (Pearce et al 1994).

Bleecker: In the USA it is common to administer β-agonists continuously for the treatment of acute asthma. Is it safe to do this for salbutamol, or could there be reason to worry because of the risk of an overdose?

Beasley: The crucial point is to give oxygen during continuous administration because this greatly reduces the risks associated with high dose β-agonist use.

Holgate: I would like to change the topic towards mortality trends. I have become aware of how asthma deaths in the inner-city areas in the USA have driven interests and policies in asthma management. What is the general consensus on what is driving asthma deaths in inner-city environments?

Weiss: The first important point is that the mortality rates in the inner-city areas in the USA are some of the highest in the world. Primarily, they affect both African American children and adults. The combination of a number of factors is probably driving these high mortality rates. On the one hand, these people are exposed to many adverse environmental factors — such as cockroaches, gas stoves, agents that cause respiratory infection, poor nutrition and passive smoking — and on the other hand, they receive inadequate health care. In the USA 75 million people have no health insurance. Therefore, for these people, asthma treatment consists of the administration of β-agonists in emergency rooms, so that instead of getting inhaled inflammatory treatment, they get episodic treatment with outmoded care.

Holgate: In your opinion, what is the crucial factor in your list? Which one would have the greatest impact in intervention trials?

Weiss: Improved health care and use of anti-inflammatory drugs. We've done a cohort study in which we've examined the effect of medication use on hospitalizations. We have showed that even for low dose inflammatories, such as beclomethasone, three canisters prescribed per year decreased the hospitalization rate in this population by 50%.

Busse: In a group of three-year-old children in our Head Start Programme, the incidence of asthma is about 20%. They all have access to health care through various government agencies, but only 5% were given anti-inflammatories.

Bleecker: We evaluated hospitalizations and found that the most frequent admissions to the paediatric wards were for asthma (about 35–40%) and most of these children had missed their outpatient visits during the past year.

Weiss: We also found that those who saw a physician were less likely to be hospitalized.

Woolcock: One point which has not been mentioned is that in western children up to the age of 15 years there is a higher death rate in males compared to females, then after that age the reverse is true. However, there are two exceptions: in Japan and in Blacks in the USA the mortality in males is much greater than in females in all age groups. We cannot interpret these observations until we know the prevalences of asthma in inner-city male and female Caucasians and Blacks.

Beasley: The situation is more complex than this because the male : female asthma mortality ratio has changed throughout the century: deaths were more common in males until about 1930, then female rates were higher until about 1960. Since then, deaths in males have been more common.

Another point I would like to make is that comparing the prevalence data together with the mortality data will be more informative, especially when making comparisons between countries. In this way, a more accurate indication of the case fatality rate can be achieved.

Sears: The results of the Finnish study (Haahtela et al 1990) suggest that most of the rising trends in asthma occur at the mild end; therefore, we need a way of determining the prevalence of more severe asthma and comparing this with mortality data. With very few exceptions, deaths occur in patients with the more severe asthma.

Woolcock: I disagree. In our studies the increases have occurred across the spectrum of severity.

Strachan: Although we're looking at mortality in the five to 34 age group, because it's thought to be a clean diagnostic group, many of those deaths are in the 20–34 age group. Most data on the prevalence of asthma relate to the less than 25-year-old age group, reiterating the desperate need for both temporal and geographical data on the prevalences and severities of different types of asthma in young adults. Amongst 1000 British children aged between five and 14, we would currently expect only one death from asthma in 250 years.

Holgate: I would like to bring up the subject of environmental factors. In England and Wales asthma deaths in the under 40-year olds peak in the summer months when pollen allergens are at their peak (Campbell et al 1997) and yet hospital admissions for asthma peak in the autumn and spring months, presumably as a result of virus infections as well as possible increases in dust mite allergens (Johnston et al 1996).

Boushey: O'Hollaren et al (1991) have found that most asthma deaths in patients sensitive to *Alternaria* occur in summer, when the levels of *Alternaria* are highest. This suggests that aeroallergens can be an important risk factor. The city in the USA with the third highest asthma mortality rates is, surprisingly, Fresno, an agricultural city in California, where the mortality rate is highest in the spring. The outdoor antigen levels in the Fresno area are the second highest in the United States. Farming in this area also involves use of large amounts of insecticides, and some physicians practising in the community have speculated that the increased level of organophosphates in the environment may contribute to the increased number of hospital admissions. This suggested association needs to be studied. A final point is that a confounding factor in the interpretation of seasonal variations of asthma is the seasonal pattern of viral infections. For example, hospitalizations for asthmatic attacks in children rise at the beginning of school terms, when viruses are transmitted.

Holgate: But what is interesting in our 10-year study (Campbell et al 1997) is that, even in young adults, the peak hospital admissions for asthma do not coincide with the times when the deaths are occurring.

Britton: Inman & Adelstein (1969), who first drew attention to the isoprenaline epidemic, showed marked seasonality in adult deaths in the UK. These peaked in autumn, which was precisely when the viral-induced episodes of asthma seemed to occur in children. Therefore, what you described is a large change in the UK.

Holgate: Yes, this change in the younger age group is interesting. In the older age group (i.e. the over 60-year olds) there are diagnostic difficulties due to the overlap with chronic obstructive pulmonary disease. Nevertheless, in contrast to the younger age group, asthma mortality peaks in the winter and early spring when virus infections are presumably an important factor (Johnston et al 1996).

H. R. Anderson: We also know that mortality is higher at the weekends and on public holidays, and the most plausible explanation for this is not environmental — these are periods when hospital staff change over, and so it is likely that changes in patient care are involved.

Busse: But wouldn't this then be extended to other diseases? Do you know of any data on that?

H. R. Anderson: I don't know of any, but I suspect that it would be the case.

Holgate: Is there any evidence that the worldwide outdoor allergen loads have changed, perhaps as a result of changes in farming practices, during the last 20 years?

Burney: In the UK the grass is being cut earlier in the season and there haven't been any significant increases in the levels of pollen, but then pollen is not the only risk factor.

Brostoff: There has actually been a considerable reduction in June peak pollen counts over the last 15–20 years, so the incidence of hay fever is actually inversely proportional to the levels of pollen (R. R. Davies, personal communication 1996).

Boushey: Changes in farming practices may not be the only important cause of changes in atmospheric allergens. For example, the Lung Association of San Francisco has tried to discourage the city from using the New Zealand olive tree for decorative planting. This tree has been a favourite in ornamental gardens in cities, possibly because it's so hardy, but its pollens are allergenic. I do not cite this to suggest that decorative trees are important causes of shifts in asthma prevalence, but rather to suggest that the focus should be on identifying potent allergens in the places inhabited by large populations.

Beasley: I would like to mention the asthma epidemic in Barcelona. It was only through detailed epidemiological studies that the cause of this epidemic was identified. One wonders how many other environmentally caused epidemics have occurred throughout the world but have not been identified because the exposures have been somewhat less, or have not been as carefully studied (Picardo 1992).

Woolcock: The only true epidemic of asthma that I know of occurred in the south-eastern highlands of New Guinea. This started in about 1972 and ended in 1987. Those affected were all adults, they were all highly atopic and they all had extremely severe disease, indeed a large number of people died. There have been no new cases since, even though house dust mites etc. are still there, suggesting that some other factor(s) was involved.

Holgate: Could you speculate on what might be behind this?

Woolcock: It is possible that this group of people are genetically different because this is the group of people who had kuru. However, there is no apparent explanation.

References

Beasley R, Windom H, Pearce N, Burgess C, Crane J 1991 Asthma mortality and inhaled beta agonist therapy. Aust NZ J Med 21:753–763

Campbell M J, Cogman GR, Johnston SL, Holgate ST 1997 Age-specific seasonality and trends in asthma mortality in England and Wales 1983–1992. Br Med J, in press

Clark RB, Allal C, Friedman J, Johnson M, Barber R 1996 Stable activation and desensitization of beta 2-adrenergic receptor stimulation of adenylyl cyclase by salmeterol: evidence for quasi-irreversible binding to an exosite. Mol Pharmacol 49:182–189

Cockroft DW, McPaarland CP, Britto SA, Swystun VA, Rutherford BC 1993 Regular inhaled salbutamol and airway responsiveness to allergen. Lancet 342:833–837

Cockroft DW, O-Byrne PM, Swystun VA, Bhagat R 1995 Regular use of inhaled salbuterol and the allergen-induced late asthmatic response. J Allergy Clin Immunol 96:44–49

Crane J, Burgess C, Pearce N, Beasley R 1993 The β-agonist controversy: a perspective. Eur Respir Rev 15:475–482

Green SA, Cole G, Jacinto M, Innis M, Liggett SB 1993 A polymorphism of the human beta-2 adrenergic receptor within the 4th transmembrane domain alters ligand binding and functional properties of the receptor. J Biol Chem 168:23116–23121

Haahtela T, Lindholm H, Björkstén F, Koskenvuo K, Laitinen LA 1990 Prevalence of asthma in Finnish young men. Br Med J 301:266–301

Inman WHW, Adelstein AM 1969 Rise and fall of asthma mortality in England and Wales in relation to use of pressurised aerosols. Lancet I:279–285

Johnston SL, Pattemore PK, Sanderson G et al 1996 The relationship between upper respiratory infections and hospital admissions for asthma: a time–trend analysis. Am J Resp Crit Care Med 154:654–660

Lemoine H, Overlack C 1992 Highly potent beta-2 sympathomimetics convert to less potent partial agonists as relaxants of guinea pig tracheae maximally contracted by carbachol: comparison of relaxation with receptor binding and adenylate cyclase stimulation. J Pharmacol Exp Ther 261:258–270

Lemoine H, Overlack C, Kohl A, Worth H, Reinhardt D 1992 Formoterol, fenoterol and salbutamol as partial agonists for relaxation of maximally contracted guinea pig tracheae: comparison of relaxation with receptor binding. Lung 170:163–180

O'Hollaren MD, Yunginger JW, Offord KP et al 1991 Exposure to an aeroallergen as a possible precipitating factor in respiratory arrest in young patients with asthma. N Engl J Med 324:359–363

Pearce N, Beasley R, Crane J, Burgess C 1994 Epidemiology of asthma mortality. In: Holgate S, Busse W (eds) Asthma and rhinitis. Blackwell Scientific, Oxford, p 58–69

Picardo C 1992 Barcelona's asthma epidemics: clinical aspects and intriguing findings. Thorax 47:197–200

Reishaus E, Innis M, MacIntyre N, Ligget SB 1993 Mutations in the same gene encoding the β2-adrenergic receptor in normal and asthmatic subjects. Am J Resp Cell Mol Biol 8:334–339

Sears MR 1997 Epidemiological trends in asthma. Can Respir J, in press

Taylor DR, Sears MR 1994 The β2-agonist controversy. Observations, explanations and relationship to asthma epidemiology. Drug Safety 11:259–283

General discussion II

Holgate: I would like to discuss whether the removal of every house dust mite will have any effects on the prevalence and severity of asthma.

Martinez: There are good data available showing that there are areas in the world where house dust mites are rare, but where the prevalence of asthma is as high as or higher than places in which they are abundant (Peat et al 1995). There are two possibilities: (1) a battery of allergens have to be removed in order for these people not to become sensitized and thus not to develop asthma; or (2) these people develop asthma and also become sensitized, which makes their asthma worse, i.e. a kind of positive feedback loop. However, detailed experiments on withdrawal should be done because it is possible that if a particular allergen in a particular area is removed none of the other allergens in the battery may be as 'asthmagenic' and these people may develop less severe illnesses.

Holgate: That is not what the data currently suggest.

Warner: This problem also worries me because we may be able to reduce the levels of house dust mites, but cat allergen is the most potent allergen — sensitization can be achieved with 10 pg — and we may never be able to reduce the levels of cat allergen to below this level.

Nelson: I would like to mention the asthma risk study in Denver that was done by David Mrazek and Mary Klinnert (personal communication 1996), who studied 150 children whose mothers had asthma. These children were re-evaluated at six years old, and 16.6% of them had classic asthma, even though there are no house dust mites in Denver.

Martinez: Another important aspect is illustrated in a paper by Malcolm Sears (Sears 1989), i.e. that not only are certain allergens important, but also the highest prevalences and severities occur in those people who are plurisensitized — the prevalence of asthma in people who are sensitive to seven allergens is 70%, whereas this decreases significantly in those who are sensitized to three allergens or less.

Weiss: We really don't understand the development of the human IgE system. I find it difficult to see how just eliminating a single or even a couple of antigens will decrease the prevalence or severity of asthma, given that it is such a complex disease and so many factors are involved. I'm rather pessimistic about these kinds of intervention trials.

Holt: But you can't jump too far in that direction because it's still possible that the missing link might be allergen-driven inflammation. In other words, one could develop sensitization to house dust mites, for example, which then sets up the inflammatory milieu that eventually causes permanent phenotypic changes in airway tissues.

Strachan: We should also think about inflammation-driven allergen exposure. In other words, if the airways are inflamed and permeable will that lead to a greater risk of allergy sensitization?

Platts-Mills: There's no evidence that more allergen is absorbed through an inflamed nose. The simple view is that inflammation results in increased uptake, but differential processing in inflamed noses is a possibility that has not been resolved. In this situation one would predict that once someone got hay fever they were at a dramatically increased risk of becoming sensitized to other allergens, e.g. house dust mites, and that's not true.

Burney: In van Niekerk's study in the Transkei inflammation and allergens were almost certainly present but broncho-constriction wasn't found (van Niekerk et al 1979). Therefore, I'm not convinced this is a satisfactory explanation. It may be true in animal models but it's not what's driving the increase in sensitization in this case. Similarly, bringing up the subject of air pollution, when I was young in London, almost every child had 'catarrh', which is surely a form of airway inflammation, but very few had hay fever or asthma.

Holt: One point which has been lost from the immunotoxicology literature is that the nature of the dose–response curve linking mucosal inflammation with T cell sensitization is biphasic and not linear.

Britton: The answer to the question about single allergen removal lies in the study that Thomas Platts-Mills did at Northwick Park, where people were admitted into hospital and achieved low levels of allergen exposure. It was not a controlled study but nevertheless the effect of rigorously excluding allergens to a practical level was insignificant.

Platts-Mills: No, the changes in histamine reactivity were eightfold and they were clinically significant as judged by exercise tolerance, symptoms and requirement for medicine (Platts-Mills et al 1982). Let me address this directly. When allergic children in Europe are taken to Davos in Switzerland they get better. They are taken out of their houses into an environment where there are no carpets, there are no animals and there's very little mould outside. Their diet also changes and they are made to exercise. This is good evidence that a protocol based on reducing allergen load can have a dramatic effect on asthma.

Holgate: So is there a consensus that intervention studies on house dust mites alone or house dust mites with cats are worthwhile procedures? Perhaps only primary sensitization in pregnancy or within the first few years of life can be realistically achieved for only one or two allergens.

Burney: In my opinion, from the evidence that Thomas Platts-Mills has raised, these studies are worthwhile. However, all the evidence indicates that it is not just sensitization to house dust mites that is increasing but also an increased sensitization to many other allergens. Therefore, it may not be a worthwhile intervention procedure, unless early sensitization to the house dust mite increases the probability of sensitization to other allergens.

Martinez: These studies will be useful because they will give us an answer either way.

Warner: We are currently performing a study in Southampton of house dust mite and cat allergen avoidance during pregnancy and the first year of life. This will address both the issue of primary prevention of allergic disease in children and tertiary prevention in their parents. To be enrolled in the study one of the parents must have allergic asthma and the mother must be less than 18 weeks pregnant. Allergen reduction measures are implemented in the home before the important stage of 22 weeks gestation when the first fetal T cell responses to allergens are seen and will continue with careful monitoring until the baby is one year of age. We hope that this will provide us with more information about the window of sensitization and the most important time period for allergen avoidance to prevent allergic disease, and at the same time we may be able to evaluate the effect of a multi-system avoidance regimen on already-existing disease in the parents.

References

Peat JK, Toelle BG, Gray EJ et al 1995 Prevalence and severity of childhood asthma and allergic sensitisation in seven climatic regions of New South Wales. Med J Aust 163:22–26

Platts-Mills TAE, Tovey ER, Mitchell EB, Mooszoro H, Nock P, Wilkins SR 1982 Reduction of bronchial hyper-reactivity during prolonged allergen avoidance. Lancet II:675–678

Sears MR, Herbison GP, Holdaway MD, Hewitt CJ, Flannery EM, Silva PA 1989 The relative risks of sensitivity to grass pollen, house dust mite and cat dander in the development of childhood asthma. Clin Exp Allergy 19:419–424

van Niekerk CH, Weinberg EG, Shove SC, Heese H de V, van Schalkwyk DJ 1979 Prevalence of asthma: a comparative study of urban and rural Xhosa children. Clinical Allergy 9:319–324

Inferences from occupational asthma

Paul Cullinan and A. J. Newman Taylor

Imperial College of Science, Technology & Medicine, National Heart & Lung Institute, 1b Manresa Road, London SW3 6LR and Royal Brompton Hospital, Sydney Street, London SW3 6LR, UK

Abstract. Occupational asthma — asthma induced by an agent inhaled at work — provides a valid model for the examination of the more general environmental causes of asthma. In many instances, definable populations exposed to a novel allergen in the workplace at concentrations that are relatively easily measured develop IgE-associated asthma and characteristic eosinophilic bronchitis. Carefully designed epidemiological studies suggest that the incidence of IgE antibody and asthma is highest in the first one to two years of exposure; and that the risk is directly related to the intensity of airborne allergen exposure. The relationship between exposure and outcome is modified both by concurrent cigarette smoking and by genotype, although the details of this latter interaction remain unclear. Symptoms, airway hyper-responsiveness and airway inflammation may persist for several years after avoidance of exposure to the initiating agent. If the relevance of the model is accepted then these insights require testing and further investigation, both within the field of occupational asthma and, by extension, in the wider field of asthma in the general environment.

1997 The rising trends in asthma. Wiley, Chichester (Ciba Foundation Symposium 206) p 160–172

Occupational asthma is asthma induced by an agent inhaled at work. Typically, but not invariably, it is a type I immunological response to an airborne allergen, associated with the production of specific IgE. Other patterns of occupational asthma include those caused by some low molecular weight agents (e.g. the diisocyanates or colophony fume) in which specific IgE cannot be reliably detected; and the recently recognized irritant-induced asthma (or reactive airways dysfunction syndrome), which can follow single, high exposures to respiratory irritants such as chlorine. It is interesting to speculate how frequently these last mechanisms may occur outside the workplace, and whether virus infections may initiate asthma through similar mechanisms, but they will not be discussed further here.

Around 300 compounds have been reported to cause hypersensitivity-induced occupational asthma. The majority of these are 'complete' allergens, often of high molecular weight, such as animal- or plant-derived proteins; asthma among research workers exposed to the excreta of laboratory animals, or among bakers working with flour and enzymic additives, are particularly common in the UK (Meredith 1993). Alternatively, low molecular weight agents, importantly acid anhydrides and the

160

complex salts of platinum, can act as haptens stimulating an immunological response when bound covalently to host proteins; specific IgE to the hapten–protein conjugate can be detected in those with occupational asthma from these chemicals.

There are a number of prior reasons why the study of occupational asthma might provide useful insights into general environmental factors in the disease. First, the phenotype of occupational IgE production and asthma is relatively specific — and especially so in those situations where the epitopic structure of the causative allergen is well understood. Second, workplace exposures are generally to allergens not encountered elsewhere; the study of the development of asthma in occupational groups therefore allows the study of the ontogeny of allergen-specific immunity following novel exposure. Third, exposed populations can be clearly delineated allowing relatively easy access to entire (and therefore representative) study populations. Fourth, the techniques of measuring allergen exposure in the occupational setting are well developed and, with many occupational tasks being stereotyped, it is possible to allocate personal exposure measures to individuals. A number of groups have shown that it is possible to measure airborne allergen concentrations in a variety of occupational settings, including research laboratories (rat and mouse urinary allergens [Gordon et al 1994]), flour mills and bakeries (flour [Sandiford et al 1995] and fungal α-amylase) and hospitals (latex [Swanson et al 1984]). Consistently, this has not been possible in domestic environments where aeroallergen levels are probably lower; indeed, the much higher exposures often encountered in the workplace are one reason why observations there should be generalized with care. It is worth noting too that occupational asthma occurs in subjects with fully developed immune systems, whereas much sensitization outside the workplace probably primarily occurs in infancy and possibly before — on the background of immune immaturity.

Timing of the response

Most population-based studies of occupational asthma have been of a cross-sectional nature; where these have included an assessment of allergen exposure, this has been simultaneous with the measurement of disease frequency. The potential for bias in such a design is well known, stemming largely from survivor effects, whereby affected persons tend to move out of situations of high exposure (the 'healthy worker effect') leading to distortion (downwards) in the measured frequency of disease and in its relationship with allergen exposure. A few studies, however, have examined full cohorts of employees across a period of time, allowing observation of the timing of the development of sensitization and asthma. In a historical cohort of workers in the platinum-refining industry exposed to immunologically potent, complex halide salts of platinum, the incidence of specific IgE measured serially by skin prick testing was highest in the first 18 months of employment (Venables et al 1989; see Fig. 1). A similar pattern has been observed in those working with small laboratory animals (Gross 1980) and in those exposed to toluene diisocyanate (Butcher et al 1977). While it is

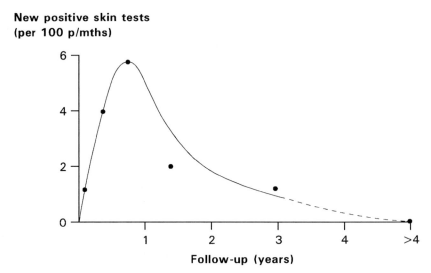

FIG. 1.   The incidence of positive skin prick tests to complex platinum salts in a cohort of platinum refinery workers. Dashed line represents an extrapolation of the data.

certainly possible for occupational asthma to develop many years after first exposure — as in some bakers — the risk appears to be highest in the early period (Herxheimer 1973). As a result of these observations, we have proposed that the risk of developing specific IgE and asthma is greatest in the first one to two years of exposure to a novel allergen.

This proposal has two implications outside the workplace. First, the search for an aetiology in individual cases of asthma should be concentrated on new exposures in the year or two prior to the onset of disease. Second, the study of the causes of asthma in populations is likely to be most fruitful when focused on periods of environmental change. These include, most obviously, birth but also changes in workplace exposures, movement to new environments (e.g. changes in home) and the introduction of new allergens into the environment (e.g. pet ownership and in the case of the Barcelona soybean epidemic).

Exposure–response relationships

Epidemiological studies of occupational asthma have frequently included measurements of the intensity of allergen exposures. These may either be: indirect, based on self-reported occupational tasks, for example; or direct, such as those where single allergen exposures have been assayed. They may also be derived from static or personal monitors, be applied on an individual or group basis, and made across whole work shifts (leading to average values) or only during specific tasks. Many of these techniques arise from the long experience of measuring dust and fibre exposures in the occupational field. A number of studies have reported a direct relationship between allergen exposure and specific sensitization or symptoms consistent with occupational asthma. Workers in a British bakery, for example, who had ever been exposed to high dust levels (a surrogate for high flour allergen exposure), had an increased prevalence of bronchial hyper-responsiveness and respiratory symptoms (Musk et al 1989). Among detergent enzyme workers, those in high intensity job categories had a higher incidence of specific IgE to alcalase (Juniper et al 1977). More recently, a gradient of increasing prevalence of work-related respiratory symptoms and of specific IgE across three categories of exposure to airborne rat urinary protein was observed in a group of employees newly exposed to laboratory animals (Cullinan et al 1994). There have been fewer studies of exposure–response relationships in low molecular weight occupational asthma, although Barker et al (1995) have demonstrated an increasing risk of sensitization to trimellitic anhydride, with increasing intensity of maximum exposure. These findings provide support for the observation that the risk of childhood asthma is related to the concentration of allergen exposure soon after birth (Sporik et al 1990): the risk of developing specific IgE and asthma is directly related to the intensity of exposure to the initiating allergen; this relationship is modified by genetic status and by concurrent cigarette smoking.

By establishing studies in which the relationship between allergen exposure and disease can be examined, it has also been possible to assess the influence of potentially modifying exposures. Concurrent cigarette smoking has been shown to increase the risk of sensitization and asthmatic symptoms in a variety of work forces, including snow-crab processors (Cartier et al 1984), those exposed to tetrachlorophthalic anhydride (Venables et al 1985) and ispaghula (Zetterstrom et al 1981), and the platinum refinery group mentioned above (Venables et al 1989). In a single study of laboratory animal workers (Cullinan et al 1994) the effect of smoking was found to interact with allergen exposure. The mechanism behind this interaction is unclear but it may reflect direct injury to the bronchial mucosa by cigarette smoke and greater access of inhaled allergens to submucosal, antigen-recognizing cells. Zetterstrom et al (1985), for example, have shown in rat models that tobacco smoke potentiated the IgE response to inhaled, but not ingested, allergen. Whether cigarette smoke exerts such an influence outside the workplace and whether other inhaled irritants have a similar effect are unknown. The model of occupational asthma implies, however, that the most sensitive means to examine the effect of inhaled irritants — including traffic-generated pollutants — on the induction of asthma would be through their potential interaction with airborne allergens.

Atopy, as conventionally determined, probably reflects an innate, non-specific immune responsiveness to environmental allergens. Occupational asthma associated with specific IgE production, caused by both inhaled proteins and haptens (e.g. platinum salts and acid anhydrides, but not diisocyanates), occurs more frequently in atopic subjects, and the risk for developing specific IgE tends to be greater still. Among laboratory animal workers we have shown an interaction between atopic

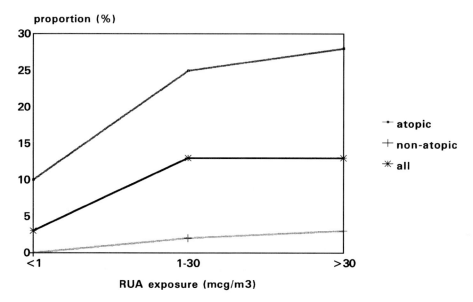

FIG. 2.   Laboratory animal workers: frequency of positive skin prick tests to rat urinary extract by intensity of exposure (to rat urinary aeroallergen [RUA]) and atopic status. mcg, microgram.

status and allergen exposure (Fig. 2), which is consistent with an increasing effect of atopy at higher exposures (Cullinan et al 1994).

The specificity of immune responsiveness is determined (and restricted) by HLA class II genotype. Since a number of agents responsible for occupational sensitization and asthma probably have a single epitope, and with increasing understanding of the protein structure of more complex agents, this is likely to be a fruitful field for the study of HLA associations in asthma. In a case-referent analysis of sensitization among workers exposed to a variety of acid anhydrides, an association between the HLA-DR3 genotype and specific IgE to trimellitic, but not phthalic, anhydride was identified (Young et al 1995). This is an observation which requires replication in similarly exposed populations but further analysis suggests that the relationship between HLA type and specific IgE in this group was strongest at lowest allergen exposures (Fig. 3).

Outcome

It is a frequent clinical observation that some patients with occupational asthma do not improve, or not entirely, once they are removed from the source of the causative allergen. A number of published case-series studies have borne this out and are summarized in Table 1. Their findings should be interpreted with some care since they are based on cases attending specialist clinics and are therefore selected, to some

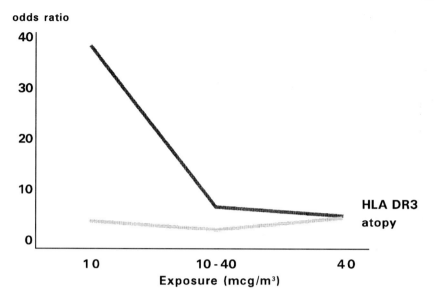

FIG. 3. Trimellitic anhydride workers: risk estimates for HLA-DR3/atopic status and positive skin prick tests to trimellitic anhydride antigen by maximum intensity of exposure. mcg, microgram.

extent, on the basis of their continuing disease. None the less, they confirm the potential for the persistence, perhaps in a sizeable proportion, of persistent asthmatic symptoms and bronchial hyper-responsiveness after exposure to the initiating agent has ceased. The mechanism for this is unknown but among patients with

TABLE 1 **Persistence of asthmatic symptoms and bronchial hyper-responsiveness in selected follow-up studies of occupational asthma**

| Agent | n | Persistent disease | | | |
		Follow-up (years)	Symptoms (%)	BHR[a] (%)	Reference
Colophony	20	1–4	90	50	Burge et al 1982
Snow-crab	31	4–6	100	84	Hudson et al 1985
Isocyanates	50	≥4	82	67	Losewicz et al 1987
	12	≥2	67	64	Paggiaro et al 1990
Western red cedar	75	1–9	49	76	Chan-Yeung et al 1987
TCPA[b]	6	4–5	100	100	Venables et al 1987

[a]BHR, bronchial hyper-responsiveness. Not all subjects tested.
[b]TCPA, tetrachlorophthalic anhydride.

diisocyanate-induced asthma it is associated with persistent airway inflammation characterized by eosinophil and lymphocyte infiltration (Paggiaro et al 1990, Saetta et al 1992).

Following cessation of occupational exposure, serial measurements of specific IgE and asthmatic symptoms were made in a small group of women sensitized to tetrachlorophthalic anhydride (Venables et al 1987). Over four years of follow-up, specific IgE declined exponentially with a half-life of about one year, confirming the absence of continuing exposure, but asthmatic symptoms and bronchial hyper-responsiveness persisted in almost all subjects. These findings have been confirmed over a further eight years of follow-up. In a similar study of snow-crab processors, specific IgE levels decreased over five years in a loglinear manner, with a half life of approximately 20 months (Malo et al 1988). Symptoms, FEV_1 (forced expiratory volume in one second) and bronchial hyper-responsiveness improved over the initial two years but failed to recover further: asthma, airway hyper-responsiveness and specific IgE may persist long after exposure to the initiating allergen has ceased.

If this observation can be generalized beyond the occupational field then it suggests that agents other than that responsible for the initiation of asthma may be responsible for the persistence of symptoms; continuing allergen exposure is not necessary for the persistence of airway inflammation. As a corollary, current exposures may not be relevant in the search for an aetiology.

Summary

If one accepts that occupational asthma is a useful model and that insights from its study can, with validity, be generalized to the study of the environmental determinants of asthma outside the workplace, then progress in two directions is necessary. First, studies of occupational asthma should be directed towards the confirmation and exploration of these inferences, and be designed on more sound principles than has often been the case to date. Of particular interest will be the analysis of the inter-relationships between allergen exposure and specific genotype.

TABLE 2 Barcelona soybean epidemic: risk factors associated with the development of soybean asthma

Factor	Level	Odds ratio	95% confidence interval
Age	45–64	1.9	1.1–3.6
	>64	2.8	1.4–6.0
Residence	<4 km from source	1.8	1.0–3.9
Atopy		3.0	1.7–5.3
Smoking	Past	1.8	0.9–3.7
	Present	2.3	1.2–4.6

Arguably, the studies involving cases of occupational asthma will provide the most powerful tool for studies of this kind .

Second, these insights need to be tested and expanded in the field of asthma outside the workplace. A successful illustration of this has been the more detailed case-referent analyses of the Barcelona soybean epidemic (Sunyer et al 1992), conducted specifically to test the hypotheses derived from the study of occupational asthma. This outbreak was an apparently clear example of novel allergen exposure across an entire population, with the consequent development of specific IgE-associated asthma. Although the latent period between first allergen exposure and the onset of disease has not been clearly established, it is believed that the great majority of cases developed within one to two years of the start of soybean unloading. An exposure–response relationship was established with subjects living nearer to the allergen source being at increased risk (Table 2); and the positive relationships with atopy and smoking, predictable from the experience with occupational asthma, were confirmed. We have since set up a large birth cohort to examine the same hypotheses.

References

Barker RD, van Tongeren M, Harris JM, Venables KM, Newman Taylor AJ 1995 Work-related symptoms and specific sensitisation in a cohort of workers exposed to acid anhydrides. Thorax 50:441P

Butcher BT, Jones RN, O'Neil C et al 1977 Longitudinal study of workers employed in the manufacture of toluene diisocyanate. Am Rev Respir Dis 66:213–216

Cartier A, Malo JL, Forrest F et al 1984 Occupational asthma in snow-crab-processing workers. 74:261–269

Cullinan P, Lowson D, Nieuwenhuijsen MJ et al 1994 Work-related symptoms, sensitisation and estimated exposure in workers not previously exposed to laboratory rats. Occup Environ Med 51:589–592

Gordon S, Tee RD, Nieuwenhuijsen M, Lowson D, Harris J, Newman Taylor AJ 1994 Measurement of airborne rat urinary allergen in an epidemiological study. Clin Exp Allergy 24:1070–1077

Gross MK 1980 Allergy to laboratory animals; epidemiologic, clinical and physiologic aspects and a trial of cromolyn in its management. J Allergy Clin Immunol 66:158–165

Herxheimer H 1973 The skin sensitivity to flour of bakers' apprentices. Acta Allergol 28:42–49

Juniper CP, How MJ, Goodwin BFJ, Kinshott AK 1977 *Bacillus subtilis* enzymes: a seven-year clinical, epidemiological and immunological study of an industrial allergen. J Soc Occup Med 27:3–12

Malo J-L, Cartier A, Ghezzo H, LaFrance M, McCants M, Lehrer SB 1988 Patterns of improvements in spirometry, bronchial hyperresponsiveness and specific IgE antibody levels after cessation of exposure in occupational asthma caused by snow-crab processing. Am Rev Respir Dis 138:807–812

Meredith S 1993 Reported incidence of occupational asthma in the United Kingdom. J Epidemiol Community Health 47:459–463

Musk AW, Venables KM, Crook B et al 1989 Respiratory symptoms, lung function and sensitisation to flour in a British bakery. Br J Ind Med 46:636–642

Paggiaro PL, Paoletti P, Bacci E et al 1990 Eosinophils in bronchoalveolar lavage (BAL) of patients with toluene diisocyanate (TDI) asthma after cessation of work. Chest 98:536–542

Saetta M, Maestrelli P, Di Stefano A et al 1992 Effect of cessation of exposure to toluene diisocyanate (TDI) on bronchial mucosa of subjects with TDI-induced asthma. Am Rev Respir Dis 145:169–174

Sandiford CP, Niewuwenhuijsen MJ, Tee RD, Newman Taylor AJ 1995 Measurement of airborne proteins involved in Baker's asthma. Clin Exp Allergy 24:450–456

Sporik R, Holgate ST, Platts-Mills TAE, Cogswell JJ 1990 Exposure to house dust mite allergen (*Der p* 1) and the development of asthma in childhood: a prospective study. N Engl J Med 323:502–507

Sunyer J, Anto JM, Sabria J et al 1992 Risk factors of soybean epidemic asthma: the role of smoking and atopy. Am Rev Resp Dis 1098–1102

Swanson MC, Agarwal MK, Yuninger JW, Reed CE 1984 Guinea pig-derived allergens. Clinico-immunologic studies, characterisation, airborne quantization and size distribution. Am Rev Respir Dis 129:844–849

Venables KM, Dally MB, Burge PS, Pickering CAC, Newman Taylor AJ 1985 Occupational asthma in a steel-coating plant. Br J Ind Med 42:517–524

Venables KM, Topping MD, Nunn AJ, Howe W, Newman Taylor AJ 1987 Immunologic and functional consequences of chemical (tetrachlorophthalic anhydride)-induced asthma after four years of avoidance of exposure. J Allergy Clin Immunol 8:212–218

Venables KM, Dalley MB, Nunn AJ et al 1989 Smoking and occupational allergy in workers in a platinum refinery 299:939–942

Young RP, Barker RD, Pile KD, Cookson WOCM, Newman Taylor AJ 1995 The association of HLA-DR3 with specific IgE to inhaled acid anhydrides. Am J Resp Crit Care Med 151:219–221

Zetterstrom O, Osterman K, McHardo L, Johansson SG 1981 Another smoking hazard: raised serum IgE concentration and risk of occupational allergy. Br Med J 283:1215–1217

Zetterstrom O, Nordvall SL, Bjorksten B, Ahlstedt S, Stelander M 1985 Increased IgE antibody responses in rats exposed to tobacco smoker. J Allergy Clin Immunol 75:594–598

DISCUSSION

Holt: This work illustrates some of the unique features of occupational asthma and in particular the dose–response curve. One could almost have predicted the relationship between specific IgE responses and the HLA-DR3 haplotype on the basis of David Marsh's work on ragweed, which showed that you will almost certainly find HLA restriction if you're looking at a single epitope (Marsh et al 1980). The apparently anomalous decrease in sensitization as the dose curve increases also makes sense. Environmental exposure to conventional inhaled allergens is in the nanogram or picogram zone, so the nature of the regulatory mechanisms that are available to the immune system there are really restricted to immune deviation. However, in occupational allergen exposure, exposure levels wander up into areas of the dose curve that we normally only associate with food allergens, and at such exposure levels options exist both for the induction of T cell anergy and T cell deletion. One could therefore speculate that individuals with the HLA-DR3 haplotype are the ones that can present the antigen most efficiently, and if there's consistent presentation of that antigen eventually the immune response will delete those specific T cells.

Cullinan: I agree but we are cautious because we are dealing with an acutely exposed group of people.

Kay: There may be separate mechanisms in occupational asthma depending on the nature of the agents to which workers are exposed. On the one hand, there are proteinaceous materials, such as urinary proteins and colophony fume, which give classical IgE-mediated, early- and late-phase reactions similar to those observed with inhalant allergens. On the other hand, highly reactive small molecules such as toluene diisocyanate (TDI) do not seem to produce an IgE response, and patients challenged with TDI often give an isolated late-phase reaction. This supports the T cell hypothesis of asthma and is therefore rather intriguing. TDI sensitization may also serve as a model of intrinsic asthma. TDI is almost a model of intrinsic asthma, in which an antigen is causing an isolated late-phase response and very severe asthma. We also have evidence for chronic T cell activation, i.e. biopsies of many patients with TDI asthma have shown that these individuals have many activated T cells.

Cullinan: Some of the examples you used were not the best examples. Colophony fume and plicatic acid are low molecular weight antigens and it's not possible to show an IgE response with any convincing regularity.

Paré: People exposed to plicatic acid in western red cedar sawdust may have a positive skin test but this is not related to symptoms. Plicatic acid is similar to TDI in that an isolated late-phase response is most often observed, but in about 20% of the cases an acute response is observed as well.

Kay: The examples I used may not be the best, but what is your opinion of the concept?

Cullinan: It is an interesting concept. Isocyanates are probably the commonest cause of most cases of occupational asthma in most developed countries, yet it's difficult to find an IgE response that reflects this. However, the Italians have shown quite a close HLA association with isocyanates, suggesting that specific antigen presentation is occurring.

Holgate: In the limited bronchial biopsy and lavage studies that have been undertaken (Saetta et al 1992a,b), it is surprising that the immunopathology does not appear to differ much from that in all other 'forms' of asthma.

Platts-Mills: Some years ago at Northwick Park we looked at the IgE antibody response to rat urine with Ann Cockcroft (Cockcroft et al 1981). Strikingly, there was a strong correlation between IgE antibody to the urinary protein and symptoms, and also a fairly good correlation between IgG antibody and estimated exposure. We were hoping to find some evidence for people who have symptoms and an immune response that did not include IgE, but we didn't find any. We interpret those results as showing that for whole proteins, T helper cell type 2, IgG and IgE responses are associated with occupational asthma, and that responses which do not include IgE are not.

Cullinan: This is a circular argument because we tend not to define occupational asthma unless they have specific IgE responses.

Warner: I have a question about particle size. When I was working in the field of laboratory animal allergy in 1987 there was a suggestion that different-sized particles in this model might lead to the differential timing of the onset of symptoms. Have there been any further developments on this issue?

Cullinan: No, we haven't managed to make any more headway on this. What appears to happen in this timing event, which is something we can't wholly explain, is that some people develop symptoms before they develop a systemic IgE response. Generally, they also appear to develop eye and nose symptoms before chest and skin symptoms.

Boushey: I suggest that if we want to examine occupational asthma in people with immature immune systems we should look at children who are taken to day-care centres. Day-care centres almost always have pets, so that the rhythm of exposure is similar to that of adults who work from nine to five.

Brostoff: I have a related point on occupational exposure to animals. I have frequently seen children who are not allergic to their own cat but are allergic to their neighbour's cat. If such children then leave home to go to university, for example, when they return they become allergic to their own cat. Therefore, all cats are not the same, and it is unclear how this tolerance is manifested. This reminds me of when Jack Pepys first talked about chemical allergy in platinum workers. When many of these people were taken away from their work their lung function continued to decline and this decline was worsened by other chemical exposures. He put forward the theory that the reaction was to the carrier and not to the hapten, i.e. it was an altered host protein problem. Have there been any follow-up studies of this work?

Cullinan: One has to be careful with these follow-up studies. The studies that I presented, with the exception of the snow-crab workers, were all of low molecular weight agents. The general opinion in our clinical experience is that sensitization to low molecular weight agents is worse than being sensitized to a biological protein. For example, when allergic laboratory animal workers cease exposure on changing profession they seem to do very well.

Strachan: I would like to explore the concept of a 'window of vulnerability', which is a phrase that has been coined by Anthony Newman Taylor and linked to the development of sensitization earlier in life (Cullinan & Newman Taylor 1994). I don't personally see how one gets from the graph of incidence by the time since starting work to the window of vulnerability. Instead, I perceive the pattern of a point-source epidemic when everyone is exposed and that there is a variable latent period before people respond. This is not the same as a window of vulnerability, during which, as I understand it, one's chances of becoming sensitized are influenced by other factors. This has a bearing on the question of prevention because if house dust mite allergen exposure were to be delayed until the age of 35, what would happen when those people are exposed to their first house dust mite at the age of 35? The occupational examples would suggest that they would still be vulnerable to sensitization.

Beasley: The studies from Australasia indicate that with the appropriate environmental exposure, adults will develop asthma later in life. For example, the prevalence of asthma increases twofold in Asian populations within 10 years of migrating to Australia. This suggests that this window of vulnerability may extend for the rest of one's life.

Holt: An analogous observation, from an immunological perspective, is that upon initial exposure to an allergen not encountered previously, it's common for everyone to make IgE, but this immune response is usually deleted over time. Those individuals who fail to down-regulate this response will express the disease in the long term. Therefore, in this context the window of vulnerability for environmental factors is related to early exposures.

Martinez: You mentioned that people who develop long-term sensitization have IgE at the beginning, but soybean sensitization occurs almost exclusively in people who already have asthma. This suggests that something in the way they react to the environment, whether it be a genetic factor or an event early in life, was present when they were exposed. Also, very few children were sensitized to soybean: it occurred mainly in adults. Therefore, there is something about this exposure that differs to those observed with other allergens.

Weiss: Cigarette smoking rather than atopy influences susceptibility to occupational asthma, which brings us back to the problem that in the real world we're dealing with a multiple exposure problem, and it's extremely difficult to isolate any of the factors involved.

Burney: There is an elegant paper on the first of the great epidemics, which was the first reported epidemic associated with exposure of the general public to castor bean allergen in North America (Figley & Elrod 1928). This paper includes the information needed to calculate the time from people arriving in the locality to the time they started to develop asthma symptoms. If these data are plotted a log normal distribution of incubation times is obtained that is exactly as one would expect with a point-source epidemic. The median incubation time is about four years, but the longest incubation time is 22 years. This last observation is not an outlier but part of the distribution. Although there might appear to be a window of vulnerability because of the heavy concentration of cases in the first four years, and the long tail of cases thereafter, this is illusory. The distribution in time is no different from any other standard 'incubation' period curve. I know of no epidemiological evidence that supports the window of vulnerability concept.

Holgate: Could you comment on the effect of adult virus infections in an occupational setting?

Cullinan: We have tried to measure viral infections at work but we have run into difficulties similar to those encountered in the general environment. It is possible that viruses have different effects in mature and immature immune systems.

Holgate: Could you also comment on the concept of the disease persisting and evolving after the antibody response has disappeared? Is it possible that factors involved in disease progression operate independently of those which initiate it, as we hypothesize in other forms of asthma linked to aeroallergen exposure?

Cullinan: Yes, I'm sure this is the case because many patients tell us that they become reactive to non-specific stimuli.

Potter: Could you comment on the rising trends of occupational asthma caused by latex?

Cullinan: There have been 29 reported cases in the UK, but we're probably further behind the USA and other countries in Europe in recognizing the extent of the problem. Merret et al (1997) have looked at about 5000 blood donors and found that 2–3% of them had raised IgE levels to extracts of latex. They haven't determined how these people have been exposed to latex. It is possible that they encounter it in the general environment. Half of the reported cases of latex asthma have been health care workers.

Potter: It has been estimated that 10% of theatre workers are sensitized to latex, and that the development of clinical latex allergy, and particularly asthma, is on the increase in the developed world.

Cullinan: The highest estimate I have come across is 17%.

References

Cockroft A, Edwards J, McCarthy P, Anderson N 1981 Allergy in laboratory animal workers. Lancet I:827

Cullinan P, Newman Taylor AJ 1994 Asthma in children: environmental factors. Br Med J 308:1585–1586

Figley KD, Elrod RH 1928 Asthma due to castor bean dust. J Am Med Assoc 90:79–82

Marsh DG, Hsu SH, Hussain R, Meyers DA, Freidhoff LR, Bias WB 1980 Genetics of human immune responses to allergens. J Allergy Clin Immunol 65:322–332

Merret TG, Keckwick R, Merret J, Burns D, Unver E 1997 Prevalence of IgE antibody responses to latex among a UK donor population. Clin Exp Allergy, in press

Saetta M, Di Stefano A Maestrelli P et al 1992a Airway mucosal inflammation in occupational asthma induced by toluene diisocyanate. Am Rev Respir Dis 145:160–168

Saetta M, Maestrelli P, Di Stefano A et al 1992b Effect of cessation of exposure to toluene diisocyanate (TDI) on bronchial mucosa subjects with TDI-induced asthma. Am Rev Respir Dis 145:169–174

The role of domestic allergens

Thomas A. E. Platts-Mills, Richard B. Sporik, Martin D. Chapman and Peter W. Heymann

University of Virginia Asthma and Allergic Diseases Center, Box 225, Charlottesville, VA 22908, USA

Abstract. The documented increase in asthma has been almost entirely in perennial asthma and a large proportion of the cases are allergic to one of the common allergens found all year round in houses, i.e. house dust mites, cats, dogs or cockroaches. In population and case-control studies sensitization to one of these allergens is the strongest risk factor for asthma (adjusted odds ratios ≥ 4). Using monoclonal antibody-based assays for the major indoor allergens it has been shown that sensitization to house dust mites is directly related to the concentration of Group 1 mite allergen in dust. This led to the hypothesis that increases in mite allergen secondary to changes in houses were responsible for increases in asthma. However, asthma has also increased in areas of the world where mites do not flourish. In these dry areas sensitization to one of the other indoor allergens is the major risk factor for asthma. Although sensitization of asthmatics reflects the concentration of allergens in their houses, these measurements of exposure do not accurately predict severity of symptoms. Other factors that can contribute to the symptoms of asthma may also have increased. In particular, diesel particulates, ozone, β2-agonists, endotoxin and rhinovirus infection have each been shown to enhance the inflammatory response to inhaled allergens. Increases in asthma must relate to some aspect of our predominantly sedentary indoor lifestyle; this could be either increased exposure to allergens or an increase in factors that enhance the response of the lungs to foreign proteins.

1997 The rising trends in asthma. Wiley, Chichester (Ciba Foundation Symposium 206) p 173–189

As we approach the end of the second millennium, most people in western countries spend the bulk of their lives indoors. Thus, a large proportion of the protein they inhale is derived from indoor sources. During the last 40 years of the 20th century there has been a truly remarkable increase in perennial asthma. In keeping with studies from as early as 1921, many or most of the children and young adults with asthma have immediate hypersensitivity to house dust or one of its components. There are two questions that stem from these observations: (1) what role do domestic or indoor allergens play in asthma among allergic individuals; and (2) can increased exposure to indoor allergens explain increases in prevalence or morbidity of asthma? If increases in exposure to allergens indoors do not explain the increase in asthma we have to assume that the increase has been caused by some other change that acts selectively on allergic individuals.

As recently as 1980 the extracts of house dust used for skin testing were undefined black liquids and there was no method of measuring or standardizing their contents. The major cat allergen (*Fel d* 1) was first purified in 1974 and this lead to techniques for measurement (Ohman et al 1974). House dust mites were recognized as a major source of allergens in house dust by Voorhorst et al (1969). They also developed the techniques for growing mites. However, the first mite allergen was not purified until 1980 (Chapman & Platts-Mills 1980). This was followed fairly rapidly by the development of monoclonal antibodies, immunoassays, cloning of cDNA and full sequencing of many of the proteins that are present in house dust (Chapman et al 1987, 1988, Chua et al 1988, Arruda et al 1995) (Table 1). Today the immunochemistry, molecular biology and immunology of the inhaled proteins associated with perennial asthma is well defined. Most importantly, there are sensitive accurate assays for the major allergens using monoclonal antibodies that can measure as little as 0.1 $\mu g/g$ of dust or 1 ng/m^3 airborne. These assays have made it possible to quantitate exposure in the houses of patients. Furthermore, it has been possible to start defining the thresholds for exposure that influence the risk of sensitization or symptoms of asthma. In Table 1 the major sources of indoor allergens are given as house dust mites, domestic animals (cat and dog) and the German cockroach. Clearly there are many other antigen sources — such as moulds, mouse urine, guinea pigs and bacteria in carpets — but these are less well defined and on a population basis probably less important. Some of these can be the most important allergen in individual houses. Each allergen source gives rise to a wide variety of proteins, many of which are enzymes. Measurement of one or two major allergens from each source is used as an index of exposure. We assume that other less well-defined indoor allergens play a role in asthma that is similar to the major sources that are well defined.

Ideally, measurements of exposure to the common allergens found in domestic houses would define the size of particles carrying airborne allergen as well as the quantity of each protein entering the different parts of the respiratory tract. Currently, it is possible to measure the quantity of airborne proteins and to estimate the mass median diameter of the particles carrying allergen in houses. However, these measurements are time consuming and technically demanding (Tovey et al 1981a, Luczynska et al 1990, Swanson et al 1989). Thus, at present all epidemiological data are based on measurements of allergen in dust obtained from reservoirs in the house (Platts-Mills et al 1992). Although any fabric can act as a reservoir, the major sites are carpets, mattresses, pillows, bedding and all upholstered furniture. For animal dander these sites are truly a reservoir, whereas for house dust mite proteins the reservoirs are also the primary sites for mite growth. Measurements of protein in reservoirs assumes that there is a consistent relationship between the floor or bedding dust and the quantity inhaled. At present the evidence is confusing but certain aspects of the relationship can be recognized.

(1) Antigens derived from house dust mites are only detectable in the air when a room is disturbed. In keeping with this, their apparent size is $\geqslant 10\,\mu m$ in diameter. Calculations of the size and quantities of mite allergen airborne suggest that

TABLE 1   Structural and functional properties of indoor allergens

Source	Allergen[a]	Molecular mass (kDa)	Function	Sequence[b]
House dust mite				
Dermatophagoides spp.	Group 1	25	Cysteinen protease	cDNA
	Group 2	14	Unknown	cDNA
	Group 3	30	Serine protease	Protein
	Der p 4	60	Amylase	Protein
	Der p 5	14	Unknown	cDNA
	Der p 6	25	Chymotrypsin	Protein
	Der p 7	22–28	Unknown	cDNA
Euroglyphus maynei	Eur m 1	25	Cysteine protease	PCR
Blomia tropicalis	Blo t 5	14	Unknown	cDNA
Lepidoglyphus destructor	Lep d 1	14	Unknown	None
Mammals				
Felis domesticus	Fel d 1	36	Possibly uteroglobin	PCR
Canis familiaris	Can f 1	25	Unknown	cDNA
Mus musculus	Mus m 1	19	Calycins, PBPs	cDNA
Rattus norvegicus	Rat n 1	19	Calycins, PBPs	cDNA
Cockroach				
Blattella germanica	Bla g 1	20–25	Unknown	None
	Bla g 2	36	Aspartic protease	cDNA
	Bla g 4	21	Calycin	cDNA
	Bla g 5	36	Glutathione transferase	cDNA
Periplaneta americana	Per a 1	20–25	Unknown	None
	Per a 3	72–78	Unknown	None
Fungi				
Aspergillus fumigatus	Asp f 1	18	Cytotoxin (mitogillin)	cDNA

[a]New nomenclature proposed by the World Health Organization/International Union of Immunological Sciences committee.
[b]Method given for full sequence determination, where available. Protein sequences are incomplete, usually N-terminal or internal peptide sequences have been determined.
PBPs, pheromone-binding proteins.

exposure occurs during disturbance in a house or while breathing close to a source (e.g. pillows) and involves inhaling relatively few, i.e. 20–100, large particles/day (Tovey et al 1981a, b, Platts-Mills & Chapman 1987).

(2) Airborne cat allergens have been studied by several groups. The major allergen (*Fel d* 1) remains airborne for long periods of time and part of this allergen is

carried on relatively small particles, i.e. $\leqslant 5\,\mu$m in diameter. Thus, exposure can occur continuously but it is increased during disturbance (Luczynska et al 1990, Swanson et al 1989).

(3) For each allergen source the highest concentration in dust is found in a different site. Thus, mite allergens are most often at a maximum in bedding, domestic animal allergens in living rooms and cockroach allergens in dust derived from kitchens. In most studies the highest concentration found in the house has been taken as the index of exposure; however, there is no clear evidence about where or how the maximum amount is inhaled. Furthermore, relative exposure at different sites, e.g. kitchens compared to beds, may not be the same for different age groups.

(4) Measurement of the concentrations of major allergens in samples of dust obtained from reservoirs (i.e. μg/g of dust) is the best accepted assessment of exposure for studies that involve large numbers of houses.

In most humid parts of the world immediate or weal and flare skin test responses to house dust can be explained by the presence of an immune response including IgE antibodies against specific proteins produced by house dust mites of the genus *Dermatophagoides*. The relationship between serum IgE antibodies and specific skin responses to the same protein is close (r values 0.7–0.8); either can be used as a marker of immediate hypersensitivity, which is the only form of sensitivity that has been associated with asthma. On the other hand, there are plenty of studies which associate asthma with sensitivity to allergens other than house dust mites. Indeed, the principle appears to be that any foreign protein source that can become airborne will induce immediate hypersensitivity, and that prolonged exposure to any of these proteins may give rise to asthma. With every source that has been studied in detail, IgE antibodies are found to multiple proteins from that source. Thus, determining the presence of sensitization either by skin tests or *in vitro* serum assays is best done with an extract containing all the proteins produced by that source.

Is the association between indoor allergens and asthma causal?

Before considering whether changes in indoor allergens explain the increase in prevalence of asthma, we will first consider the evidence that indoor allergens are causally related to asthma. The basis for evaluating causality with exposure to a non-infectious agent was outlined by Bradford Hill, who proposed a series of criteria and suggested that if they were met then causality should be assumed (Hill 1965). We have discussed in detail the applicability of these criteria to house dust mites as a cause of asthma (Sporik et al 1992), and only the main points are addressed here.

The strength and consistency of the association

The relevant association is that between sensitization to indoor allergens and asthma (Smith et al 1969, Sporik et al 1990, 1995, Sears et al 1989). For house dust mite sensitization this association is extremely strong with adjusted odds ratios for asthma from four to more than 10 (Peat et al 1990, Woolcock & Peat 1997, this volume). In areas of the world where house dust mites do not flourish because of low humidity, sensitization to other allergens has been associated with asthma, e.g. animal dander in New Mexico (Sporik et al 1995) or cockroaches in the major cities of the northeastern USA (Rosenstreich 1996, Call et al 1992, Gelber et al 1993).

Is there a dose–response relationship between exposure and the disease?

Over the last 10 years a series of cross-sectional and prospective studies have established that there is a dose–response relationship between exposure to mite allergens and sensitization (Platts-Mills et al 1992). For children who are atopic, as defined by family history or by skin tests to outdoor allergens, there is an apparent threshold at $2\,\mu g$ Group 1 mite allergen/g dust (Kuehr et al 1994). In communities where most of the houses contain greater than $2\,\mu g$ of these proteins, house dust mite sensitization will be common (i.e. $>50\%$) among the asthmatic children. Since sensitization is associated with asthma and there is a dose–response relationship between exposure and sensitization, it was logical to expect a dose–response relationship between exposure and the symptoms of asthma. In some studies there is an association; however, in many studies this relationship is not obvious even if the analysis is restricted to allergic patients (Platts-Mills et al 1995). The main conclusion is that many different factors can contribute to inflammation and symptoms and that this obscures a simple dose–response relationship between exposure to allergens and symptoms (Fig. 1).

Experimental studies

Provocation experiments.   Bronchial provocation with allergens can induce both immediate and late decreases in FEV_1 (forced expiratory volume in one second). The late response includes an inflammatory response and has most of the characteristics of an exacerbation of asthma. Furthermore, the eosinophil-rich inflammation that occurs at 12–24 h correlates with increased bronchial hyper-reactivity (BHR).

Avoidance studies.   The idea that removing asthmatics from their houses would be beneficial was first studied by Storm van Leuwen who used a 'climate chamber' in Holland (Van Leuwen et al 1927). In studies carried out between 1960 and 1990 it has consistently been shown that children moved to a high altitude sanatorium improve clinically, and that most of them demonstrate progressive decreases in BHR (Boner et al 1985). In London when young adults who were allergic to house dust mites were admitted to an allergen-free unit, they experienced improvement in symptoms, decreased medication requirement and significant reductions in BHR. Those studies involved a decrease in exposure to *Der p* 1 from $13.4\,\mu g/g$ to $\leqslant 0.2\,\mu g/g$ (Platts-Mills et al 1982). Most recently, Boner and his colleagues in Verona have demonstrated that children taken out of their houses showed parallel decreases in BHR and

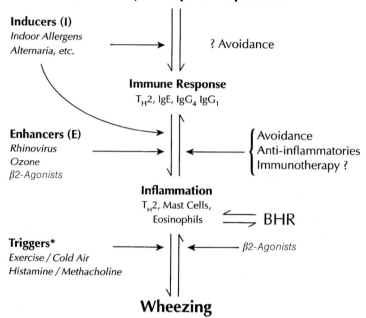

FIG. 1.   Inducers are those foreign proteins or allergens that can give rise to an immune response characterized by T helper (T_H) 2 cells, IgE and IgG antibodies. Continued exposure to inducers (predominantly indoors) gives rise to characteristic eosinophil-rich inflammation in the lungs and to the associated bronchial hyper-reactivity (BHR). The inflammatory response of the lungs to foreign proteins varies from patient to patient and can be up-regulated by a variety of enhancers. Once the lungs are inflamed and hyper-reactive, wheezing can be induced by a variety of non-specific enhancers.

'inflammation' as judged by eosinophils in induced sputum (Boner et al 1985). The conclusion of the experimental studies is that the lung inflammation characteristic of asthma can be induced by provoking the lungs with allergen and can be reduced by decreasing exposure to indoor allergens.

Plausibility

Given: (1) that patients who have immediate hypersensitivity to indoor allergens will develop the symptoms and pathology of asthma when their lungs are exposed to allergen; (2) that there is an excellent dose–response relationship between exposure and sensitization; (3) that full avoidance of indoor allergens can lead to improvement of the disease; and (4) that most patients are living in houses which contain allergen; it is logical to assume a cause and effect relationship between indoor allergen exposure and asthma. The major problems with the argument are that the quantities of allergen used for bronchial provocation are not commonly present in the air of houses, and that there is not a good dose–response relationship between the measured concentration of allergen in reservoirs in houses and symptoms. The best explanation of the available evidence is that chronic (i.e. weeks and months) of allergen exposure results in inflammation of the lungs which in turn is related to increased non-specific BHR. However, the severity of symptoms is related to a wide range of other factors that can either trigger attacks directly or enhance the inflammatory response to allergens.

The relevance of enhancers and triggers

Until 1970 it was generally assumed that asthma was a physiological condition of the lungs and, in keeping with this view, all the agents that increased symptoms were grouped together as triggers (Altounyan 1970). In many textbooks, exposure to cats, rhinovirus infections, passive smoke, cold air and stress were listed together as triggers of asthma. Given the evidence that inhaled foreign proteins can induce an immune response characterized by IgE antibodies and antigen-specific lymphocytes of the T helper (Th) 2 phenotype, it seems logical to classify these agents as causes or perhaps less judgementally as inducers. Over the last 10 years it has been demonstrated that many other agents which are associated with attacks of asthma can increase the inflammatory response to inhaled allergens. The distinction here is that these agents do not produce an immune or inflammatory response on their own. The clearest examples of this group are rhinoviruses, ozone, β2-agonists, endotoxins and diesel particulates (Diaz-Sanchez et al 1994). These agents can be described as enhancers. There is excellent evidence from cross-sectional studies in the emergency room (Duff et al 1993, Rakes et al 1995) and prospective studies of children that rhinoviruses can induce attacks of asthma (Johnston et al 1995). In the emergency room studies carried out in Charlottesville, the combination of a positive PCR result for rhinovirus and IgE antibody to common indoor allergens was strongly associated with asthma. Direct challenge studies with rhinoviruses do not induce either episodes of asthma or an eosinophil response in the nose (Fraenkel et al 1994). Thus, the likely explanation is either that rhinoviruses can increase the inflammatory response to inhaled allergens (Calhoun et al 1994, Busse et al 1997, this volume) or that patients with inflammation and intercellular adhesion molecule 1 up-regulation in the respiratory tract make a different response to rhinovirus infection. At present, there is no evidence that rhinoviruses can induce an immune response of the Th2 or IgE antibody type.

The evidence about β2-agonists is important because of the widespread use of these inhalers. Following the initial data from New Zealand suggesting that fenoterol could increase BHR, there were several studies giving positive and negative answers as to whether other β2-agonists could produce a similar effect. However, recently Cockcroft and his colleagues in Saskatchewan have shown that regularly inhaled β2-agonists can up-regulate the late response to allergen challenge (Cockcroft et al 1995).

This result is important because it implies that $\beta 2$-agonists could have a cumulative negative impact in some cases, but no such effect in many others.

The important feature of the enhancers is that they go a long way to explaining how you can have an epidemic of asthma in which most of the patients are allergic to common indoor allergens and yet not be able to find a dose–response relationship between allergen exposure and the severity of symptoms. The concept of enhancers also offers another point in the equation, where changes in lifestyle or environment could have contributed to the increased prevalence and morbidity of asthma.

Does increased exposure to indoor allergens explain the increase in asthma?

Given the strong correlation between house dust mite sensitization and asthma, it was logical to ask whether changes in houses could have contributed to and/or caused the increases in asthma. In some areas of the world there have been dramatic changes in houses and behaviour that would be expected to increase exposure to house dust mites. Thus, in New Zealand and England houses have become warmer, are less well ventilated and have more fitted carpets. Humidity has probably not increased, since in both countries humidity has always been high. That children are spending more time indoors is undoubted, but whether four hours extra indoors represents a significant increase in inhaled allergen compared to 18 h including eight hours asleep on a pillow is not clear. It is also possible that lying on the floor or on a sofa allows increased inhalation of foreign protein but this has not been quantitated. The evidence that sensitization to indoor allergens other than house dust mites is associated with asthma in areas where there has also been an increase is very important. Any argument that increases in asthma are a consequence of increased exposure to indoor allergens would have to postulate increased cockroach allergens in inner cities in the USA and increased exposure to cat or dog allergens in northern Sweden or the mountain states of the USA. Overall, it seems unlikely that increases in the concentration of these other allergens have been sufficient to explain the observed increases in asthma. An alternative explanation is that decreased ventilation has led to increased exposure to all indoor allergens. However, this doesn't explain increased asthma in Atlanta or Hong Kong, where the temperature is generally hot and windows remain open.

Our current analysis of increased exposure would say that sensitization to indoor allergens has increased in parallel with the increases in perennial asthma and that many of the changes in lifestyle could have increased exposure to indoor allergens. However, if increased exposure to allergens was really the central cause of the increase we would expect to see a clear relationship between exposure and severity of disease. In most studies this has not been clear. Thus, it seems likely that there is at least one other factor that has increased which is acting as an enhancer of the response to indoor allergens.

What has really changed from 1960 to 1995?

Given the observed increases in asthma, it is important to step back and ask what changes could have had an influence. Because the response is complex none of the major changes should be ignored. Thus, we are looking for changes that could influence: (i) the immune response to common environmental proteins; (ii) the inflammatory response in the lungs; or (iii) the severity of airflow obstruction either judged by objective measurements or symptoms.

Diet

Several different dietary changes have been associated with increased asthma, including high salt diet, low intake of oily fish, and increased levels of colourings and preservatives. However, changes in westernized diet are much more complex because there has been a wide range of changes in methods of growing and preserving foods. Two examples are: (i) the use of hormones to accelerate growth of cattle; and (ii) use of potent insecticides and acaricides to prevent the growth of plant parasites and storage mites in grain. Decreased mite antigens in grain and thus decreased oral mite antigen in food could have changed the immune response to inhaled allergen. At present, although it is likely that dietary changes have influenced the prevalence and severity of asthma, the changes do not appear to be sufficient to explain the phenomena.

Introduction of broad-spectrum antibiotics

The purification of penicillin in Oxford by Florey and Chain in 1942 led to a complete revolution in the treatment of childhood infections. By 1965 the regular use of broad-spectrum antibiotics was routine for tonsillitis, strep throat, otitis media and bronchitis. The result was a dramatic decrease in chronic suppurative infections and rheumatic fever. However, bacterial antigens can induce interleukin 12 production, which tends to drive immune responses towards the Th1 phenotype. Thus, it is possible that the changes in the pattern of bacterial infections in childhood have allowed increased immune responses to inhaled allergens which are predominantly of the Th2 phenotype.

Changes in housing

These have been discussed above as possible causes of increased exposure to indoor allergens. However, it remains possible that chemical or other exposures indoors have enhanced the response to inhaled allergens. In addition, carpets are an important source of endotoxin which may act as an enhancer.

Increased sedentary time

Televisions were introduced around 1950 and have become steadily more pervasive. Progressive improvements in the quality of the picture, the number of channels and remote controls have been associated with truly astonishing viewing hours. Repeated surveys have confirmed that school-age children are watching an average of three hours of television per day. It is obvious that viewing represents a decrease in exercise, and it has recently been confirmed that there is a direct correlation between obesity and the number of hours spent watching (Gortmacher et al 1996). Prior to 1960 there were many communities where it was normal for children to walk to school and to play outside for two to three hours after school. Today children travel to school by bus or car, and they sit watching television or computers for three hours in the evening.

Sitting and watching a hypnotic light box could impact the lungs in other ways. Certainly prolonged sitting is associated with 'snacking', i.e. a high salt diet, but in addition, prolonged sitting still may represent an abnormally long period of shallow breathing. It is possible that prolonged periods of tidal breathing alter the response of the lungs to inhaled antigens, or that regular activity protects the lungs. What is clear is that there has been a major decrease in activity/exercise in almost all westernized communities.

Conclusions

The increase in asthma worldwide is predominantly in perennial asthma. In many areas where an increase has been documented, sensitization to house dust mite antigens is the single strongest risk factor for asthma. This is true in England, New Zealand, Australia, Japan and the southeastern USA.

In areas where humidity is low, sensitization to other indoor allergens has been shown to be significantly associated with asthma.

On the basis of the strength of the epidemiological associations, the results of challenge studies and avoidance studies, it is reasonable to assume that there is a causal relationship between exposure to indoor allergens and asthma.

While many of the changes in houses from 1960 to 1990 may have increased the concentration of allergens in dust or the exposure to these allergens, there are good reasons for not accepting this increase as the primary cause of the increased prevalence of asthma: (a) the lack of a simple dose–response between exposure to indoor allergens and symptoms or severity of symptoms; and (b) the observations that increases in asthma are associated with sensitization to domestic animals, German cockroach allergens and *Alternaria* as well as house dust mites of the genus *Dermatophagoides*.

Increased symptoms of asthma or inflammation of the lungs can also be produced by several factors that enhance the response to inhaled allergens. These include human rhinovirus, endotoxin, β2-agonists, ozone and diesel particulates. Although exposure to some of these inducers has increased, none of them appear to explain the extent of the phenomenon.

Many other changes in lifestyle could contribute to asthma, including changes to diet, other effects of changes in housing and the pervasive effects of television. Sitting still for three hours per day may change the response of the lung as well as increasing exposure. Alternatively, activity may simply be essential for the normal function of the lungs. We are still faced with a worldwide epidemic of asthma among children who are sensitized to indoor allergens and spend most of their lives indoors.

References

Altounyan RE 1970 Changes in histamine and atropine responsiveness as a guide to diagnosis and evaluation of therapy in obstructive airways disease. In: Pepys J, Frankland SW (eds) Disodium chromoglycate in allergic airways disease. Butterworth, London, p 47–53

Arruda LK, Vailes LD, Mann BJ et al 1995 Molecular cloning of a major cockroach (*Blattella germanica*) allergen, *Bla g* 2. J Biol Chem 270:19563–19568

Boner AL, Niero E, Antolini I, Valletta EA, Gaburro D 1985 Pulmonary function and bronchial hyperreactivity in asthmatic children with house dust mite allergy during prolonged stay in the Italian Alps (Misurina 1756 m). Ann Allergy 54:42–45

Busse WW, Gern JE, Dick EC 1997 The role of respiratory viruses in asthma. In: The rising trends in asthma. Wiley, Chichester (Ciba Found Symp 206) p 208–219

Calhoun WJ, Dick EC, Schwartz LB, Busse WW 1994 A common cold virus, rhinovirus 16, potentiates airway inflammation after segmental antigen bronchoprovocation in allergic subjects. J Clin Invest 94:2200–2208

Call RS, Smith TF, Morris E, Chapman MD, Platts-Mills TAE 1992 Risk factors for asthma in inner-city children. J Pediatr 121:862–866

Chapman MD, Platts-Mills TAE 1980 Purification and characterization of the major allergen from *Dermatophagoides pteronyssinus* antigen P1. J Immunol 125:587–592

Chapman MD, Heymann PW, Wilkins SR, Brown MJ, Platts-Mills TAE 1987 Monoclonal immunoassays for the major dust mite (*Dermatophagoides*) allergens, *Der p* 1 and *Der f* 1, and quantitative analysis of the allergen content of mite and house dust extracts. J Allergy Clin Immunol 80:184–194

Chapman MD, Aalberse RC, Brown MJ, Platts-Mills TAE 1988 Monoclonal antibodies to the major feline allergen *Fel d* 1. II. Single step affinity purification of *Fel d* 1, N-terminal sequence analysis, and development of a sensitive two-site immunoassay to assess *Fel d* 1 exposure. J Immunol 140:812–818

Chua KY, Steward GA, Thomas WR et al 1988 Sequence analysis of cDNA coding for a major house dust mite allergen, *Der p* 1. J Exp Med 167:175–182

Cockcroft DW Obyrne PM, Swystun VA, Bhagat R 1995 Regular use of inhaled albuterol and the allergen-induced late asthmatic response. J Allergy Clin Immunol 96:44–49

Diaz-Sanchez D, Dotson RA, Takenaka H, Saxon A 1994 Diesel exhaust particles induce local IgE production *in vivo* and alter the patterns of IgE messenger RNA isoforms. J Clin Invest 94:1417–1425

Duff AL, Pomeranz ES, Gelber LE et al 1993 Risk factors for acute wheezing in infants and children: viruses, passive smoke, and IgE antibodies to inhalant allergens. Pediatrics 92:535–540

Fraenkel DJ, Bardin PG, Sanderson G, Lampe F, Johnston SL, Holgate ST 1994 Immunohistochemical analysis of nasal biopsies during rhinovirus experimental colds. Am J Resp Crit Care Med 150:1130

Gelber LE, Seltzer LH, Bouzoukis JK, Pollart SM, Chapman MD, Platts-Mills TAE 1993 Sensitization and exposure to indoor allergens as risk factors for asthma among patients presenting to hospital. Amer Rev Resp Dis 147:573–578

Gortmacher SL, Must A, Sobol AM, Peterson K, Colditz GA, Dietz WH 1996 Television viewing as a cause of increasing obesity among children in the United States, 1986–1990. Arch Ped Adol Med 150:356–362

Hill AB 1965 The environment and disease: association or causation. Proc R Soc Med 58:295–300

Johnston SL, Pattemore PK, Sanderson G et al 1995 Community study of role of viral infections in exacerbations of asthma in 9–11-year-old children. Br Med J 310:1225–1228

Kuehr J, Frischer T, Meinert R et al 1994 Mite exposure is a risk for the incidence of specific sensitization. J Allergy Clin Immunol 94:44–52

Luczynska CM, Li Y, Chapman MD, Platts-Mills TAE 1990 Airborne concentrations and particle size distribution of allergen derived from domestic cats (*Felis domesticus*): measurements using cascade impactor, liquid impinger and a two site monoclonal antibody assay for *Fel d* 1. Am Rev Resp Dis 141:361–367

Ohman JL, Lowell FC, Bloch KJ 1974 Allergens of a mammalian origin. III. Properties of a major feline allergen. J Immunol 113:1668–1677

Peat JK, Salome CM, Woolcock AJ 1990 Longitudinal changes in atopy during a 4-year period: relation to bronchial hyperresponsiveness and respiratory symptoms in a population sample of Australian schoolchildren. J Allergy Clin Immunol 85:65–74

Platts-Mills TAE, Chapman MD 1987 Dust mites: immunology, allergic disease, and environmental control. J Allergy Clin Immunol 80:755–775

Platts-Mills TAE, Tovey ER, Mitchell EB, Moszoro H, Nock P, Wilkins SR 1982 Reduction of bronchial hyperreactivity during prolonged allergen avoidance. Lancet II:675–678

Platts-Mills TAE, Thomas WR, Aalberse RC et al 1992 Dust mite allergens and asthma: report of a 2nd international workshop. J Allergy Clin Immunol 89:1046–1060

Platts-Mills TAE, Sporik RB, Wheatley LM, Heymann PW 1995 Is there a dose–response relationship between exposure to indoor allergens and symptoms of asthma? J Allergy Clin Immunol 96:435–440

Rakes GP, Arruda E, Ingram JM et al 1995 Human rhinovirus in wheezing children: relationship to serum IgE and nasal eosinophil cationic protein. J Allergy Clin Immunol 96:280

Rosenstreich DL 1996 Relationship between sensitization, allergen levels, and asthma morbidity in inner-city children. Am J Resp Crit Care Med 153:255A

Sears MR, Herbison GP, Holdaway MD, Hewitt CJ, Flannery EM, Silva PA 1989 The relative risks of sensitivity to grass pollen, house dust mite and cat dander in the development of childhood asthma. Clin Exp Allergy 19:419–424

Smith JM, Disney ME, Williams JD, Goels ZA 1969 Clinical significance of skin reactions to mite extracts in children with asthma. Br Med J 1:723–726

Sporik R, Holgate ST, Platts-Mills TAE, Cogswell J 1990 Exposure to house dust mite allergen (*Der p* 1) and the development of asthma in childhood: a prospective study. N Engl J Med 323:502–507

Sporik RB, Chapman MD, Platts-Mills TAE 1992 House dust mite exposure as a cause of asthma. Clin Exp Allergy 22:897–906

Sporik R, Ingram JM, Price W, Sussman JH, Honsinger RW, Platts-Mills TAE 1995 Association of asthma with serum IgE and skin-test reactivity to allergens among children living at high altitude: tickling the dragon's breath. Am J Resp Crit Care Med 151:1388–1392

Swanson MC, Campbell AR, Klauk MJ, Reed CE 1989 Correlations between levels of mite and cat allergens in settled and airborne dust. J Allergy Clin Immunol 83 :776–783

Tovey ER, Chapman MD, Wells CW, Platts-Mills TAE 1981a The distribution of dust mite allergen in the houses of patients with asthma. Am Rev Resp Dis 124:630–635

Tovey ER, Chapman MD, Platts-Mills TAE 1981b Mite faeces are a major source of house dust allergens. Nature 289:592–593

Van Leuwen S, Einthoven W, Kremer W 1927 The allergen proof chamber in the treatment of bronchial asthma and other respiratory diseases. Lancet I:1287–1289

Voorhorst R, Spieksma FThM, Varekamp N 1969 House dust mite atopy and the house dust mite *Dermatophagoides pteronyssinus* (Troussart, 1897). Stafleu's Scientific, Leiden
Woolcock AJ, Peat JK 1997 Evidence for the increase in asthma worldwide. In: The rising trends in asthma. Wiley, Chichester (Ciba Found Symp 206) p 122–139

DISCUSSION

Nelson: You mentioned that house dust mites were not present in northern Sweden but Wickman et al (1993) have found them. Therefore, are you equally sure about the reports of lack of physical activity?

Platts-Mills: I am confident about the lack of physical activity because I have heard detailed descriptions from Bo Lundback and others. He said that before television children in northern Sweden, as in most other countries, spent much of their leisure time playing outside, but that has changed with the advent of television.

Holgate: Are we absolutely certain that there are no house dust mites in northern Scandinavia?

Strachan: Mite allergens have been detected in Sweden but the levels are orders of magnitude lower than those in western and southern Europe (Nordvall et al 1988). I don't know what the levels are in Finland.

Platts-Mills: Working with Bo Lundback we have recently analysed dust samples from Kiruna in northern Sweden and we found no mite allergen (i.e. $< 0.4 \mu g/g$) in any of the samples.

H. R. Anderson: In spite of this the prevalence of asthma is similar in different parts of Sweden (Bjornsson et al 1994).

Boushey: The prevalence of asthma in Finland is very low. It is possible that there are degrees of predisposition and, because the levels of mites are low, asthma only occurs in those most strongly prediposed to develop it. If this is correct, then the low levels of house dust mites measured do not exclude the house dust mite as the responsible indoor allergen.

Platts-Mills: In a community with many indoor pets I suspect that pet allergens will be the dominant indoor allergen for the whole community, rather than house dust mite allergens.

Busse: What is the relationship between house dust mites and allergic rhinitis? Are house dust mites a risk factor for allergic rhinitis or are they more dominant allergens for lower airway disease?

Platts-Mills: There are patients coming into my clinic who are dominantly sensitive to house dust mites and who are complaining of perennial rhinitis. Some of them get better either when they're treated with immunotherapy or when you give them allergen avoidance advice. Therefore, I believe that chronic allergic rhinitis is related to house dust mites, and that some of this is associated with asthma. However, there are many asthmatics who deny any nasal symptoms but are clearly allergic to house dust mites.

Busse: Ragweed is not a major allergen for lower airway disease, but it causes a lot of upper airway problems. I have the impression that house dust mite-sensitive individuals either have lower airway disease that dominates their symptomatology or don't have upper airway disease. Is there any evidence on this issue?

Platts-Mills: The problem relates to perennial exposure. Nasal symptoms appear to be less prominent in cases of continuous exposure. However, eyes react quite differently because a certain particle velocity is required to make an impact, and this velocity is not achieved indoors. Therefore, conjunctivitis as a symptom of hay fever is an outdoor phenomenon, although it is possible to get rhinitis from indoor allergens. In addition, it is likely that asthma is favoured in some way by chronicity of exposure.

Sears: Seven years ago we reported that the house dust mite was the dominant allergic risk factor for asthma in children in New Zealand (Sears et al 1989), whereas hay fever is more clearly related to outdoor allergen sensitization (Sears et al 1993).

Platts-Mills: It depends on how you define hay fever in the questionnaire. If you include conjunctivitis then you will definitely identify pollen-sensitive individuals.

Sears: We asked whether they had had hay fever, which included the symptoms of sneezing and itching of the nose and eyes.

Magnussen: In Germany cats have played a predominant role in indoor allergen exposure. Would immunotherapy against cats be useful in this case?

Platts-Mills: Most of us believe that immunotherapy for asthma is possible. However, I'm not convinced that it is a useful treatment for the whole population. This approach will have to wait until a treatment is developed that is less likely to cause anaphylaxis, and therefore safer for routine use, and preferably more effective. We believe that the future lies in whole cloned molecules, with the IgE determinants removed by site-directed mutagenesis, rather than in peptides (Smith & Chapman 1995).

Busse: Is there any evidence that obese individuals have a higher propensity to develop airway hyper-responsiveness?

Paré: Obese people have a lower functional residual capacity, i.e. they breathe with a slightly lower lung volume. The supine position also lowers the functional residual capacity. If one performs a methylcholine challenge in an individual who is supine they're more responsive than if they are sitting. Therefore it is possible that obese persons have a higher level of responsiveness, but as far as I'm aware this has not been tested.

Woolcock: We have also been interested in obesity. When Jenny Peat includes weight in her regression analysis, it is not a significant risk factor; however, asthmatic children have a higher calorie intake than non-asthmatic children. We do not know if asthmatic children watch television for more hours than non-asthmatic children, but this would be of interest. Asthmatic children may have a different metabolism, so that despite a greater caloric intake they do not become obese.

Britton: I have a point about the social class gradients in disease. One implication of your results is that people in low socioeconomic groups are more obese and spend more time watching television.

Platts-Mills: That's true in the USA, both obesity and increased hours watching television have been shown to be more common among low socioeconomic groups. However, I did not mean to suggest that obesity and asthma are directly linked, it is more likely that they are both consequences of the same changes in behaviour.

Britton: But in the UK allergic diseases are high social class phenomena. There is an increased prevalence of infection in the first year of life in low social classes, but allergic diseases later on in childhood and adolescence are associated with the higher social classes.

Platts-Mills: We don't know enough about asthma in the African American population in the south of the USA prior to 1950 when children walked to school and their parents worked outside. We don't have records of asthma prevalence comparable to those available from other areas. When the rural population from the south moved to Detroit to make motor cars, they started to live in apartments, took buses to school and spent longer indoors. This may be the first time a low socioeconomic population has been described as a group most at risk from asthma.

Martinez: I would like to caution against making generalizations. In Puerto Rico the prevalence of asthma is higher than in any other part of the USA — 20% of the population of Puerto Rico have asthma — yet the prevalence of obesity is low. The Puerto Ricans are healthy and they spend much of their time outdoors.

Platts-Mills: But the levels of indoor allergens in Puerto Rico are high.

Holgate: We have to be fairly pragmatic because in different environments across the world there are likely to be different factors operating. No one could convince me that in Tristan da Cunha watching television accounts for all, or indeed any of, the cases of asthma.

Paré: Thomas Platts-Mills mentioned that in a cross-sectional study a dose–response relationship did not exist between exposure and symptoms, yet there is a dose–response relationship between exposure and sensitization. It follows, therefore, that the degree of sensitization shouldn't correlate with the symptoms, yet we were shown data suggesting that the degree of sensitization, as assessed by skin tests, did relate to symptoms. Can you clarify this issue, because it is relevant to preventative studies? Are there any data which suggest that decreasing exposure decreases sensitization?

Platts-Mills: Ann Woolcock has shown in her studies in Australia that if you know the mean mite allergen level in the houses within a community you can predict the prevalence of mite sensitization among asthmatic children in that community (see Woolcock & Peat 1997, this volume). Studies in Europe and the USA support this, and they all indicate that there is a threshold of $2\,\mu g$ of Group 1 house dust mite allergen/g house dust. If the mean level is above that, there are significant associations with sensitization and asthma. This threshold may have biological significance because it represents about 100 mites/g house dust, and that may be the level below which the house dust mite colonies don't thrive very well.

Sensitized individuals have IgE on mast cells in their lungs. We know that it is possible to provoke them if you give them enough house dust mite allergen. Data from the National Jewish Hospital in Denver in the 1970s showed that provided enough allergens were given to skin test positive patients they all wheezed in the end (Cavanaugh et al 1977). However, this relationship varies enormously, so that some of the sensitized individuals never develop symptoms and some develop symptoms easily. Therefore, this overrules a dose–response relationship within a small population, but not necessarily in a large one. Chan-Yeung et al (1995) showed that a dose–response relationship to symptoms was present in Winnipeg and Vancouver. However that study was comparing Vancouver, which is wet, with Winnipeg, which is not.

Potter: In Soweto the levels of *Der p* 1 are less than 2 μg in 74% of homes, and yet house dust mites sensitivity occurs in 45% of childhood asthmatics (Davis et al 1994). Therefore, in my opinion, a value of 2 μg is too high. Sensitization is occurring at much lower levels. The situation is quite different, however, in the South African coastal areas where mean levels of *Der p* 1 antigens in bedding are typically between 20 and 30 μg/g of dust and high levels of exposure occur (Potter et al 1996).

Platts-Mills: One explanation of this could be that the methods for assessing these levels are not yet adequately standardized, or that we need to make different measurements of exposure.

Kay: There may be a certain degree of complementarity between your data and ours. You have shown a relationship between exposure and sensitization, and between sensitization and asthma symptoms, but you don't observe a relationship between exposure and asthma symptoms. We have found a correlation between interleukin (IL)-4 expression and IgE levels but not between IL-4 and symptoms. In contrast, IL-5 correlates with symptoms but not atopy. Furthermore, nasal corticosteroids down-regulate IL-4 but not IL-5 mRNA in allergic rhinitis (Masuyama et al 1994). This contrasts with asthma, where there is a dramatic decrease in IL-5 levels, as well as a substantial decrease in IL-4 levels, after prednisolone treatment (Robinson et al 1993). Perhaps the missing link between atopy and asthma symptoms is IL-5 and subsequent eosinophil recruitment. If you could measure IL-5 levels in your sensitized individuals you may be able to define a clearer relationship between exposure and asthma symptoms.

References

Bjornsson E, Plaschke P, Norrman E 1994 Symptoms related to asthma and chronic bronchitis in three areas of Sweden. Eur Resp J 7:2146–2153

Cavanaugh M J, Bronsky EA, Buckley JM 1977 Clinical value of bronchial provocation testing in childhood asthma. J Allergy Clin Immunol 59:41–47

Chan-Yeung M, Manfreda J, Ward H et al 1995 Mite and cat allergen levels in homes and severity of asthma. Am J Resp Crit Care Med 152:1805–1811

Davis G, Luyt D, Prescott R, Potter PC 1994 House dust mites in Soweto. Curr Allergy Clin Immunol 7:16–17

Masuyama K, Jacobson MR, Rak S et al 1994 Topical glucocorticosteroid (fluticasone propionate) inhibits cytokine mRNA expression for interleukin-4 (IL-4) in the nasal mucosa in allergic rhinitis. Immunology 82:192–199

Nordvall SL, Eriksson M, Rylander E, Schwartz B 1988 Sensitization of children in the Stockholm area to house dust mites. Acta Paediatr Scand 77:716–720

Potter PC, Davis G, Maujra A, Luyt D 1996 House dust mite allergy in southern Africa. Clin Exp Allergy 26:132–137

Robinson DS, Hamid Q, Ying S et al 1993 Prednisolone treatment in asthma is associated with modulation of bronchoalveolar lavage cell interleukin-4, interleukin-5 and interferon-gamma cytokine gene expression. Am Rev Respir Dis 148:401–406

Sears MR, Herbison GP, Holdaway MD, Hewitt CJ, Flannery EM, Silva PA 1989 The relative risks of sensitivity to grass pollen, house dust mite and cat dander in the development of childhood asthma. Clin Exp Allergy 19:419–424

Sears MR, Burrows B, Flannery EM, Herbison GP, Holdaway MD 1993 Atopy in childhood. I. Gender and allergen-related risks for development of hay fever and asthma. Clin Exp Allergy 23:941–948

Smith AM, Chapman MD 1996 Reduction in IgE binding to allergen variants generated by site-directed mutagenesis: contribution of disulfide bonds to the antigenic structure of the major house dust mite allergen, Der p 2. Mol Immunol 33:399–405

Wickman M, Nordvall SL, Pershagen G, Korsgaard J, Johansen N 1993 Sensitization to domestic mites in a cold temperate region. Am Rev Respir Dis 148:58–62

Woolcock AJ, Peat JK 1997 Evidence for the increase in asthma worldwide. In: The rising trends in asthma. Wiley, Chichester (Ciba Found Symp 206) p 122–139

Air pollution and trends in asthma

H. Ross Anderson

Department of Public Health Sciences, St. George's Hospital Medical School, Cranmer Terrace, London SW17 0RE, UK

Abstract. There is considerable concern about possible links between ambient air pollution and the upward trend in asthma. This chapter reviews the mechanistic and epidemiological evidence concerning air pollution and asthma and examines the hypothesis that trends in asthma could be explained by air pollution. It is concluded that existing evidence is not sufficient to link air pollution with the initiation of asthma in healthy subjects. Although there is better evidence that air pollution can provoke or aggravate asthma, it probably plays a minor role at a public health level, in comparison with other factors. It is therefore unlikely that trends in asthma could be explained by air pollution. Furthermore, correlations between some air pollutants and asthma over time are not consistent with the hypothesis. The possibility of a specific effect of motor vehicle pollution needs further investigation but this factor is unlikely to be the main cause of the worldwide increase in asthma.

1997 The rising trends in asthma. Wiley, Chichester (Ciba Foundation Symposium 206) p 190–207

There is considerable evidence that asthma and other atopic diseases such as allergic rhinitis and eczema have increased over the past few decades. In many countries atopic diseases constitute the commonest chronic disease group in children and in countries such as Australia and the UK asthma is the commonest reason for emergency hospital admission and use of medications.

Progress has been made in understanding the basic pathological and biological mechanisms of asthma, and asthma is now considered to be best characterized pathologically as an allergic inflammation which in turn causes airway obstruction and increased bronchial reactivity. Of the currently known risk factors for asthma, the strongest are a family history of atopy and the occurrence of other atopic diseases such as hay fever and eczema. Many other risk factors have been identified but none have been sufficient to explain why asthma prevalence varies markedly across regions or why its prevalence has increased.

There has been much speculation concerning the possible role of ambient air pollution as a cause of the increase in asthma and there is a widespread assumption by the public and many health professionals that there is a definite and substantial link between the two. This attitude is understandable in view of the known sensitivity of asthmatics to inhaled irritants, and it has been further enhanced by an increasing public concern about environmental pollution and the effects of increased traffic and urbanization in general. This chapter reviews the evidence linking asthma to outdoor air pollution and focuses on the question of whether trends in asthma could be due to changes in ambient air pollution.

The chapter begins by outlining the mechanistic or basic scientific evidence, based on animal and some human experimental studies, for a plausible link between asthma and air pollution. This is followed by a review of the epidemiological evidence that air pollution may initiate or provoke asthma in ambient conditions. It concludes by examining the hypothesis that trends in asthma have been influenced by trends in the scale or composition of ambient air pollution. Due to restrictions on space, no exhaustive bibliography is provided. The reader is directed to a number of recent reviews of asthma and air pollution, especially the report of the UK Department of Health Committee on the Medical Effects of Air Pollutants (Department of Health 1995a), together with various other reviews of this subject (British Society for Allergy and Clinical Immunology 1995, Wardlaw 1993, Burr 1995), as well as to general reviews of the epidemiology of asthma (Burney 1992, Burr 1993, Strachan 1995a,b).

Potential mechanisms

The main measured outdoor pollutants that have been connected with respiratory effects are particles, sulfur dioxide (SO_2), nitrogen dioxide (NO_2) and ozone. Laboratory studies have shown that all of these are capable of causing pathological or physiological effects on various elements of the respiratory system (Table 1) (Department of Health 1991, 1992, 1993, 1995b,c, American Thoracic Society 1996). Potentially, many of these effects could affect processes involved with the initiation or provocation of asthma (Table 2). Initiation of asthma refers to the development of asthma in an individual who has previously been free of the disease; this could be either through direct toxicity or through an enhancement of the sensitization process. Similarly, the provocation of asthma in those who already have the underlying disease could be caused by direct toxicity or by reducing the stimulatory threshold for allergens or other irritants.

TABLE 1   Pathological effects of air pollution on the airways and lungs

Tissue/cells	Effect
Epithelium	Cell death, denudation
Mucosal vasculature	Leakage of fluid
Inflammatory cells	Stimulation
	Inflammatory mediators released

The existence of plausible mechanisms derived from animal studies does not necessarily mean that ambient air pollution has an effect on humans. Human chamber studies have been important in demonstrating the acute effects (or lack of) of individual pollutants on symptoms, physiological variables (such as bronchial responsiveness) and pathology. They have also been able to explore the possible interactions between different pollutants and between pollutants and allergens (Department of Health 1995c). Table 3 summarizes what has been learnt from human experimental studies about the effects of pollutants at ambient concentrations. The strongest evidence relates to ozone, which at ambient levels appears to be capable of causing toxic effects on the respiratory tract. Although there is considerable individual variation in the response to ozone, there is no consistent evidence that, in general, asthmatics are

TABLE 2   Potential effects of air pollution on asthma

Type of asthma	Effect
Asthma initiated in previously healthy persons	Direct toxic effects Effect on sensitization process
Existing asthma: provocation of symptoms	Direct effect on bronchial responsiveness Reduction in stimulatory threshold to allergens or inhaled irritants

TABLE 3   Effects of ambient concentrations of air pollutants in human chamber studies

Air pollutant	Effect	Are asthmatics more sensitive than healthy subjects?
Ozone	Inflammation of airways	Possibly
	Restriction of inspiration	No
	Increase in bronchial responsiveness	Possibly
	Enhancement of response to allergens	Yes
Sulfur dioxide	Increase in airway resistance in asthmatics	Yes
Nitrogen dioxide	Evidence for any effect inconsistent	Possibly
	Enhancement of response to allergens	Yes
Particles	Little known about effects	Not known
	Acid aerosols increase bronchial responsiveness	Possibly
Mixtures	Combined effects additive not interactive	Not known

affected more than healthy subjects. In chamber studies, ambient concentrations of SO_2 tend not to have effects even on asthmatics, although at higher levels asthmatics are definitely more sensitive than healthy subjects. The results of NO_2 studies are conflicting. Very little is known about the effects of particles because these are difficult to study in a chamber situation. However, it is likely that acid aerosols cause increased bronchial responsiveness. Chamber studies indicate that prior exposure to air pollution may enhance the response to a subsequent challenge with allergen (Jörres et al 1996). It needs to be emphasized that chamber studies do not simulate the pattern of ambient exposure and that subjects are confined to adults (for ethical reasons).

Indirect epidemiological evidence

This relates mainly to the effects on asthma of active and passive smoking and of indoor pollution due to unflued combustion associated with cooking and heating. These sources of pollution have certain components in common with outdoor air pollution, the main ones being NO_2, particles and carbon monoxide. There is increasing evidence that active smoking affects the incidence and severity of asthma. Passive smoking seems to have little effect on the incidence of wheezing illness after early childhood, but it does aggravate a proportion of the asthmatic population. In a meta-analysis of all studies to date, gas cooking was associated with a small increase in respiratory symptoms, including those of asthma (Hasselblad et al 1992). It is not clear whether the NO_2 component is the responsible agent but in using such evidence to draw inferences about the likely effects of outdoor NO_2 it should be noted that peak levels of NO_2 in kitchens with gas cookers frequently exceed World Health Organization outdoor standards (Department of Health 1993).

Low levels of asthma have been reported from some developing countries where the population is exposed to high concentrations of wood smoke from domestic fires (Anderson 1978). Recently, it has been reported that asthma is less common in southern Bavarian rural homes which use wood for heating (von Mutius et al 1996). Such observations indicate that there is no necessary adverse effect of air pollution on asthma. It is less likely that wood smoke has a direct protective effect than that it is a marker for some other factor, such as 'hygiene'.

Epidemiological approaches to the investigation of asthma and air pollution

There are two main types of population study relating to the association between asthma and air pollution. One type is referred to here as 'temporal', meaning that time relationships between cause and effect are the focus of interest. When the time interval is fairly short (days, weeks or months) such evidence is relevant to the short-term effects of air pollution on persons who already have the asthmatic disease; this is termed variously as the inciting, provocation, precipitation or aggravation of asthma. The other approach is termed 'spatial' and exploits area variations in exposure to air pollution or in asthma to see if they are associated with one another. The health outcome indicator in such studies is usually period prevalence, a measure that reflects incidence, prognosis and severity. Less commonly it is possible, by using cohort studies, to measure incidence itself; these have the advantage of enabling better control for confounding factors such as smoking. Spatial studies give some indication of the role of air pollution in the initiation or induction of the asthmatic disease in individuals who were previously healthy.

Population studies of temporal associations between asthma and air pollution

Seasonal associations

One of the most universal factors affecting exacerbations of asthma is season. If air pollution were an important cause of asthma symptoms a seasonal correlation would be expected. Where this has been investigated there seems to be little or no association with air pollution. In particular, the marked autumn peak in asthma that occurs in many countries is not associated with a seasonal increase in any of the known pollutants.

Air pollution episodes

The health effects of various air pollution episodes have been investigated in several countries (Department of Health 1995c). Some episodes involved pollution mixtures from the burning of coal (particles, SO_2 and acid aerosols) and more recently there have been investigations of winter episodes characterized by high levels of NO_2, and of summer episodes characterized by high levels of ozone. In none of these studies has there been an unequivocal effect on asthma; most effects have occurred among older persons with chronic cardiorespiratory disease. In the historic London fog of 1952 it was remarked that asthmatics tended not to be seriously affected (Ministry of Health 1954). Many years later in the NO_2 episode in London in 1991 asthma admissions were not obviously affected (Anderson et al 1995).

Asthma epidemics

Asthma epidemics occur from time to time and air pollution has often been blamed. However, where appropriate investigations have been carried out such episodes have usually been explained by an increase in aeroallergens. An example would be the association between soybean allergen from dockside silos in Barcelona and asthma epidemics in that city (Anto et al 1989). During some of these epidemics, air pollution was raised to a moderate degree but this is probably because local atmospheric conditions associated with poor dispersal of allergens were also associated with a build up of air pollutants. During a recent epidemic of asthma in England in June 1994, there was little evidence of an increase in air pollution.

Daily time-series studies in individuals with asthma (panel studies)

This is a potentially powerful method of investigating the short-term effects of air pollution on individuals but surprisingly few such studies have been done in asthmatic subjects. Most studies in healthy individuals show that ambient pollution may cause small effects on lung function not associated with symptoms. It is possible that such effects, if experienced by an asthmatic, might increase the level of symptoms. Some panel studies of asthmatics have observed an increase in daily symptoms and medications in association with particulate and photo-oxidant air pollution, although the effects are generally small and there is considerable individual variability (Department of Health 1995a).

Daily time-series studies at an aggregated level

In these studies daily counts of hospital or emergency room admissions for asthma are correlated with daily air pollution levels in the area or city concerned, controlling for known confounders such as weather and temperature. Significant positive associations have been reported from the USA and Europe (Dockery & Pope 1994). The pollutants concerned include particles (such as PM10, Black Smoke and acid aerosol), SO_2, ozone and NO_2, with poor consistency across centres (Department of Health 1995a). Where significant effects are observed, these tend to be of a similar size to those observed with admissions for other respiratory conditions, suggesting that asthmatics are not especially sensitive. Within the range of pollutants experienced in a city, the effect of air pollution is to increase admissions by less than 5%.

Population studies of geographical variations in asthma and air pollution

Geographical variations in air pollution and asthma

These attempt to determine whether the prevalence of asthma symptoms is related to exposure to outdoor pollution. In interpreting such studies it is important to keep in mind that prevalence reflects incidence (i.e. the initiation of asthma), prognosis and severity (i.e. the provocation or aggravation of asthma). Although many studies have reported a correlation between air pollution and the prevalence of respiratory symptoms (such as cough and phlegm), and diagnoses such as bronchitis, the evidence relating to symptoms more specific for asthma is weaker and inconsistent. One problem is that many studies have compared only two areas and lack the statistical power to draw inferences from the results. In addition, there has often been inadequate control of potential confounders such as the indoor environment and smoking. More helpful are analyses of larger numbers of areas. Such studies in the UK have concluded that regional variations in air pollution appear to bear no relation to asthma prevalence in children or adults and that variations in asthma prevalence bear no clear relation to outdoor pollution (Department of Health 1995a). Indeed, the epidemiology of asthma within the UK is marked by a lack of regional variation (Strachan et al 1994), and even in unpolluted areas, such as the Isle of Skye, the prevalence of asthma compares with that in polluted conurbations (Austin et al 1994). From what is known about the spatial distribution of asthma in other countries, such as Australia, the same conclusion can be drawn (Robertson et al 1992).

A better indication of the effects of air pollution on the incidence of asthma may be obtained by comparing the cohorts distinguished by different lifetime exposures to air pollution. A study of this type compared the incidence of asthma in Seventh Day Adventists living in California according to estimates of lifetime exposure to photochemical oxidants and particles. The cumulative risk of physician-diagnosed asthma was increased in those with more exposure to particles and ozone, but the covariation of these makes it difficult to single out one or other of these pollutants (Greer et al 1993).

Comparison of urban with rural environments

A specific variant of the spatial approach is the comparison of urban and non-urban areas. The urban/rural differentials in pollution have changed over time. Up until the 1970s, urban pollution was dominated by domestic, industrial and power generation sources, with lower levels in rural areas. Nowadays, whole regions share in the exposure to ozone and SO_2. While traffic is most intense in the towns, NO_2 and fine particles may travel considerable distances from the towns into the rural areas. The evidence for the UK suggests that there is no urban excess in asthma prevalence or asthma mortality. This is in contrast with the urban excess in asthma prevalence and mortality in the USA. However, this has been attributed not to urban air pollution but to lifestyle, and socioeconomic and health care factors (Weitzman et al 1990).

Exposure to traffic

Because pollution from traffic is causing most concern, a number of studies have investigated the relationships between proximity to traffic and asthma symptoms, asthma admissions and lung function. A number of these have reported significant associations, after taking into account possible confounders such as passive and active smoking, gas cooking and social factors (Wjst et al 1993). Proximity to heavy commercial traffic appears to be especially important. Although the effects are generally small, and could, in the case of asthma diagnosis or symptoms, be explained by reporting bias, there is a clear case for further investigation of this phenomenon.

Correlation of asthma trends with air pollution

From the types of evidence reviewed above, it is concluded that although it is plausible that ambient air pollution might have a role in the initiation of asthma, there is little evidence to suggest that this happens at a public health level. The role of air pollution in the provocation of asthma is more plausible and there is little doubt that this is one factor in the short-term epidemiological patterns of asthma exacerbations. However, at the public health level the effect is probably small and cannot be responsible for the main temporal features of asthma such as seasonality and day-to-day variations. At the same time, there are many other competing explanations for the pattern of occurrence of asthma; these include allergens, infections, weather, psychological factors, indoor air pollutants and diet (Seaton et al 1994). Supporting evidence for some of these is also weak or inadequate, but in the present state of knowledge it would seem unlikely that air pollution could be responsible for the trends in asthma.

Trends in asthma

Trends in asthma have been reviewed extensively (Burr 1987, Burney 1992, Anderson 1993, Strachan 1995a, Department of Health 1995a). Serial prevalence surveys in children in the UK, Switzerland, USA, Australasia and Taiwan all point to an increase. There is less evidence relating to adults but asthma has increased in military recruits in Finland, Switzerland and Israel and in adults in Western Australia. There is also evidence for an increase in other manifestations of atopy such as eczema and hay fever. A recent review of the UK evidence (Department of Health 1995a) concluded that the prevalence of asthma in children had increased by about 50%. Trends in various indicators of asthma in children are shown in Fig. 1. The increase in

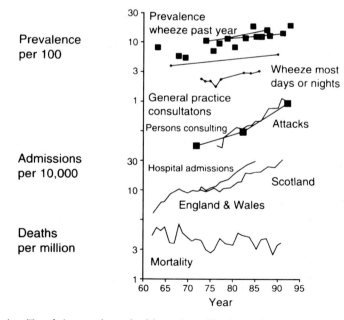

FIG. 1.   Trends in prevalence, health service utilization and mortality from asthma in children aged between five and 14 in the UK from 1962 to 1992.

diagnosed asthma has been greater than that of asthma symptoms because of changes in diagnostic practice. The greatest relative increase has been in the utilization of health services for asthma. In England and Wales, asthma admissions increased more than 10-fold in children from 1962 to 1992, and similar rises have been reported from other English-speaking countries. Increases have also occurred in primary care consultations and in the use of medicines. A substantial but unquantifiable proportion of the change in utilization is likely to have been due to medical care rather than epidemiological factors.

Trends in pollution

For the UK, details of urban and rural air pollution have been reviewed (United Kingdom Photochemical Oxidants Review Group 1987, Quality of Urban Air Review Group 1993, 1996). The correlation of asthma with air pollution over time is not straightforward because there is inadequate information about trends in community exposure to air pollution. National inventory data do, however, show a clear trend in total emissions of respiratory pollutants and in their sources. In the UK emissions of SO_2 have declined, with the largest proportion now coming from power generation. These stations tend to be fewer in number and located away from main cities; however, their emissions are from high stacks and consequently disseminate over wide areas. Emissions of Black Smoke have declined markedly with the largest contribution now coming from road transport, especially diesel vehicles. These changes have been reflected in marked falls in measured levels of SO_2 and Black Smoke, especially in cities (Fig. 2).

Emissions of nitrogen oxides are mainly from vehicles, which increased until the early 1990s. They are projected to fall as a result of catalytic converters and then

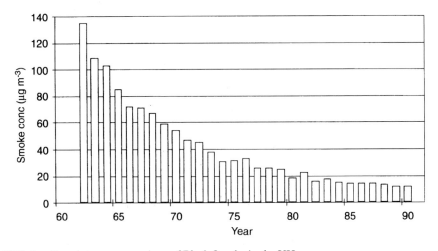

FIG. 2.   Trends in concentrations of Black Smoke in the UK.

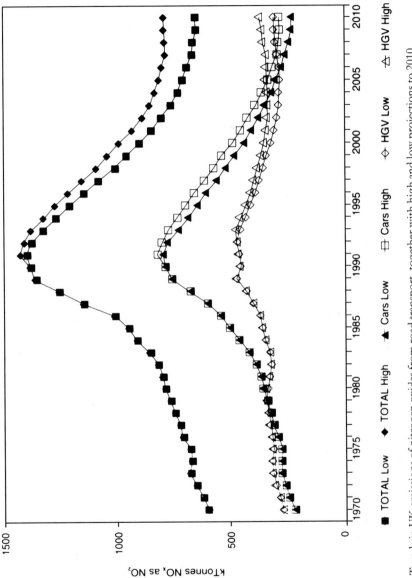

FIG. 3. Trends in UK emissions of nitrogen oxides from road transport, together with high and low projections to 2010.

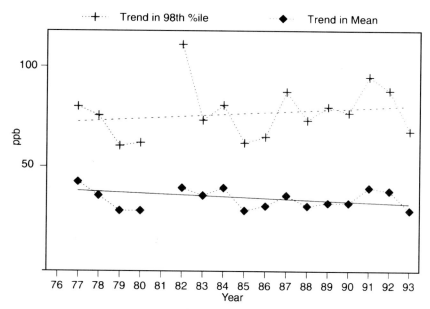

FIG. 4.   Trends in concentrations of nitrogen dioxide in central London from 1977 to 1993. ppb, parts per billion.

flatten out in the next century as vehicle volume increases (Fig. 3). Data on long-term trends in urban ambient levels of NO_2 are confined to London, where there has been no significant upward trend (Fig. 4), perhaps due to traffic saturation. There is, however, an increase in 98th percentiles, indicative of an increase in peak levels.

Ozone is a secondary pollutant formed mainly by the action of sunlight on NO_2 and oxygen in the presence of volatile organic compounds and hydrocarbons which act as catalysts and are also emitted by combustion sources such as motor vehicles and industrial processes. Because ozone is scavenged by nitric oxide (NO), levels of ozone tend to be lower in cities, and in central London the levels of ozone have fallen because of this (Fig. 5). In non-polluted areas there is evidence of an increase in baseline ozone levels and these have probably doubled over the past century. Sporadic ozone episodes are related to weather conditions and no trend towards an increase in episodes has emerged over the past 20 years.

The source of particles has changed considerably, and those which are respirable are a combination of dust, particles from diesel vehicles (mainly carbon) and chemical substances derived from NO_2 and SO_2 (sulfates, nitrates, acid aerosols) (Quality of Urban Air Review Group 1996). The fine fraction ($< 2.5\,\mu$m aerodynamic diameter) is probably distributed widely over the countryside.

Correlations between trends in asthma and individual air pollutants are therefore contradictory. There is an inverse correlation with trends in SO_2 and Black Smoke. There is no evidence for an increase in ozone exposure in populated areas and in the

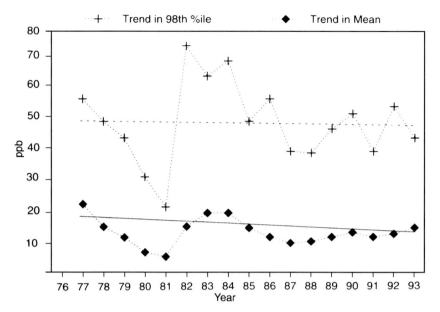

FIG. 5.   Trends in peak ozone concentrations in central London from 1977 to 1993. ppb, parts per billion.

cities exposure may have even fallen. Ambient levels of NO_2 have changed little. These observations argue against the air pollution hypothesis. Similar conclusions have been reached by workers in the USA (Lang & Polansky 1994). Certain indicators have, however, increased along with asthma. These are emissions of oxides of nitrogen, and the general trend towards increased emissions from vehicles, especially particles from diesel commercial vehicles and buses. If air pollution were responsible for the increase in asthma, this would need to be explained by some special quality of motor vehicle emissions and although this might be possible, other epidemiological evidence reviewed earlier in this chapter does not point towards traffic being an important factor. In particular, the even geographical distribution of asthma in the UK suggests that trends have been similar irrespective of ambient pollution levels.

Conclusion

From a toxicological and mechanistic viewpoint, it is plausible that air pollution could affect the biochemical and cellular processes which are relevant to asthma. There is some evidence from human chamber studies that this may occur in humans at ambient concentrations. The epidemiological evidence does not support the hypothesis that air pollution is important for the initiation of asthma at a population level. It is clear, however, that air pollution plays a role in the provocation of asthma, albeit a small one at a population level. The potential for air pollution to explain trends in asthma is therefore limited. When trends in asthma and air pollution are examined, there is no clear correlation between them. In particular, exposure to air pollution has generally declined in recent decades. On the other hand, there has been a shift towards motor vehicle pollution. Although some component of this cannot be excluded as contributing in a small way to the trend in asthma, other explanations for the trend are equally if not more plausible.

Acknowledgements

Much of the material and ideas in this chapter were derived from my participation with colleagues in the preparation of the report 'Asthma and Outdoor Air Pollution' for the Committee on the Medical Effects of Air Pollution of the Department of Health for England. I thank them, and especially Robert Maynard, who was the Scientific Secretary to the Asthma Subgroup.

References

American Thoracic Society 1996 Heath effects of outdoor air pollution. Am J Respir Crit Care Med 153:3–50

Anderson HR 1978 Respiratory abnormalities in Papua New Guinea children: the effects of locality and domestic wood smoke pollution. Int J Epidemiol 7:63–72

Anderson HR 1993 Is asthma really increasing? Paediatr Resp Med 1:6–10

Anderson HR, Limb ES, Bland JM, Ponce de Leon A, Strachan DP, Bower JS 1995 The health effects of an air pollution episode in London, December 1991. Thorax 50:1188–1193

Anto JM, Sunyer J, Rodriguez-Roison R, Suarez-Cervera M, Vasquez L 1989 Community outbreaks of asthma associated with inhalation of soybean dust. N Engl J Med 320:1097–1102

Austin JB, Russell G, Adam MG, Mackintosh D, Kelsey S, Peck DF 1994 Prevalence of asthma and wheeze in the Highlands of Scotland. Arch Dis Child 71:211–216

British Society for Allergy and Clinical Immunology 1995 Air pollution and allergic disease. Clin Exp Allergy 25(suppl 3)

Burney PGJ 1992 Epidemiology. In: Clark TJH, Godfrey S, Lee TH (eds) Asthma. Chapman & Hall, London, p 254–308

Burr ML 1987 Is asthma increasing? J Epidemiol Community Health 41:185–189

Burr ML 1993 Epidemiology of asthma. In: Burr ML (ed) Epidemiology of clinical allergy. Karger, Basel (Monographs Allergy Series 31) p 80–102

Burr ML 1995 Pollution: does it cause asthma? Arch Dis Child 72:377–379

Department of Health 1991 Advisory Group on the Medical Aspects of Air Pollution Episodes. First report: Ozone. HMSO, London

Department of Health 1992 Advisory Group on the Medical Aspects of Air Pollution Episodes. Second report: Sulphur dioxide acid aerosols and particulates. HMSO, London

Department of Health 1993 Advisory Group on the Medical Aspects of Air Pollution Episodes. Third report: Oxides of nitrogen. HMSO, London

Department of Health 1995a Department of Health Committee on the Medical Effects of Air Pollutants. Asthma and outdoor air pollution. HMSO, London

Department of Health 1995b Department of Health Committee on the Medical Effects of Air Pollutants. Non-biological particles and health. HMSO, London

Department of Health 1995c Advisory Group on the Medical Aspects of Air Pollution Episodes. Fourth report: Health effects of exposures to mixtures of air pollutants. HMSO, London

Dockery DW, Pope CA 1994 Acute respiratory effects of particulate air pollution. Ann Rev Public Health 15:107–132

Greer JR, Abbey de Burchette RJ 1993 Asthma related to occupational and ambient air pollutants in nonsmokers. J Occup Med 35:909–915

Hasselblad V, Eddy DM, Kotchmar DJ 1992 Synthesis of environmental evidence: nitrogen dioxide epidemiology studies. J Air Waste Manag Assoc 42:662–671

Jörres R, Nowak D, Magnussen H 1996 The effect of ozone exposure on allergen responsiveness in subjects with asthma or rhinitis. Am J Respir Crit Care Med 153:56–64

Lang DM, Polansky M 1994 Patterns of asthma mortality in Philadelphia from 1969 to 1991. New Engl J Med 331:1542–1546

Ministry of Health 1954 Reports on public health and medical subjects no. 95: Mortality and morbidity during the London fog of December 1952. HMSO, London

Quality of Urban Air Review Group 1993 Urban air quality in the United Kingdom. Department of the Environment, Bradford

Quality of Urban Air Review Group 1996 Airborne particulate matter in the United Kingdom. University of Birmingham, Birmingham

Robertson CF, Bishop J, Dalton M et al 1992 Prevalence of asthma in regional Victorian schoolchildren. Med J Aust 156:831–833

Seaton A, Godden D, Brown K 1994 Increase in asthma: a more toxic environment or a more susceptible population? Thorax 49:171–174

Strachan DP 1995a Time trends in asthma and allergy: ten questions, fewer answers. Clin Exp Allergy 25:791–794

Strachan DP 1995b Epidemiology. In: Silverman M (ed) Childhood asthma and other wheezing disorders. Chapman & Hall, London, p 7–31

Strachan DP, Anderson HR, Limb ES, O'Neill A, Wells N 1994 A national survey of asthma prevalence, severity, and treatment in Great Britain. Arch Dis Child 70:174–178

United Kingdom Photochemical Oxidants Review Group 1987 Ozone in the United Kingdom. Department of the Environment, London

Von Mutius E, Illi S, Nicolai T, Martinez F 1996 Relation of indoor heating with asthma, allergic sensitisation, and bronchial responsiveness: survey of children in Southern Bavaria. Br Med J 312:1448–1450

Wardlaw AJ 1993 The role of air pollution in asthma. Clin Exp Allergy 23:81–96

Weitzman M, Gortmaker S, Sobol A 1990 Racial, social, and environmental risks for childhood asthma. Am J Dis Child 144:1189–1194

Wjst M, Reitmeir P, Dold S et al 1993 Road traffic and adverse effects on respiratory health in children. Br Med J 307:596–600

DISCUSSION

Busse: Is there any evidence that air pollutants can act as additive risk factors for asthma?

H. R. Anderson: One of the problems with the daily hospital admissions studies is that although one can put more than one pollutant into the model, it becomes very muddy statistically and interactions may be difficult to determine, especially when one is working at the limits of detectability. Chamber studies will probably give us the best clue as to the possibility of interactions; my understanding of chamber study evidence is that an additive model would be the most feasible to adopt for public health purposes.

Nelson: Your data that air pollution is generally decreasing and asthma is increasing are convincing. However, you have not taken into account that the levels of diesel exhaust particulates, which act as an adjuvant and cause increased sensitization, are increasing.

H. R. Anderson: That's a fair comment. All I can say is that in a time-series study of asthma admissions in London, where we also put aeroallergens into the model, we couldn't find any evidence for an interaction. We measured levels of particles in the UK mainly by measuring the levels of Black Smoke particles, which are now largely due to diesel exhaust in urban areas. Although the levels of Black Smoke particles have decreased, the contribution to particle levels from road transport in both absolute and relative terms is increasing. Furthermore, the fine and ultra fine fractions, which we can't measure widely at the moment, are probably spread widely around the countryside. We now have the capacity to test the diesel particle–aeroallergen interaction hypothesis at a public health level.

Martinez: Your data can be compared with those from East and West Germany because the enormous burden of exposure to particulates in Leipzig is associated with less asthma and less bronchial responsiveness than in Munich (von Mutius et al 1994).

H. R. Anderson: The East and West German comparison is, in a sense, a cross-section of what has happened in the UK: in both cases traditional pollutants are associated with less asthma.

Magnussen: We have now reinvestigated the same groups of subjects in the different areas of Germany as their lifestyles are beginning to unify (Heinrich et al 1996). So far, we have found that in Hamburg, for example, the proportion of adults aged 20–44 years who have a positive skin prick test has remained almost the same over the last four years, whereas in Erjurt, which is in East Germany, the proportion is increasing. We will be testing these subjects again twice in the next 10 years.

I also have another comment. In our last series of chamber studies we found that responsiveness of the airways to allergen increased by a 1.8 doubling concentration with 3 h of intermittent exercise and 250 ppb ozone (Jörres et al 1996). I'm not sure what this means in terms of epidemiology but I'm sure that ozone is an important factor in increasing asthma symptoms.

H. R. Anderson: I agree.

Nelson: You indicated that there was a higher level of pollution in East Germany. Are you referring to industrial pollution? Because surely traffic pollution is greater in West Germany.

Magnussen: The East German air pollution studies were mainly based on measuring the levels of particles, which are decreasing at present. However, the concentration of NO_2, which is an index of traffic-related pollution, did not differ considerably between East and West Germany.

Martinez: I would like to add to that the data that Erika von Mutius and I recently published on children living in rural areas of Bavaria (von Mutius et al 1996). We found that children who were exposed to coal or wood stoves at home were significantly less likely to have a positive skin test to allergens, bronchial hyper-responsiveness or asthma than those who were not exposed to wood or coal in their homes.

Weiss: There's a certain amount of ecological evidence that particulate air pollution decreases the risk of asthma. However, how is exposure to particulates or wood smoke, for example, translated into an immunological effect?

Holt: Experiments with animal models have shown that interfering with the function of lung macrophages, either by administration of toxic particulates or by particulate overload, can disturb local immunoregulation, leading to selective stimulation of T helper 2 cell-dependent immune responses (Thepen et al 1992).

Holgate: The opposite side of this is that many of these pollutants, including particulates, are oxidants. By interacting with the airway epithelium, probably through the transcription factor NFκB, they generate chemokines and cytokines, up-regulate a range of vascular adhesion molecules (Manning et al 1994) and, therefore, produce an inflammatory reaction.

Holt: Bengt Björkstén and colleagues have looked at primary allergic sensitization and how it relates to air pollution. They found that associations are not observed unless the population is stratified. That is, if the high risk group is first identified then factors such as environmental tobacco smoke and industrial air pollution show a more significant association with primary sensitization (Björkstén 1994).

Kay: It is possible that pollen counts may be misleading as an index of outdoor allergen exposure. For example, the large increase in asthma admissions that was associated with thunderstorms was preceded by a large burst of pollen 48 h previously (Murray et al 1994). Most of the people affected were atopic and highly sensitive to grass pollen, raising the possibility that allergens are leaching out of pollen grains such that their dispersal is independent of the actual pollen grain count. Therefore, the measurements of allergen exposure may be inaccurate. Linked to this is the issue of diesel fumes combining with allergenic material to produce particularly potent sensitizing agents.

H. R. Anderson: To investigate this hypothesis using epidemiological methods, we need daily data over three or four years which we can analyse using time-series methods. All we have at the moment are pollen counts not pollen grain counts.

Magnussen: Ozone is clearly an initiator of inflammatory reactions. The lag period between inhalation of ozone and the cellular reaction is between four and 24 h. Therefore, it is possible that ozone together with pollen increases the response, so that the pollen count alone is not an appropriate measure of inflammation (Peden et al 1995).

Woolcock: But exposure to ozone causes symptoms, it does not cause asthma.

Burney: If one looks at people who are skin test positive to grass, the period when they experience most symptoms is in the summer, suggesting that exposure to grass pollen is an important exposure, at least in this group.

Strachan: The most likely explanation for this asthma outbreak in June 1994 is that it occurred in a group of highly pollen-sensitive individuals, many of whom had not suffered asthmatic symptoms before, and whose symptoms were triggered for the first time in response to a thunderstorm and shortly after a high pollen count. It was probably caused by abnormal dispersal and/or disruption of pollen that enabled it to be inhaled more deeply into the airway than it would normally be. Therefore, I agree with your point in general, but there are situations where pollen allergy could cause asthma attacks.

Nelson: Several investigators have shown that grass ragweed antigens are carried on small particles or even in vapour form throughout the pollen season (Spieksma et al 1990, Schumacher et al 1988, Agarwal et al 1984, Habenicht et al 1984). Also, the study at the Mayo clinic by Welsh et al (1987) showed that in some patients there is a progressive development of asthma symptoms throughout the pollen season, and Reid et al (1986) have shown that in northern California epidemics of asthma occur during the grass pollen season. Therefore, we shouldn't deny that plant products, although perhaps not pollen grains, can cause asthma.

Holgate: Creating symptoms is one thing, creating a new disease is an entirely different matter.

References

Agarwal MK, Swanson MC, Reed CE, Yunginger JW 1984 Airborne ragweed allergens: association with various particle sizes and short ragweed plant parts. J Allergy Clin Immunol 74:687–693

Björkstén B 1994 Risk factors in early childhood for the development of atopic diseases. Allergy 49:400–407

Habenicht HA, Burge HA, Mullenberg ML, Solomon WR 1984 Allergen carriage by atmospheric aerosol. II. Ragweed–pollen determinants in submicronic atmospheric fractions. J Allergy Clin Immunol 74:64–67

Heinrich J, Richter K, Magnussen H, Wichmann HE 1996 Do asthma and asthma symptoms in adults already converge between East and West Germany? Am J Respir Crit Care Med 153:856A

Jörres R, Nowak D, Magnussen H 1996 The effect of ozone exposure on allergen responsiveness in subjects with asthma or rhinitis. Am J Respir Crit Care Med 153:56–64

Manning AM, Anderson DC, Bristol JA et al 1994 Transcription factor NF-κB: an emerging regulator of inflammation. Ann Rep Med Chem. Acad press, San Diego, CA, p 235–244

Murray V, Venables K, Laing-Morton T, Partridge M, Thurston J, Williams D 1994 Epidemic of asthma possibly related to thunderstorms. Br Med J 309:131–132

Peden DB, Setzer RW, Devlin RB 1995 Ozone exposure has both a priming effect on allergen-induced responses and an intrinsic inflammatory action in the nasal airways of perennially allergic asthmatics. Am J Respir Crit Care Med 151:1336–1345

Reid MJ, Moss RB, Hsu Y-P, Kwasnicki JM, Commerford TM, Nelson BL 1986 Seasonal asthma in northern California: allergic causes and efficacy of immunotherapy. J Allergy Clin Immunol 78:590–600

Schumacher MJ, Griffith RD, O'Rourke MK 1988 Recognition of pollen and other particulate aeroantigens by immunoblot microscopy. J Allergy Clin Immunol 82:608–616

Spieksma FTM, Kramps JA, van der Linden AC et al 1990 Evidence of grass pollen allergenic activity in the smaller micronic atmosphere aerosol fraction. Clin Exp Allergy 20:273–280

Thepen T, McMenamin C, Girn B, Kraal G, Holt PG 1992 Regulation of IgE production in presensitized animals: *in vivo* elimination of alveolar macrophages preferentially increases IgE responses to inhaled allergen. Clin Exp Allergy 22:1107–1114

von Mutius E, Martinez FD, Fritzsch C, Nicolai T, Roell G, Thiemann HH 1994 Prevalence of asthma and atopy in two areas of West Germany and East Germany. Am J Respir Crit Care Med 149:358–364

von Mutius E, Illi S, Nicolai T, Martinez FD 1996 Relation of indoor heating with asthma, allergic sensitisation and bronchial responsiveness: survey of children in south Bavaria. Br Med J 312:1448–1450

Welsh PW, Stricker WE, Chu C-P et al 1987 Efficacy of beclomethasone nasal solution, flunisolide, and cromolyn in relieving symptoms of ragweed allergy. Mayo Clin Proc 62:125–134

The role of respiratory viruses in asthma

William W. Busse, James E. Gern and Elliot C. Dick

University of Wisconsin Medical School, JS/220 Clinical Science Center, 600 Highland Avenue, Madison, WI 53792–3244, USA

Abstract. Respiratory infections are common causes of increased asthma for patients of all ages. Current evidence indicates that viral, and not bacterial, infections are the most important respiratory illnesses which increase the severity of asthma. Of the respiratory viral infections associated with increased asthma, rhinoviruses, i.e. the cause of common colds, have proven to be the virus most often found in association with increased asthma severity. Although the association between rhinovirus infections and asthma is most dramatically illustrated in children, asthma patients of all ages can be affected and the attacks of asthma can be severe. Studies to establish the mechanisms by which rhinoviruses enhance asthma severity have begun to focus on how this virus promotes allergic inflammation. We have found that experimental rhinovirus infections enhance airway responsiveness and, perhaps most importantly, the likelihood that a late allergic reaction will occur to an antigen challenge. Furthermore, using bronchoscopy and segmental antigen challenge, we have found that rhinovirus infections promote mast cell release of histamine and the recruitment of eosinophils to the airways. These data support the concept that rhinovirus infections act to promote allergic inflammation and by this mechanism increase both the likelihood of asthma occurring and the severity of wheezing.

1997 The rising trends in asthma. Wiley, Chichester (Ciba Foundation Symposium 206) p 208–219

Respiratory viral infections are important causes of wheezing for many patients with asthma (Stark & Busse 1991, Pattemore et al 1992, Bardin et al 1992, Johnston et al 1993). In young healthy infants, respiratory syncytial virus (RSV) and parainfluenza virus infection cause wheezing episodes that may be recurrent in some individuals (Martinez et al 1988). Moreover, these episodes are more frequent in boys but become less of a problem by the second year of life. An apparent major factor in episodes of RSV-induced wheezing is the existence of small, underdeveloped airways in young male infants. As the child grows older, the airway size increases, and the mechanical occlusion of the airway associated with the viral infection becomes less of a problem. There are, however, individuals who experience recurrent episodes of wheezing with colds and go on to develop persistent asthma. Individuals with this susceptibility usually have a family history of allergic diseases (Martinez et al 1995).

In older children and young adults, respiratory infections continue to be a cause of wheezing, but the causative virus is different. Duff and colleagues at the University of

TABLE 1   Odds ratios for wheezing among children with a positive radio-allergosorbent test (RAST), virus culture or elevated cotinine level (data from Duff et al 1993)

Risk factor	Odds ratio	
	Age < 2 years	Age > 2 years
RAST	+/−	4.5
Virus	8.2	3.7
Cotinine (⩾10 ng/ml)	4.7	0.6
RAST and virus	+/−	10.8

Virginia (Duff et al 1993) evaluated children who presented to an emergency room with acute episodes of wheezing. In children less than two years of age, nearly 70% of those presenting with wheezing had virus growing on culture of their airway secretions; RSV was the major infection associated with wheezing in these young children. In contrast, children greater than two years of age with wheezing had virus cultured in only 31% of such episodes, and the respiratory virus detected in these children was rhinovirus. To further evaluate this situation, the investigators calculated the odds ratio for wheezing in these two groups of children (Table 1). For children less than two years of age, the existence of a respiratory infection and passive exposure to smoke was an important risk factor for wheezing. In children greater than two years of age, in contrast, allergy and the presence of virus were the risk factors associated with wheezing. These studies indicate an age-dependent relationship between the infecting virus and the possibility that the coexistence of allergic disease is a major risk factor for children over two years of age to wheeze with respiratory infections.

Sebastian Johnston and colleagues at Southampton evaluated 108 children, aged nine to 11 years, over a 13-month period (Johnston et al 1995). In this study population episodes of increased asthma or symptoms of an upper respiratory infection were noted by the subjects and evaluated by measurements of lung function and collection of airway secretions for virus culture and virus RNA. The investigators found that over 80% of the wheezing episodes in these children were associated with viral respiratory infections. Furthermore, reverse transcriptase (RT)-PCR techniques demonstrated that rhinovirus was noted in 60% of the wheezing episodes. The observations by Johnston and his co-workers indicate the importance of respiratory infections, particularly rhinovirus, to asthma exacerbations, and that in some patients these episodes can be severe.

These, and other studies, underscore the importance of viral respiratory infections to exacerbations of wheezing in infants and children. It is also apparent that the virus associated with these wheezing episodes is age dependent. Furthermore, there is evidence that the coexistence of allergic disease becomes an important risk factor, along with rhinovirus infections, when children are over two years of age. The following discussion will examine the effect of rhinovirus infection on airway function and review the known mechanisms by which rhinovirus infections can promote the possibility of wheezing with colds and the development of allergic inflammation.

Mechanisms of rhinovirus-induced wheezing

A number of mechanisms have been proposed to explain how respiratory viruses induce asthma. These include:

(1) damage to airway epithelium;
(2) reflex bronchospasm from upper airway inflammation;
(3) aspiration of upper airway inflammatory mediators;
(4) local airway generation of pro-inflammatory cytokines;
(5) enhanced recruitment of inflammatory cells to the airway;
(6) enhanced inflammatory mediator release; and
(7) generation of virus-specific IgE antibodies.

Although all of these factors likely play some role in wheezing with respiratory infections, it is our hypothesis that respiratory viruses, including rhinovirus, generate cytokines which then up-regulate existing airway inflammation and thus increase the likelihood that asthma will occur.

To begin to address the effect that rhinoviruses may have on airway inflammation, Lemanske et al (1989) evaluated the effect of a rhinovirus infection on bronchial responsiveness and the airway response to inhaled allergen in 10 individuals with allergic rhinitis. In these subjects, the experimental rhinovirus infection increased airway responsiveness to inhaled histamine. The immediate airway response to inhaled antigen was also enhanced and it paralleled changes in airway responsiveness. More importantly, Lemanske et al (1989) observed that the frequency of late allergic reactions to inhaled allergen increased during the acute rhinovirus infection. Prior to the rhinovirus infection, one of 10 subjects had a late allergic reaction. At the time of the acute rhinovirus infection, eight of the 10 subjects had a late allergic reaction to an allergen challenge. Furthermore, when evaluated four weeks after recovery from the viral respiratory infection, five of the seven individuals continued to have a late allergic reaction. These observations suggest that one mechanism by which respiratory viruses promote airway hyper-responsiveness and the possibility wheezing is through an enhancement of those factors that cause the development of late allergic reactions, a model for allergen-driven inflammation.

In a subsequent study from our institution, Calhoun et al (1994) used bronchoscopy and segmental challenge of the airway with antigen to evaluate the effects of a rhinovirus infection allergic inflammatory in the airway. In this study, subjects were seen on three separate occasions: (1) pre-cold; (2) during acute respiratory infection;

and (3) four weeks post-infection. During each study period, the subjects had two bronchoscopies. At the first bronchoscopy, antigen was introduced into the airway and lavage was performed immediately afterwards. This approach evaluates the effect of antigen on the acute allergic response that is characterized by mast cell activation and mediator release. Forty-eight hours later bronchoscopy was repeated, and the same airway segments were identified and re-lavaged. The timing of this procedure allowed us to measure those features associated with late allergic reactions, i.e. the inflammatory response. When bronchoscopy and antigen challenge were conducted during the acute rhinovirus infection, mast cell histamine release to antigen was increased. More importantly, eosinophil recruitment measured 48 h after antigen challenge was also greater during the acute rhinovirus infection. The increase in eosinophil recruitment was still detected four weeks after the acute respiratory infection. These studies suggest that an experimental rhinovirus infection of the upper airway promotes allergen-driven allergic responses in the lower airway and this enhancement in the response to antigen is seen predominantly in those features associated with the late allergic inflammatory response, i.e. eosinophils.

To expand upon these observations and the influence of respiratory infections on bronchial inflammation, Fraenkel et al (1995) experimentally infected subjects with rhinovirus to evaluate its effect on lower airway histology. During the rhinovirus infection, the infected subjects had an increase in airway responsiveness. Lower airway biopsies were also obtained and analyses revealed a number of interesting changes. First, there was an increase in CD3+ cells infiltrating the submucosa; these changes were found in both asthmatic and normal subjects. Moreover, airway mucosal eosinophilia was increased at the time of the viral respiratory infection and persisted for weeks beyond the infection, but only in those subjects with asthma. These observations imply that eosinophil function and its involvement in allergic inflammation is influenced by viral respiratory infections. The increase in eosinophils could contribute to airway inflammation and, with these changes, a heightened level of bronchial responsiveness and tendency to wheeze.

Mechanisms of rhinovirus-induced airway inflammation

The above observations raise the possibility that rhinoviruses can enhance or promote the development of allergic inflammation. A number of *in vitro* models have been developed to evaluate the consequences of rhinovirus interactions with immune cells. In one series of experiments, airway macrophages were isolated by bronchoalveolar lavage and then incubated with either RV16 or culture fluid. In these experiments, Gern et al (1996) found that RV16 caused macrophages to generate tumour necrosis factor (TNF)-α and interleukin (IL)-1β. The generation of these cytokines occurred in the absence of rhinovirus replication within the airway macrophages. The release of these particular pro-inflammatory cytokines could have a profound effect on airway epithelium and increase the expression of adhesion markers, e.g. intercellular adhesion molecule (ICAM)-1, and function of inflammatory cells present in the lung.

To extend these observations and further elucidate the effect of rhinovirus on cell function, we incubated peripheral blood mononuclear cells with RV16. When supernatants were collected 22 h following incubation with RV16, increased concentrations of interferon (IFN)-α were detected. Although IFN-γ is important in host defence against viral respiratory infections, it can also activate lymphocytes as indicated by an increase in the expression of CD69.

Finally, we evaluated the effect of RV16 incubation with peripheral blood mononuclear cells on markers of cell activation. Peripheral blood mononuclear cells were incubated for 22 h with rhinovirus and then evaluated by flow cytometry. The rhinovirus exposure caused CD3$^+$ lymphocytes to increase their expression of the early activation marker, CD69. Furthermore, when the CD3$^+$ CD69$^+$ cells were isolated by flow cytometry, and evaluated by RT-PCR, an increased expression of mRNA for IFN-γ was noted.

Collectively, these *in vitro* studies indicate that rhinoviruses can activate lymphocytes and cause the generation of cytokines, which, under appropriate circumstances, can have pro-inflammatory actions. Furthermore, when rhinoviruses interact with macrophages, these cells produce and secrete TNF-α and IL-1β. These cytokines can up-regulate epithelial expression of ICAM-1. Since ICAM-1 is the major receptor for rhinoviruses, rhinoviruses may have a greater likelihood to infect and perpetuate the process. IFN-α is also generated by RV16 activation of monocytes and thus cytokines can act upon T lymphocytes to increase their CD69 expression. Activation of the subpopulation of CD3$^+$ CD69$^+$ cells is associated with an increased expression of mRNA encoding IFN-γ, which can then have a pro-inflammatory effects upon eosinophils, as well as increasing adhesion proteins on airway epithelium.

Finally, in preliminary studies, we have evaluated the possibility that eosinophils may have a direct role in the immune response to rhinoviruses. In a series of experiments, we found small amounts of rhinovirus bound to unactivated eosinophils. When eosinophils were activated by IFN-γ, in contrast, and when they expressed more ICAM-1 receptors, rhinovirus binding was increased. Further, when rhinoviruses and eosinophils were incubated with peripheral blood mononuclear cells, lymphocyte proliferation occurred. These studies strongly suggest that eosinophils can act as antigen-presenting cells for rhinoviruses and can also activate lymphocytes. It has not been determined whether the activated lymphocytes generate a unique cytokine profile.

Summary

Rhinovirus infections are major causes of wheezing. From *in vivo* studies, rhinoviruses have been shown to increase features of allergic inflammation, i.e. expression of the late allergic reaction, release of mast cell mediators and recruitment of eosinophils to the airways. Moreover, there is *in vitro* evidence that rhinoviruses cause lymphocytes and macrophages to generate a variety of pro-inflammatory cytokines. Given these observations, we hypothesize that rhinovirus infections change the cytokine milieu of the lower airway; if allergen exposure occurs in this 'new' inflammatory setting, the likelihood for and intensity of allergic inflammation is greater. In the patient with existing asthma, the end result will be enhanced inflammation and asthma.

Acknowledgement

This work was supported by grants AI 26609 and HL44098 from the National Institutes of Health.

References

Bardin PG, Johnston SL, Pattemore PK 1992 Viruses as precipitants of asthma symptoms. II. Physiology and mechanisms. Clin Exp Allergy 22:809–822

Calhoun WJ, Dick EC, Schwartz LB, Busse WW 1994 A common cold virus, rhinovirus 16, potentiates airway inflammation after segmental antigen bronchoprovocation in allergic subjects. J Clin Invest 94:2200–2208

Duff AL, Pomeranz ES, Gelber LE et al 1993 Risk factors for acute wheezing in infants and children: viruses, passive smoke, and IgE antibodies to inhalant allergens. Pediatrics 92:535–540

Fraenkel DJ, Bardin PG, Sanderson G, Lampe F, Johnston SL, Holgate ST 1995 Lower airways inflammation during rhinovirus colds in normal and in asthmatic subjects. Am J Respir Crit Care Med 151:879–886

Gern JE, Dick EC, Lee WM et al 1996 Rhinovirus enters but does not replicate inside monocytes and airway macrophages. J Immunol 156:621–627

Johnston SL, Bardin PG, Pattemore PK 1993 Viruses as precipitants of asthma symptoms. III. Rhinoviruses: molecular biology and prospects for future intervention. Clin Exp Allergy 23:237–246

Johnston SL, Pattemore PK, Sanderson G et al 1995 Community study of role of viral infections in exacerbations of asthma in 9–11-year-old children. Br Med J 310:1225–1228

Lemanske RF Jr, Dick EC, Swenson CA, Vrtis RF, Busse WW 1989 Rhinovirus upper respiratory infection increases airway hyperreactivity and late asthmatic reactions. J Clin Invest 83:1–10

Martinez FD, Morgan WJ, Wright AL, Holberg CJ, Taussig LM, Group Health Medical Associates Personnel 1988 Diminished lung function as a predisposing factor for wheezing respiratory illness in infants. N Engl J Med 319:1112–1117

Martinez FD, Wright AL, Taussig LM et al 1995 Asthma and wheezing in the first six years of life. N Engl J Med 332:133–138

Pattemore PK, Johnston SL, Bardin PG 1992 Viruses as precipitants of asthma symptoms. I. Epidemiology. Clin Exp Allergy 22:325–336

Stark JM, Busse WW 1991 Respiratory virus infection and airway hyperreactivity in children. Pediatr Allergy Immunol 2:95–110

DISCUSSION

Brostoff: What is the mechanism for turning off inflammation?

Busse: At the moment we've been more interested in establishing the mechanism by which respiratory viruses turn on inflammation. One reason why asthmatic subjects may have more difficulty with rhinovirus infection is because they express more intercellular adhesion molecule (ICAM)-1 on their epithelium. Furthermore, they may have more inflammatory cells in the airway. These pre-existing conditions may make these individuals more likely to shift from being non-symptomatic to symptomatic.

Holgate: We have developed a technique using *in situ* PCR applied to bronchial biopsies to find out which cells contain the viral genome, and we have found that most of the rhinovirus-positive cells are epithelial cells (Bates et al 1997). Viral mRNA is not present in eosinophils or in T cells, and only the occasional monocyte/macrophage contains viral mRNA. Purely from this observation alone, we could conclude that, although the lower airway can be infected, the epithelium itself is sufficient to drive the inflammatory response towards an exacerbation of asthma.

Busse: I agree. The epithelium is the primary target for the rhinovirus.

Boushey: I also agree that the epithelial cell may be the pivotal cell mediating the airway changes caused by the rhinovirus. The nasal lavage from children with natural rhinovirus infection or from people with induced rhinovirus infection contains increased levels of interleukin (IL)-6 and IL-8. IL-8 is a potent chemoattractant of polymorphonuclear leukocytes (PMNs). The sputum produced spontaneously by patients with acute asthma contains many PMNs in addition to eosinophils, and Sur et al (1993) have shown that the airways of people dying within a few hours of the onset of the attack contain many PMNs. Therefore, the asthmatic attacks provoked by viral infection may involved not just an amplification of the attraction of eosinophils but also alteration and activation of PMNs.

Busse: Part of this may be explained by the time at which samples are taken.

Platts-Mills: In Bill Busse's study of rhinovirus infection without allergen challenge, increased numbers of eosinophils in the lung were not observed. In contrast, Fraenkel et al (1995) did see an up-regulation of eosinophils in the lung.

Busse: But these experiments are different. We measured the numbers of eosinophils in bronchial lavage fluid and did not observe an increase without allergen challenge. In contrast Fraenkel et al (1995) analysed bronchial biopsies.

Platts-Mills: Fraenkel et al (1994) described studies of nasal biopsies, in which they injected rhinoviruses into the nose but didn't observe eosinophil up-regulation there either acutely or later on. Why did they see up-regulation of eosinophils in the lung (Fraenkel et al 1995) but not in the nose, when clearly the primary impact of the rhinovirus is in the nose?

Holgate: Because these are people suffering from asthma. If we had looked at subjects with allergic rhinitis we may have observed eosinophil recruitment and activation in the nasal mucosa. In our experience rhinovirus infection leading to the common cold is accompanied either by no overall nasal leukocyte response (Fraenkel et al 1994) or a neutrophilia (Teran et al 1997).

Martinez: Are these reactions exclusive to the lung or the nose? Have you looked at peripheral blood eosinophils?

Busse: We observed an increase in eosinophils in lavage fluid but not in the circulation. However, we did not look at the function of airway eosinophils.

Holgate: We have obtained similar results with human peripheral blood basophils at the peak of the common cold in asthmatics, not only in response to IgE-dependent stimulation but also to ligation of CD49 and CD29a of the very late antigen (VLA)-4 receptor (whose natural ligand is either fibronectin or vascular adhesion molecule 1) (Thomas et al 1995). However, we have not yet looked at the same stimuli when applied to eosinophils.

Busse: It is possible that corticosteroids decrease airway inflammation and thus make it less likely for a viral infection to increase airway injury and hence asthma.

Holgate: We gave nine- to 11-year-old wheezy children 400 µg beclomethasone dipropionate as a dry powder or matched placebo daily for six months and looked at the frequency, magnitude and duration of virus-induced episodes of upper and lower respiratory symptoms, and also at the peak expiratory flow rate (Doull et al 1997). Despite having clear effects on growth (Doull et al 1995), inhaled corticosteroids had only a minor effect in reducing the magnitude of the episodes, with no effect on the frequency or duration. The reported beneficial effect of rapid corticosteroids on virus-induced asthma episodes has crept into the literature with remarkably little evidence in the form of clinical trials to support the practice.

Boushey: I have also recently searched for literature supporting the worldwide practice of doubling the dose of inhalant steroids for asthma. I could only find two studies that analysed this specifically (Lahdensuo et al 1996, Wilson & Silverman 1990). It seems to be a recommendation based on slender evidence.

Holt: What are the differences in the pathology of rhinovirus infection between asthmatics and non-asthmatics?

Holgate: The only difference that we observed was that there was a persistence of eosinophilia in the asthmatics (Fraenkel et al 1995). This was not the case for neutrophils or T cells in the lower airway: the levels of these cells increased and then decreased in both asthmatics and non-asthmatics. We did not look at the levels of cytokines.

Martinez: Is anything known about the influence of viruses on apoptosis of eosinophils?

Holgate: No, not as far as I am aware.

Busse: One point to bear in mind is that you have only looked at small pieces of tissue from large areas, so one should be wary of making generalizations. Larger biopsies from the nose have not demonstrated any effect of rhinovirus on airway histopathology. Most studies suggest that rhinoviruses do not cause inflammatory changes in the epithelium.

Boushey: That is what is so interesting. It's difficult to find cells that are infected, and the rhinovirus seems to have little inflammatory effect, so the key may lie in defining how the inflammatory response is amplified in the asthmatic airway.

Holgate: In nasal lavages of both atopic and non-atopic people, we found that there were large increases in all of the chemokines that we studied. These included IL-8, monocyte chemotactic protein-1α and macrophage inflammatory protein-1α, in addition to other cytokines — IL-1β (but not IL-1α) tumour necrosis factor (TNF)-α, γ-interferon (IFN-γ), granulocyte macrophage colony-stimulating factor (GM-CSF) and IL-6. Of these products, atopics had greater and more prolonged elevations of IL-6, TNF-α and GM-CSF (Teran et al 1997, Lau et al 1996).

Kay: I would like to ask Bill Busse to clarify T cell sensitization in his model. You suggested that eosinophils act as antigen-presenting cells (APCs), inducing the proliferation of T cells. On the other hand, you seemed to suggest that your observations were immunologically non-specific.

Busse: There was an increased expression of CD3$^+$ CD69$^+$ lymphocytes following inoculation of mononuclear cells with rhinovirus. This suggests that the cellular response to rhinovirus may be specific (i.e. that a few clones respond to the virus) or non-specific (i.e. that cells are activated as a consequence of the mononuclear generation of cytokines).

Kay: Don't you think this is surprising, considering the frequency of rhinovirus infection?

Busse: These *in vitro* results suggest that viruses are recognized by APCs and that this non-specifically initiates a response which includes cytokine generation. Such a possibility may explain why patients experience chest symptoms within 48 h.

Britton: Is there any evidence of a change in the exposure to virus infections which may explain the rising prevalence of asthma?

Burney: Or that may explain the different prevalences in different places? Because the general understanding is that viral infections, in contrast to bacterial infections, don't vary greatly between places.

Holgate: I am not totally certain about this because the human rhinoviruses that cause most of the common colds are so fastidious. The studies have not yet been done because the PCR technology required has only just been developed. PCR-based virus identification has to be linked with epidemiology to find out more about the behaviour of these viruses.

Paré: Does allergic inflammation make viral infection worse, vice versa or both? In other words, does the up-regulation of ICAM-1 result in a persistence of virus and more lower airway infection with virus? Have you done quantitative PCR analysis to determine whether the viral infection is more persistent in asthmatics?

Busse: We have not conducted these experiments.

Holgate: What one can demonstrate in cultured epithelial cells is that if a small amount of cytokine is introduced, such as TNF-α or IFN-γ, the cells become more sensitive to infection at much lower doses of virus than otherwise would be the case. Once a few viruses penetrate the cell, then through mechanisms yet to be defined, they up-regulate the expression of ICAM-1 (Papi et al 1996), the receptor for the major subtype of rhinovirus. The presence of these cytokines at biologically active concentrations in asthmatic airways would render the epithelial cells more susceptible to occupation by rhinovirus. Another interesting point we've shown in these *in situ* PCR experiments is that the basal cells seem to be infected in preference to the suprabasal cells. If, on account of epithelial disruption as occurs in asthma, the basal cell population is more exposed to the environment than in the case of non-asthmatics, then these cells are likely to be more easily occupied by virus. Also, in the presence of cytokines ICAM-1 is more easily expressed on basal cells than on suprabasal cells.

Platts-Mills: Canonica et al (1995) have shown that natural exposure to allergen up-regulates ICAM-1 expression. Do you have similar results?

Holgate: We have only looked at this using image analysis on immuno-histochemistry, which is not ideal. The best way of quantifying the amount of product on the surface of a cell is to do immunogold labelling and count the number of gold grains using an electron microscope. This has not been done with virus infection *in vivo*.

Potter: You showed that if your cells are incubated with rhinovirus there is an increased IL-1β expression *in vitro*. Have you measured the levels of IL-1β in the nasal lavage of asthmatics who are infected with rhinovirus? In the mouse model it is possible to activate T helper (Th) 2 cells directly through the IL-1β receptor. This is not the case for Th1 cells because they do not have the IL-1β receptor. Therefore, the demonstration of elevated levels of IL-1β in nasal fluids may explain the eosinophilia.

Busse: No, we have not done this.

Holgate: We have found high levels of IL-1β, but not IL-1α, in nasal lavage fluid, so there is a definite selection of cytokines.

Heusser: Have you looked for the production of IL-4 and IL-5 by these clones?

Busse: We observed variable responses among the generated clones. Some secrete IFN-γ.

Heusser: There seems to be a certain amount of bystander activation occurring because only a small fraction of these cells are specific. However, the majority of cells express the activation marker.

Busse: I agree, but I don't have any additional information.

Boushey: When the intensity and duration of nasal symptoms following rhinovirus inoculation in atopic and non-atopic subjects are compared, no difference is found among the subjects naïve to the virus. In atopic subjects who have antibody titre to that specific strain, however, the symptomatic response is greater than in non-atopic subjects (Bardin et al 1994).

Holgate: I would like to raise the issue of indoor air pollution. There is some literature beginning to emerge on the accumulation of chemical air pollutants in the home. Does anyone have any information on this?

Burney: The results we recently published on adults suggested that women who had gas stoves at home had worse lung function and more symptoms than women who had electric cookers (Jarvis et al 1996). These results were more striking than one would expect. However, this was just one study, so we should wait for more data on a much broader spectrum of the population before we jump to any conclusions. There are other isolated studies that have looked at other pollutants in the home, but again these tend to be one-off studies at the moment.

H. R. Anderson: In New Guinea, the population burn wood in their houses but the prevalence of asthma there is low, so it is quite clear that high levels of indoor pollution alone are not sufficient to initiate asthma. As far as cooking with gas is concerned, the evidence is conflicting. One of the things that could be discussed is, in view of the chamber studies showing an interaction between nitrogen dioxide and aeroallergens, whether we should look at the interaction between gas cooking and house dust mite allergens or some other aeroallergen in the home.

Strachan: Air pollution can be usefully addressed in terms of personal exposure because much of the public concern about outdoor air pollution fails to take into account what people are actually breathing in. This comes back to the discussions of lifestyle and activity. We spend about eight hours a day in bed, so we should consider this as being one of the major sources of inhaled irritants or allergens. There is also the question of what exposures do we receive during the rest of the time we spend indoors, and do these have any influence? We only have crude tools available to us. We usually measure only the reservoir or emission source but we should think more about the methods of dispersal and the possibility that particles and allergens remain airborne for longer in some circumstances than in others.

References

Bardin PG, Fraenkel DJ, Sanderson G et al 1994 Amplified rhinovirus colds in atopic subjects. Clin Exp Allergy 24:457–464

Bates P, Sanderson G, Holgate ST, Johnston SL 1997 *In situ* RT-PCR to identify rhinovirus replication in epithelial cells. British Assoc Lung Res summer meeting, 19–20 Sept 1996 (abstr), Respir Med, in press

Canonica GW, Ciprandi G, Pesce GP, Buscaglia S, Paolieri F, Bagnasco M 1995 ICAM-1 on epithelial cells in allergic subjects: a hallmark of allergic inflammation. Int Arch Allergy Immunol 107:99–102

Doull IJM, Freezer NJ, Holgate ST 1995 Growth of prepubertal children with asthma treated with inhaled beclomethasone dipropionate. Am J Respir Crit Care Med 151:1715–1719

Doull IJM, Lampe F, Smith S, Schreiber J, Freezer NJ, Holgate ST 1997 The effect of inhaled corticosteroids on episodes of viral-associated wheezing in school age children. Br Med J, submitted

Fraenkel DJ, Bardin PG, Sanderson G, Lampe F, Johnston SL, Holgate ST 1994 Immunohistochemical analysis of nasal mucosal biopsies during experimental colds. Rhinovirus 16 in atopic and non-atopic volunteers. Am J Respir Crit Care Med 150:1130–1136

Fraenkel DJ, Bardin PG, Sanderson G, Lampe F, Johnston SL, Holgate ST 1995 Lower airways inflammation during rhinovirus colds in normal and in asthmatic subjects. Am J Respir Crit Care Med 151:879–886

Jarvis D, Chinn S, Luczynska C, Burney P 1996 Association of respiratory symptoms and lung function in young adults with use of domestic gas appliances. Lancet 347:426–431

Lahdensuo A, Haahtela T, Hennale J et al 1996 Randomized comparison of guided self-management and traditional treatment of asthma over one year. Br Med J 312:748–752

Lau LCK, Corne JM, Scott SJ, Davies R, Friend E, Howarth PH 1996 Nasal cytokines in common cold. Am J Respir Crit Care Med 153:697 (abstr)

Papi A, Wilson SJ, Johnston SL 1996 Rhinoviruses increase production of adhesion molecules (CAM) and NF-κB. Am J Respir Crit Care Med 153:866 (abstr)

Sur S, Crotty TB, Kephart GM et al 1993 Sudden-onset fatal asthma. Am Rev Respir Dis 148:713–719

Teran LM, Johnston SL, Schröder J-M, Church MK, Holgate ST 1997 Relationship of interleukin-8 to neutrophil influx in naturally occurring colds in asthmatic children. Am J Respir Crit Care Med 1996, in press

Thomas LH, Corne JM, Holgate ST, Warner JA 1995 Integrin clustering causes increased histamine release (HR) from basophils of patients with symptomatic colds. FASEB J 9:1046A

Wilson NM, Silverman M 1990 Treatment of acute, episodic asthma in preschool children using intermittent high dose inhaled steroids at home. Arch Dis child 65:407–410

Prenatal origins of asthma and allergy

Jill A. Warner, Amanda C. Jones, Elizabeth A. Miles, Brenda M. Colwell and John O. Warner

Department of Child Health, University of Southampton, Level G, Centre Block, Southampton General Hospital, Tremona Road, Southampton SO16 6YD, UK

Abstract. The prevalence of asthma and related allergic disorders has increased considerably over the last 25 years. Genetic stock has not changed, so environmental factors must have influenced the phenotype. Infants who develop allergy already have an altered immune response at birth. We have investigated the development of immune responses during gestation and the effect of maternal allergen exposure during pregnancy and infant exposure in the first month of life on the development of allergy and disease. There was higher specific peripheral blood mononuclear cell proliferation to house dust mite ($P = 0.01$) and birch pollen ($P = 0.004$) in the third trimester compared with the second trimester, with the first positive responses seen at 22 weeks gestation. Maternal exposure to birch pollen after 22 weeks resulted in higher ($P = 0.005$) infant peripheral blood mononuclear cell responses to birch pollen at birth. Infants born at term, with at least one atopic, asthmatic parent, who developed allergic symptoms and positive skin prick test by one year of age had raised proliferative responses to house dust mites at birth compared to those with no symptoms ($P = 0.01$). In genetically predisposed individuals, antenatal factors, including maternal and thereby fetal exposure to allergens and maternoplacental–fetal immunological interactions, are active in determining whether an allergic predisposition is manifested as disease.

1997 The rising trends in asthma. Wiley, Chichester (Ciba Foundation Symposium 206) p 220–232

Rising trends in childhood asthma and related allergic diseases

There has been an increase in the prevalence and severity of allergic disorders and, in particular, asthma in children, though clear-cut epidemiological evidence to support this has been slow to accumulate, mainly because of a lack of an agreed definition of asthma suitable for population surveys. One study from South Wales, using identical ascertainment amongst 12-year olds showed a change in point prevalence between 1973 and 1988 from 4 to 9% for asthma, 5 to 16% for eczema and 9 to 15% for hay fever (Burr et al 1989). This increase has occurred in many countries and has been demonstrated in Finnish military conscripts (Haahtela et al 1990), Taiwanese schoolchildren (Hsieh & Shen 1988), Australian children (Robertson et al 1991) and adolescent Maories in New Zealand (Shaw et al 1990). Although diagnostic transfer might account for the increase in some of the studies, it is clearly not the case for the majority (Burr 1993). Furthermore, there have been enormous increases in hospital admissions for childhood asthma over the last eight to 10 years with no reduction in severity on admission, no increase in readmission ratio and no evidence of diagnostic transfer (Anderson 1989). A relatively small shift in population susceptibility due to changes in the environment could account for the increased frequency of disease and the even greater increased numbers experiencing severe disease.

The hereditary aspect of allergic disease was first described by Cooke & Vander Veer (1916). Analysis of their allergic patients demonstrated a familial tendency with 50% of children with one allergic parent and 80% of those with two allergic parents becoming atopic.

More recently, Ruiz et al (1991) showed that significantly more infants with an allergic mother developed allergic eczema than those with an allergic father. Cookson et al (1992) reported that the transmission of atopy at the chromosome 11q locus was detectable only through the maternal line. These studies suggest that an atopic mother can modify the development of the infant immune response towards the allergic phenotype. It is possible that this could be brought about by the antibody and cytokine profiles experienced by the fetus *in utero*.

T cells and cytokines

Based initially on studies in mice, allergen responsive T helper (Th) cell clones from allergic individuals have been shown to produce select cytokines of the interleukin (IL)-4 gene cluster encoded on chromosome 5q31, namely IL-4, IL-5, IL-6, IL-10 and IL-13 (Th2-like responses). Non-atopic Th cell clones produce IL-2, γ-interferon (IFN-γ) and tumour necrosis factor (TNF)-β (Th1-like responses) (Ricci et al 1993), whilst subtypes produce IL-3 and granulocyte macrophage colony-stimulating factor (GM-CSF) (Mossmann et al 1986). These cytokines have a wide range of effects, including the activation and recruitment of accessory cells in the allergic response — specifically mast cells, eosinophils and basophils. Both in murine models of atopy and in human allergy, it has been shown that opposing signals from Th1 cells producing IFN-γ, and Th2 cells producing IL-4 and IL-13 influence CD40-dependent IgE synthesis by B cells (Mossman et al 1986, Snapper & Paul 1987, Finkleman et al 1988, Vercelli et al 1990, Gauchat et al 1990). IFN-γ inhibits transformation to this isotype (Coffmann & Carty 1986). Of particular relevance is that when compared to adult T cells, those from neonates have a reduced IFN-γ production after polyclonal stimulation (Bryson et al 1980, Wakasugi & Virelizier 1985, Lewis et al 1986) and the same has been shown for IL-4 production (Lewis et al 1991). Holt et al (1992) have demonstrated that although the IFN-γ-producing capacity by CD4$^+$ T cell clones from babies was reduced relative to adults, it was significantly lower still in babies born to allergic families. It has also been demonstrated that IFN-γ production by cord blood mononuclear cells is reduced in those newborns with a family history of atopic disease (Rinas et al 1993).

IL-10 is a product of various cell types, including monocytes, B cells and T cells, and it is associated with the differentiation of Th2 cells. IL-10 inhibits cytokine production, particularly of IFN-γ, by T cells and natural killer cells (D'Andrea et al 1993). It has been suggested that IL-10 prevents the production of the IFN-γ-inducing cytokine, IL-12, by accessory cells. One possible mechanism for our findings of reduced IFN-γ production by neonatal T cells is an imbalance of IL-10 and IL-12 production.

Statistical analysis

The non-parametric Mann-Whitney U Test was used to compare between proliferative responses in the second and third trimesters and between mothers who had and had not been exposed to birch pollen from the 22nd week of pregnancy. The Yates corrected χ^2 test was used to compare positive and negative responders in the second and third trimesters and between mothers who had and had not been exposed to birch pollen. Spearman's rank correlation test was used to correlate gestational age with proliferative response.

T cell responses at birth and in the first year of life

We have found raised cord blood T cell proliferative responses and defective IFN-γ production to stimulation with specific allergens in babies who have subsequently developed allergic problems in relation to those allergens (Warner et al 1994), and these observations have been partly confirmed by others (Tang et al 1994). We have also found that babies born to atopic asthmatic parents who have developed allergic manifestations by one year of age have significantly lower $CD4^+ CD45RO^+$ (memory) and $CD4^+ CD25^+$ (activated) T cells in the cord blood compared with babies who were born in a similar situation but had not developed allergic disease or in babies born to non-allergic parents (Miles et al 1994). However, by six months of age these differences are lost (Miles et al 1996), presumably because the relevant T cell populations have moved into the target organs, including the lungs, under the influence of postnatal allergen exposure.

T cell development during gestation

The first lymphocytes are seen in the thymus of the developing fetus at eight to nine weeks gestation and the cortex is distinguishable from the medulla at 10 weeks. At this stage the more mature T cells in the thymus can demonstrate proliferative responses to the mitogen phytohaemagglutinin and histocompatibility antigens (Hayward 1981, Toivanen et al 1981).

T cell numbers increase in the fetal spleen and liver between the 12th and 23rd week of gestation. The migration of the T cells to the circulation occurs at about 15–16 weeks and is likely to be critical for the development of immune competence because most B cell antigen responses require T cell help (Hayward & Ezer 1974). Until recently, little

TABLE 1 Fetal peripheral blood T cell responses and cell surface markers during the gestational period 15–22 weeks

Gestation (weeks)	Proliferative response to phytohaemagglutinin	CD3$^+$ lymphocytes (%)	CD25$^+$ T cells (%)
15–16 ($n = 5$)	no	3	< 10
17–18 ($n = 9$)	yes	7	20
19–20 ($n = 8$)	yes	22	30
21–22 ($n = 5$)	yes	27	50

has been known about the functional maturity of the circulating T cells at this stage. However, we have performed fluorescence-activated cell sorter analysis of fetal T cells and shown that whilst CD25$^+$ T cells were virtually undetectable at 15 weeks gestation, at 22 weeks they were approximately 50% of the levels at full term (Table 1). Peripheral blood mononuclear cell (PBMC) proliferative responses to phytohaemagglutinin were first detected at 17 weeks. These proliferative responses continued to increase and were significantly higher in the third trimester than the second trimester ($P < 0.0001$), and they correlated with gestational age (Fig. 1). Even more importantly, we have demonstrated the same increase in proliferative response to specific inhalant and ingestant allergens, supporting the theory of intra-uterine priming (Jones et al 1996).

The fetal T cells were able to produce positive proliferative responses (greater than twice the background level) to a range of allergen sources (house dust mite, cat fur, birch tree pollen, β-lactoglobulin and ovalbumin) from 22 weeks gestation, and for each allergen the proliferation ratios correlated with gestational age. This strongly suggests that maternal allergen exposure is important in the priming of fetal T cells such that at birth they already respond to environmental allergens.

At birth, babies at high risk of developing allergy with a raised proliferative response to β-lactoglobulin and deficient IFN-γ production were those who went on to develop food-associated eczema with a positive skin prick test to milk (Warner et al 1994). Therefore, it is important to determine at what stage in pregnancy this priming occurred with its related down-regulation of IFN-γ. As we know that positive responses can be seen from 22 weeks gestation and that there are circulating T cells from 15 weeks gestation, it can be hypothesized that the second trimester of pregnancy is the vital time period. It has been shown that maternal food allergen avoidance in the third trimester of pregnancy is ineffective in the prevention of infant allergy (Falth-Magnusson & Kjellman 1992). This may be due to it having been too late and that fetal sensitization had already occurred. We have also shown that infant cells stimulated at birth with birch tree pollen showed a significantly ($P = 0.005$) higher proportion of positive responders in the group whose mothers had been exposed to

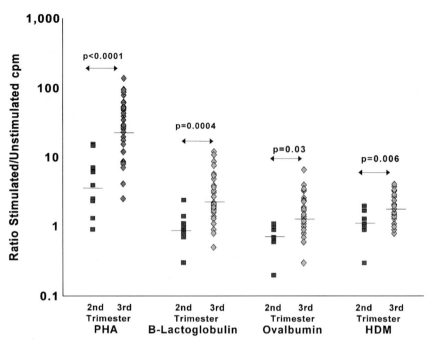

FIG. 1.   Graph showing the infant peripheral blood mononuclear cell proliferative response
ratios to phytohaemagglutinin (PHA) and allergens in the second and third trimesters of
pregnancy. Medians are shown. HDM, house dust mite.

birch pollen beyond the 22nd week of pregnancy compared to those who were not
exposed in this period. This would suggest that maternal avoidance of trigger factors
needs to be established before 22 weeks gestation to prevent fetal T cell priming.

Maternal, placental and fetal immunological interactions

We believe that there is a powerful maternal and placental influence on the fetal
immune response, which promotes or suppresses Th2-like activity, but the nature of
this influence is not known. Evidence is growing that during pregnancy the maternal
immune response becomes heavily biased towards the Th2 phenotype, with increasing
IL-4 and IL-10 during gestation being detected in the murine system. Clinically, a
picture of reduced cell-mediated immunity has been described in pregnancy
(Weinberg 1984). The benefit of this loss of cell-mediated immunity may be a
reduction in natural killer cell activity. These cells have been shown to have a role in

spontaneous abortion and may attack the trophoblast (Gendron & Baines 1988). Additionally, IFN-γ is an abortifactant, whose effect may be mediated through the activation of natural killer cells by this cytokine (Robertson et al 1992). Clearly Th1-type cell-mediated immune responses are undesirable for the maintenance of pregnancy.

To date, most evidence of the role of cytokines in pregnancy has been derived from the murine system. Dudley et al (1993) showed increasing IL-4 and decreasing IL-2 production by murine maternal splenocytes during gestation. However, very low levels of these lymphokines were detected in decidual lymphocyte cultures. Delassus et al (1994) likewise saw increases in IL-4 and IL-10, and some increase in IFN-γ in PBMC cultures from maternal blood. In the placenta, increases were seen in IL-4, but IFN-γ did not increase and IL-2 remained low.

Jones et al (1995) have shown that IL-4 is produced by the human amnion epithelium in the first and third trimester of pregnancy (second trimester not tested) and Cadet et al (1995) described the presence of mRNA coding for IL-10 at term in human placental tissue. We are currently investigating the presence of mRNAs encoding IFN-γ, IL-4, IL-5, IL-10, IL-12 and IL-13, as well as their protein products, in the fetal–placental–maternal human system in the second and third trimesters of pregnancy to determine how and when maternal and placental cellular responses affect the development and control of infant responses to allergens.

Preliminary results show that PBMCs from most fetuses spontaneously release IFN-γ during the second and third trimesters of pregnancy, but that there are some which do not release this Th1 cytokine even when stimulated with phytohaemagglutinin. By the time positive proliferative responses are seen to antigens (>22 weeks gestation) mRNA encoding the Th2 cytokines IL-4, IL-10 and IL-13 can he detected in fetal PBMCs.

We hypothesize that the role of non-specific fetal PBMC IFN-γ production is to counteract the effects of IL-4 and IL-10 produced by the placenta and/or the mother. A mechanism such as this would be essential to prevent an allergic (Th2) phenotype in all newborns. Failure of this mechanism may underlie the development of atopy.

Currently, we are not aware of any reports of the ability of maternal allergy-promoting cytokines to cross the placenta. However, amniotic fluid has been shown to contain granulocyte colony-stimulating factor, GM-CSF, TNF-α, IL-1, IL-6 and IL-8 (Stallmach et al 1995). This does not necessarily indicate passage from the mother as they may all be placentally derived; however, further investigation is needed. We have also been able to detect IL-10 in amniotic fluid, which is present in higher concentrations in atopic mothers than in non-atopic mothers.

Studies of T cell activation, specific proliferative responses to allergens, and the cytokine gene expression and cytokine release of triggered cells from terminated fetuses and premature babies are underway to determine whether commencing allergen avoidance during the second trimester of pregnancy results in the prevention of these raised responses.

Conclusions

Infants who subsequently become allergic have an altered immune response at birth, suggesting that events which occur during pregnancy can influence the development of the allergic phenotype. Raised proliferative responses to specific allergens are seen from 22 weeks gestation and these are related to maternal exposure to the triggering allergen. Fetal PBMC production of IFN-γ increases with gestational age, but some infants produce little or no IFN-γ whatever the stimulant. In light of the suggestions that successful pregnancy is a Th2 phenomenon, it may be hypothesized that these infants are at a higher risk of developing a Th2 response than those whose IFN-γ production is greater and therefore better able to balance the Th2 cytokine switch pathway. Maternal atopy is associated with increased exposure of the fetus to IL-10. Whilst the development of specific T cell responses during gestation is likely to be a normal phenomenon, set against a background of reduced fetal IFN-γ production, high maternal allergen exposure may lead to an increased risk of allergic sensitization in the infant.

Acknowledgements

The authors would like to thank The National Asthma Campaign, The British Lung Foundation, The David and Frederick Barclay Foundation, The European Society for Pediatric Allergy and Immunology, Sandoz Pharmaceuticals, Pharmacia and National Power, all of whom have provided funding for our work described in this article.

References

Anderson HR 1989 Increase in hospital admissions for childhood asthma: trends in referral, severity, and readmissions from 1970 to 1985 in a health region of the United Kingdom. Thorax 44:614–619

Bryson YJ, Winter HS, Gard SE, Fischer TJ, Stiehm ER 1980 Deficiency of immune interferon production by leukocytes of normal newborns. Cell Immunol 55:191–200

Burr ML 1993 Epidemiology of asthma. In: Burr ML (ed) Epidemiology of clinical allergy. Karger, Basel (Monographs Allergy Series 31) p 80–102

Burr ML, Butland BK, King S, Vaughan-Williams E 1989 Changes in asthma prevalence: two surveys fifteen years apart. Arch Dis Child 64:1452–1456

Cadet P, Rady PL, Tyring SK, Yandell RB, Hughes TK 1995 Interleukin 10 messenger ribonucleic acid in human placenta: implications of a role for interleukin 10 in fetal allograft protection. Am J Obstet Gynecol 173:25–29

Coffman RL, Carty JA 1986 A T-cell activity that enhances polyclonal IgE production and its inhibition by interferon-gamma. J Immunol 136:949

Cooke RA, Vander Veer A 1916 Human sensitization. J Immunol 1:201–305

Cookson WOCM, Young RP, Sandford AJ et al 1992 Maternal inheritance of IgE responsiveness on chromosome 11q. Lancet 340:381–384

D'Andrea A, Aste-Amezaga M, Valiante NM, Ma X, Kubin M, Trinchieri G 1993 Interleukin-10 (IL-10) inhibits human lymphocyte interferon-gamma production by suppressing natural killer cell stimulatory factor/IL-12 synthesis in accessory cells. J Exp Med 178:1041–1048

Delassus S, Coutinho GC, Saucier C, Darche S, Kourilsky P 1994 Differential cytokine expression in maternal blood and placenta during murine gestation. J Immunol 152:2411–2420

Dudley DJ, Chen C-L, Mitchell MD, Daynes RA, Araneo BA 1993 Adaptive immune responses during murine pregnancy: pregnancy-induced regulation of lymphokine production by activated T lymphocytes. Am J Obstet Gynecol 168:1155–1163

Falth-Magnusson K, Kjellman N-IM 1992 Allergy prevention by maternal elimination diet during late pregnancy: a five year follow-up of a randomised study. J Allergy Clin Immunol 89:709–713

Finkleman FD, Katona IM, Mosmann TR, Coffman RL 1988 IFN-γ regulates the isotypes of Ig secreted during *in vivo* humoral immune responses. J Immunol 140:1022–1026

Gauchat J-F, Lebman DA, Coffman RL, Gascan H, deVries JE 1990 Structure and expression of germline E transcripts in human B-cells induced by interleukin-4 to switch to IgE production. J Exp Med 172:463–473

Gendron RL, Baines MG 1988 Infiltrating decidual natural killer cells are associated with spontaneous abortion in mice. Cell Immunol 113:261–267

Haahtela T, Lindholm H, Björkstén F, Koskenvuo K, Laitinen LA 1990 Prevalence of asthma in Finnish young men. Br Med J 301:266–268

Hayward AR 1981 Development of lymphocyte responses and interactions in the human fetus and newborn. Immunol Rev 57:39–60

Hayward AR, Ezer G 1974 Development of lymphocyte populations in the human foetal thymus and spleen. Clin Exp Immunol 17:169–178

Holt PG, Clough JB, Holt BJ et al 1992 Genetic risk for atopy is associated with delayed post-natal maturation of T cell competence. Clin Exp Allergy 22:1093–1099

Hsieh K-H, Shen J-J 1988 Prevalence of childhood asthma in Taipei, Taiwan, and other Asian Pacific countries. J Asthma 25:73–82

Jones CA, Williams KA, Finlay-Jones JF, Hart PH 1995 Interleukin 4 production by human amnion epithelial cells and regulation of its activity by glycosaminoglycan binding. Biol Reprod 52:839–847

Jones AC, Miles EA, Warner JO, Colwell BM, Warner JO 1996 Fetal peripheral blood mononuclear cell proliferative responses to mitogenic stimulants during pregnancy. Pediatr Allergy Immunol 7:109–116

Lewis DB, Larsen A, Wilson CB 1986 Reduced interferon gamma mRNA levels in human neonates: evidence for an intrinsic T-cell deficiency independent of other genes involved in T-cell activation. J Exp Med 163:1018–1023

Lewis DB, Yu CC, Meyer J, English BK, Kahn SJ, Wilson CB 1991 Cellular and molecular mechanisms for reduced interleukin-4 and interferon-γ production by neonatal T-cells. J Clin Invest 87:194–202

Miles EA, Warner JA, Lane AC, Colwell BM, Warner JO 1994 Altered T-lymphocyte phenotype and function at birth in babies born to atopic parents. Pediatr Allergy Immunol 5:202–208

Miles EA, Warner JA, Jones AC, Colwell BM, Bryant TM, Warner JO 1996 Peripheral blood mononuclear cell proliferative responses in the first year of life in babies born to allergic parents. Clin Exp Allergy 26:780–788

Mosmann TR, Cherwinski H, Bond MW, Griedlin M, Coffman RL 1986 Two types of murine T helper cell clones. I. Definition according to profile of lymphokine activities. J Immunol 136:2348

Ricci M, Rossi O, Bertoni M, Matucci A 1993 The importance of Th2-like cells in the pathogenesis of airway allergic inflammation. Clin Exp Allergy 23:360–369

Rinas U, Horneff G, Wahn V 1993 Interferon-γ production by cord blood mononuclear cells is reduced in newborns with a family history of atopic disease and is independent from cord blood IgE levels. Pediatr Allergy Immunol 4:60–64

Robertson CF, Heycock E, Bishop J, Nolan T, Olinsky A, Phelan PD 1991 Prevalence of asthma in Melbourne schoolchildren: changes over 26 years. Br Med J 302:1116–1118

Robertson SA, Mayrhofer G, Seamark RF 1992 Uterine epithelial cells synthesise granulocyte-macrophage colony-stimulating factor (GM-CSF) and interleukin-6 (IL-6) in pregnant and non-pregnant mice. Biol Reprod 46:1069

Ruiz RGG, Richards D, Kemeny DM, Price JF 1991 Neonatal IgE: a poor screen for atopic disease. Clin Exp Allergy 21:467–472

Shaw RA, Crane J, O'Donnell TV, Porteous LE, Coleman ED 1990 Increasing asthma prevalence in a rural New Zealand adolescent population: 1975–89. Arch Dis Child 65:1319–1323

Snapper CM, Paul WE 1987 Interferon-γ and B-cell stimulatory factor-1 reciprocally regulate Ig isotype production. Science 236:944–946

Stallmach T, Hebisch G, Joller-Jemelka HI, Orban P, Schwaller J, Engelman M 1995 Cytokine production and visualised effects in the feto-maternal unit. Quantitative and topographic data on cytokines during intrauterine disease. Lab Invest 73:384–392

Tang MLK, Kemp AS, Thorburn J, Hill DJ 1994 Reduced interferon-γ secretion in neonates and subsequent atopy. Lancet 344:983–985

Toivanen P, Uksila J, Leino A, Lassila O, Hirvonen T, Ruuskanen O 1981 Development of mitogen responding T cells and natural killer cells in the human fetus. Immunol Rev 57:89–105

Vercelli D, Tabara HH, Lauener RP, Geha RS 1990 IL-4 inhibits the synthesis of IFN-γ and induces the synthesis of IgE in human mixed lymphocyte cultures. J Immunol 144:570–573

Wakasugi N, Virelizier JL 1985 Defective IFN-γ production in the human neonate. I. Dysregulation rather than intrinsic abnormality. J Immunol 134:167–171

Warner JA, Miles EA, Jones AC, Quint DJ, Colwell BM, Warner JO 1994 Is deficiency of interferon gamma production by allergen triggered cord blood cells a predictor of atopic eczema? Clin Exp Allergy 24:423–430

Weinberg ED 1984 Pregnancy-associated depression of cell-mediated immunity. Rev Infect Dis 6:814–831

DISCUSSION

Martinez: Erika von Mutius and I published an article on asthma in premature babies (von Mutius et al 1993). We found that children who had been born prematurely and had been ventilated (and who were perhaps growth retarded *in utero*) were much more likely to have asthma later in childhood than children who had been born prematurely and had not been ventilated or than children who had been born at term. What was interesting, however, was that children who had been ventilated after being born prematurely were less likely to have skin test reactivity to allergens than children who had been born at term. It is difficult to explain these results. It is possible that the lungs of these children were somehow affected by the ventilator.

Sears: You indicated that children of low birth weight or retarded intra-uterine growth are less atopic. We've looked at birth rate versus airway responsiveness

(Sears et al 1997) and found that children of low birth weight are less likely to develop asthma, which agrees with your results.

Warner: Although we must be careful to discriminate low birth weight from genuine intra-uterine growth retardation.

Sears: I would like to clarify that when saying that low birth weight children have less asthma, I am talking about long-term persistent asthma and not early childhood wheezing, which is what your study addresses. It is possible that in our studies the early non-atopic wheeze, which is not atopic persistent asthma, has disappeared by mid-childhood, and we are then finding that low birth weight children are at a reduced risk of having persistent atopic asthma.

Holt: Fiona Stanley has one of the best databases in the world on intra-uterine growth rates, and she can distinguish between the different classes of intra-uterine growth retardation. Hopefully, she'll be able to come up with some answers to these questions using her database.

Holgate: Taking the reverse argument, Godfrey et al (1994) have found that head circumference at birth is positively related to allergic disease in adults. In a separate study, so far unpublished, I. J. M. Doull has shown that head circumference also relates positively to the presence of skin tests to common allergens at the age of 11 years. A variety of other anthropometric measures, including heel–crown length and abdominal circumference, were also examined but they failed to predict the atopic phenotype. Barker and colleagues have predicted chronic obstructive lung disease, hypertension, diabetes mellitus and osteoporosis using different body size measures in infancy, and they have come up with the hypothesis that adult degenerative diseases are programmed early in life, possibly due to nutritional and hormonal influences on the developing fetus (Barker 1992).

Warner: This is a slightly different issue because they were explaining their data in terms of changes in nutrition at various points during pregnancy, whereas altered cytokine profiles may persist until the baby is born. Barker's work applies to babies where nutrition was adequate in the first trimester, but decreased in the second trimester.

Holgate: The argument seems to be that maternal nutrition is able to alter cytokine or hormone secretion by the placenta, and that brain growth, which dictates head circumference, is under the influence of these factors, particularly in the last trimester of pregnancy when head (and brain) growth is maximum.

Woolcock: In children under five years old, males are much more skin test positive than females. I know of no explanation for this. Did you also observe this?

Warner: We haven't yet looked at whether there was a different level of response between males and females.

Paré: What is the nature of the factor that is crossing the placenta to make these cells antigen specific?

Warner: This is not yet known. We don't even know what size of molecule is able to cross or the concentrations involved. We're currently setting up some trophoblast cultures to look at antigen passage across the trophoblast, and to determine whether we can detect antigenic activity on the other side. I am interested in those reports which suggest that it is possible to measure house dust mite allergens in cord blood because this would support our hypothesis that the fetus is directly exposed to allergens inhaled or ingested by the mother.

Paré: Could anything else that causes specific responses other than antigens be getting across?

Warner: Yes, we could be observing an anti-idiotypic response to maternal antibody, although in my opinion this is unlikely.

Martinez: Is it possible that some of the peptides produced by digestion of the original antigen by macrophages could cross the placenta and be specifically presented to the fetus by the antigen-presenting cells (APCs) of the fetus?

Warner: Experiments need to be set up to look first at the ability of maternal APCs to present antigen to these early fetal cells and then the ability of fetal APCs to take up specific peptides and present them to fetal T cells. If they can, then your suggestion is likely.

Holt: If an anti-idiotypic network was operative in this situation we would observe frequent responses to tetanus toxoid, given that all the mothers have tetanus toxoid-specific antibodies, but we haven't. This suggests that the antigen exposure is crucial in the induction of the fetal T cell responses.

Busse: Are the routes of antigen exposure and the eventual target organ known? Because one would anticipate that in childhood, systemic absorption of antigen would be more important whereas later in life the route of administration is from inhalation. Does the route of exposure determine target organ specificity?

Warner: This suggestion fits well with our results from the high risk babies we studied throughout their first year of life. There is a proliferative response to allergen at birth, but this systemic response significantly decreases by six months of age in those babies who go on to develop allergic disease. This must be due to a specific pattern of antigen exposure. There are results from animal models which suggest that if the antigen is inhaled those original sensitized cells move to the lung. We might be able to look at this in a SCID mouse model.

Busse: Once they're sensitized and exposed to antigen, what is the consequence?

Holgate: This is a crucial question because nearly 50% of the population is atopic. In the UK 85–90% of the atopics are house dust mite sensitive, whereas the proportion of these subjects who have clinical asthma is low. Thus, the target organ for the expression of the atopic phenotype, which in the case of asthma is the lung, is largely unexplained.

Strachan: Can fertility influence the pattern of cytokine production *in utero*?

Warner: Possibly, because it is known that many spontaneous abortions are due to an unusual cytokine production by the materno-fetal unit.

Cullinan: Have you observed any effects of maternal smoking?

Warner: We have taken urine samples from the premature babies in this study, and these are currently being analysed. However, in the high risk cohort we have shown that maternal smoking is associated with early wheeze in the first year of life but not with wheeze beyond this time point. As far as the immunology is concerned, we hope that this will be elucidated, in relation to whether maternal smoking affects cytokine production, by our study of the maternoplacental–fetal interactions in premature babies and the subsequent development of allergic disease.

Holgate: Although it has been argued that genomic imprinting is an important factor that increases the maternal influence on atopic expression in the offspring (Doull 1996), maternal environmental factors seem to dominate. Maternal smoking seems to be a particularly good example of this because it can affect the development of the lung and immune response *in utero* as well as having a deleterious effect on the baby once born through the effects of passive smoking.

Warner: Our intervention study, looking at the effects of protecting mothers from exposure to house dust mite and pet allergens from 18 weeks of pregnancy, should provide more information about the effect of maternal allergen exposure on infant immune responses. We already have an indication that they are important because the infants of mothers who were exposed to birch pollen at 22 weeks of pregnancy or beyond had significantly higher proliferative responses at birth to birch pollen than infants whose mothers were not exposed.

Holgate: Certainly, in the mouse homologues of chromosomes 5 and 11 there is no evidence for genomic imprinting (Watson et al 1995).

Platts-Mills: Most allergens are inhaled at a rate of only 10 ng per day and estimating the quantity of house dust mite allergen in the blood is rather inaccurate (10 ng/day into 5 litres is roughly 2 pg/ml). If sensitization is occurring *in utero* it is occurring with extremely low levels of allergen and we should therefore be cautious about the accuracy of the assays at such low concentrations. In contrast, we consume grams of ovalbumin per day, so it's easy to see how this could cause sensitization. Indeed, it would be surprising if children weren't sensitized to ovalbumin.

Warner: House dust mites are present in some foodstuffs. It would be interesting to measure the concentrations of house dust mite allergens present in cereals because it is possible that exposure is coming through the gastrointestinal tract as well as the respiratory tract. The Ministry of Agriculture, Fisheries and Foods have shown that mite allergen is present in grain extracts.

Platts-Mills: The quantities of storage mites are probably much lower in cereals now that cereals are treated with pirimiphos-methyl, which kills both dust mites and storage mites (Mitchell et al 1981). Previously, cereals would have been much more infested. The issue of how much allergen is getting across the placenta is important, especially if high affinity maternal IgG is present because then there may be some blocking effect or a priming effect if the mother has antibody and is allergic.

Warner: IgG itself can cross the placenta, so it is possible that antigen bound to IgG can also cross.

Heusser: Did you determine the type of the cells that produce interleukin (IL)-4? Because one of the major sources of IL-4 production in mature individuals is from basophils.

Warner: We haven't yet looked at IL-4 production in that system, but it is something that we will be doing shortly. The IL-4 in murine models has been shown to be produced by the placental cells themselves and Catherine Jones, who is now in our group, has shown positive staining of the amnion with anti-IL-4 antibody in human placenta. The cells in the placenta are largely not immune cells, but we need to determine whether the immune cells that are there can direct the cytokine production of other cell populations.

G. Anderson: It is important to determine whether the lymphocyte proliferation responses you have observed are true recall responses to an antigen recognized by the immune system *in utero*, weak primary responses that measure the ability of cells to respond to a foreign antigen or even weak mitogenic responses. The proliferative index you showed was much smaller than one would expect to observe in a true recall response to a specific antigen.

Warner: I agree. One of the issues we need to address is the level of proliferative index we consider to be positive. We are currently using a stimulation index of two times the background as positive, but our results remain the same if we use three times the background, which some other groups have used. In response to your point about these being primary responses, these are six-day cultures, so I would not expect these to be primary responses because they would take more than six days to develop. Also, if the cells are only exposed to the antigens for three days they do not respond positively, indicating that this is not a mitogenic response.

References

Barker DJP 1992 The fetal and infant origins of disease. Br Med J 25:457–463

Doull IJM 1996 Maternal inheritance of atopy? Clin Exp Allergy 26:613–615

Godfrey BK, Barker BJP, Osmond C 1994 Disproportionate fetal growth and raised IgE concentration in adult life. Clin Exp Allergy 24:641–648

Mitchell EB, Platts-Mills TAE, Pereira RS, Malkovska Y, Webster AD 1983 Basophil and eosinophil deficiency in a patient with hypogammaglobulinemia associated with thymoma. Birth Defects Orig Artic Ser 19:331

Sears MR, Holdaway MD, Flannery EM, Herbison GP, Silva PA 1997 Parental and neonatal risk factors for development of asthma, atopy and airway hyper-responsiveness. Arch Dis Child, in press

von Mutius E, Nicolai T, Martinez FD 1993 Prematurity as a risk factor for asthma in preadolescent children. J Pediatr 123:223–239

Watson M, Lawrence S, Collins A et al 1995 Exclusion from proximal 11q of a common gene with megaphenic effect on atopy. Am J Hum Genet 59:403–411

Maternal risk factors in asthma

Fernando D. Martinez

Respiratory Sciences Center, University of Arizona School of Medicine, 1501 North Campbell Avenue, Tucson, AZ 85724, USA

Abstract. There is now increasing evidence that maternal factors may play a role in the development of asthma and asthma-related syndromes in children. For years it has been known that younger mothers are more likely to have children who develop wheezing illnesses in early life. It has been suggested that the development of the lung may differ in children of younger mothers compared to that in children of older mothers, but the biology of this association is not well understood. Recent data suggest that there is a much stronger association of allergic conditions in early life with allergic disease in the mother than in the father. Maternal asthma is more strongly associated with childhood asthma than is paternal asthma. The influence of the pattern of immune responsiveness in the mother on the ontogeny of the immune system in children needs further exploration, and it may offer new clues as to the factors determining the development of asthma and allergy in children.

1997 The rising trends in asthma. Wiley, Chichester (Ciba Foundation Symposium 206) p 233–243

There is increasing interest in the possible role of maternal influences on the development of asthma. This has mainly been the result of studies showing that events occurring during fetal life may affect the developmental pathways followed by the immune system and the lung and airways both prenatally and postnatally. Complex metabolic and immune interactions are established between the mother and the fetus that we are only beginning to understand. The epidemiological data suggesting that maternal age, maternal smoking, maternal allergies and some complications of pregnancy may increase the risk of developing asthma and asthma-like symptoms during infancy and childhood are reviewed.

Maternal age

During the last 40 years several reports have indicated that maternal age is an important risk factor for postneonatal mortality. Morrison et al (1959), for example, reported that postneonatal mortality for 'respiratory diseases' was higher in mothers aged less than 20 years than in older mothers. These trends were independent of birth rank and social class. No such trends were observed for deaths attributed to 'congenital

233

malformations'. Friede et al (1987) confirmed these findings in a large sample of over two million births.

Until recently, however, no large studies of the relationship between maternal age and postneonatal morbidity were available. We recently studied the relationship between wheezing/non-wheezing lower respiratory tract illnesses (LRI) and maternal age during the first year of life (Martinez et al 1992a). For this purpose, we used data from the Children's Respiratory Study, which was designed to assess prospectively the risk factors for asthma and asthma-like symptoms in a cohort of over 1200 children living in Tucson, Arizona, USA (Taussig et al 1989). We found that the risk of having wheezing LRI during the first year of life was inversely related to maternal age. When compared with infants of mothers aged over 30 years, the odds ratios (95% confidence intervals) were: 2.4 (1.8–3.1) for infants whose mothers were less than 21 years ($P < 0.0001$); 1.8 (1.4–2.3) for infants whose mothers were aged 21–25 ($P < 0.0001$); and 1.4 (1.1–1.6) for infants whose mothers were aged 26–30 ($P < 0.001$). These results were independent of maternal education, birth rank, feeding practices (breast feeding or bottle feeding), maternal smoking, birth weight, marital status, day care use, ethnicity and gender. Non-wheezing LRI were unrelated to maternal age.

Several recent studies have addressed the issue of the relationship between wheezing illnesses and maternal age in older children. Anderson et al (1986) first reported that children of younger mothers were at a higher risk of developing asthma than children of older mothers. They studied over 8800 children from a cohort of British newborns born in 1958. They found that young maternal age (up to 20 years of age) was associated with a 40 to 80% increased risk of developing asthma by age 16. Interestingly, this increased risk was observed both for asthma that started by age seven and for asthma starting after that age. This association was independent of socioeconomic status and of feeding practices (breast feeding or bottle feeding). Schwartz et al (1990) studied a sample of the population of the United States aged six months to 11 years. They reported a significant inverse relationship between maternal age and physician-diagnosed asthma, which was independent of the child's age, race, sex and birth weight. Maternal age was also inversely related (albeit not significantly) with the prevalence of wheezing. Lewis et al (1995) studied the occurrence of wheezing by five years of age and of wheezing in the previous year at 16 years of age among children who wheezed by age five in over 15 000 British children born in 1970. They found that maternal age was unrelated to wheezing by age five. However, continued wheezing at aged 16 was approximately twice as likely among children of mothers aged 19 or less than among children of mothers age 40 or more, and this association was statistically significant and independent of social status, sex, feeding practices, maternal smoking and birth order. More recently, Strachan et al (1996) reanalysed the data derived from the 1958 British cohort previously reported by Anderson et al (1986). They were unable to confirm a significant relationship between maternal age and incidence of asthma at different ages from birth to age 33. Strachan et al (1996), however, adjusted the data for several parameters including 'pneumonia by age seven', which was a strong predictor of incidence of asthma by age 16. It is possible that this may have overcorrected the data, given the fact that Martinez et al (1992a) had found a strong association between wheezing LRI and maternal age, and wheezing LRI may have been labelled 'pneumonia' in the data of Strachan et al (1996). In addition, the size of the sample available for multivariate analysis was much smaller than the initial 8800 subjects enrolled (Anderson et al 1986), and this may have decreased the power of the analysis.

There is at present no conclusive explanation for the association between maternal age and wheezing illnesses. It has been suggested that maternal age may be a proxy for some unknown social factor not considered in some of the analyses (Martinez et al 1992a). Others have suggested that subtle aspects of the maternal–infant relationship may be influenced by maternal age. Jones et al (1980), for example, found that younger mothers were not as responsive as older mothers to their newborn infant's needs. McAnarney et al (1984, 1986) reported that maternal age was associated with less favourable behaviours when the infant was nine to 12 months old. The way in which mothering skills may affect the young child and increase the risk of wheezing illnesses and asthma is unknown. However, studies in experimental animals have suggested that stress may play a crucial role in lung development. Kida & Thurlbeck (1980) showed that mild stressful stimuli (in the case of their studies, intraperitoneal injections of saline) during crucial phases of postnatal lung development may be associated with irreversible changes in lung structure. Naeye (1981) has also suggested that young maternal age may also have subtle effects on fetal development. It is well known that younger mothers (up to 21 years of age) have children whose average birth weight is up to 200 g lower than that of older mothers (over 35 years of age) (Martinez et al 1992a). Naeye (1981) thus speculated that the growth requirements of young mothers may compete with the growth requirements of their fetuses for available nutrients. This may affect all organs, including the lungs.

The possible role of maternal age on lung development, if confirmed, could contribute to our understanding of the association between maternal age and asthma. Our group has shown that the level of airway function measured shortly after birth is an important predictor of wheezing during the first three years of life (Martinez et al 1995), and this effect was independent of other familial and socioeconomic factors. Maternal age may thus increase the risk of wheezing by altering lung development. To test this hypothesis, we studied the association between maternal age and airway function in children enrolled in the Children's Respiratory Study (Taussig et al 1989). Partial expiratory flow volume curves were assessed both at baseline and after inhalation of dry, cold air in almost 500 children at a mean age of approximately six years. Dry, cold air is known to elicit a broncho-constrictive response in subjects who have bronchial hyper-responsiveness. We found that height-adjusted maximal expiratory flow rates were significantly lower in children of younger mothers (up to 21 and 21–24 years of age) than in children of older mothers (aged over 24 years). No association was found between maternal age and response to cold, dry air (F. Martinez, unpublished observations 1996). These results support the hypothesis that children of younger and older mothers have different patterns of lung development.

Maternal smoking

Strong evidence is now available indicating that exposure to tobacco smoke products is associated with increased risk of respiratory disease in infants and children (United States Environmental Protection Agency 1995). Children of smoking mothers are two to three times as likely to develop LRI during infancy as children of non-smoking mothers (United States Environmental Protection Agency 1995). This association has been found with striking consistency in different countries and it is clearly not explained by any specific confounding factor (United States Environmental Protection Agency 1995). Although the effect has been mainly reported for maternal smoking, exposure to environmental tobacco smoke in children of non-smoking mothers has also been found to increase the risk of LRI in early life (Chen et al 1988). It is thus likely that, whereas most of the association between passive tobacco smoke and respiratory illnesses in early childhood is attributable to *in utero* exposure, postnatal exposure may be important as well.

There is also evidence indicating that maternal smoking is associated with an increased risk of developing asthma during childhood (Martinez et al 1992b, Weitzman et al 1990), but the evidence is less striking than that for an association between passive smoking and LRI in early life (Cunningham et al 1996). However, there is strong support for a role of maternal smoking (and for exposure to environmental tobacco smoke in general) in increasing the severity of asthma (Murray & Morrison 1989) and the frequency of asthmatic attacks (Evans et al 1987) in children who already have asthma.

There are several mechanisms by which tobacco smoke exposure may increase the risk of respiratory illness in childhood. Children of smoking mothers have been found to have lower levels of lung function than children of non-smoking mothers, and this has been noticed in studies performed both shortly after birth (Tager et al 1995) and during school years (Strachan et al 1990). As explained earlier, a low level of lung function is a predisposing factor for wheezing during viral infections (Martinez et al 1995). There is some evidence that exposure to environmental tobacco smoke may enhance bronchial hyper-responsiveness (Forastiere et al 1994) and increase the risk of becoming sensitized to inhaled aeroallergens (Martinez et al 1988). However, it is possible that these effects may require very high levels of exposure, which may explain why not all studies have been able to confirm these associations (Soyseth et al 1995).

Maternal allergies

There is evidence suggesting that a history of allergies and/or asthma in mothers is more strongly associated with atopic disease in their children than is paternal history (Halonen et al 1992). It is thus possible that the mother may have an influence on the child's phenotype that goes beyond genetic transmission of susceptibility. It is unlikely that this influence may be explained by a shared environment in early postnatal life because cord serum IgE levels are also higher in children of allergic mothers than in children of non-allergic mothers, an influence that is not observed in children of allergic fathers (Halonen et al 1992). It is thus likely that a mother with allergy may draw the developing fetal immune system transplacentally towards a pattern of response to environmental stimuli that predisposes to asthma and allergies.

How this may occur is not well understood. It is possible that maternal allergies may enhance antigen presentation to the immature fetal immune system. This may occur by preprocessing of antigen by maternal antigen-presenting cells, which may be necessary given the limitations of the fetal immune system in providing the accessory cell function needed to activate a T cell response (von Hoegen et al 1995). Placental immune responses, which are known to be predominately of the T helper (Th) 2 type (Lin et al 1993), may be different in allergic mothers than in non-allergic mothers, enhancing for example the early development of Th2-like responses to environmental stimuli by the fetus. Clearly, much more work needs to be done in this area of research.

Complications of pregnancy

There is intriguing new evidence suggesting that complications of pregnancy, such as antepartum haemorrhage or maternal albuminuria, may be associated with the incidence of asthma and wheezing illnesses from birth to age 33 years (Strachan et al 1996). These results require confirmation, and the mechanisms by which antepartum haemorrhage and maternal albuminuria may decrease and increase, respectively, the incidence of asthma remain obscure. Nevertheless, these reports again point towards non-specific intra-uterine influences that may interact with the child's genetic background to impact the risk of developing asthma.

Conclusions

The possible role of environmental influences on the development of asthma has (justifiably) been the subject of persistent inquiry. It has now become clear that the intra-uterine environment may play a crucial role in regulating the expression of the inherited susceptibility to asthma.

Acknowledgement

This research was supported by a Research Career Development Award for Minority Faculty (HL-03154) from the National Heart, Lung and Blood Institute.

References

Anderson HR, Bland JM, Patel S, Peckham 1986 The natural history of asthma in childhood. J Epidemiol Community Health 40:121–129

Chen Y, Li W, Yu S, Qian W 1988 Chang-Ning epidemiological study of children's health. I. Passive smoking and children's respiratory diseases. Int J Epidemiol 17:348–355

Cunningham J, O'Connor GT, Dockery DW, Speizer FE 1996 Environmental tobacco smoke, wheezing, and asthma in children in 24 communities. Am J Respir Crit Care Med 153:218–224

Evans D, Levison J, Feldman CH et al 1987 The impact of passive smoking on emergency room visits of urban children with asthma. Am Rev Respir Dis 135:567–572

Forastiere F, Agabiti N, Corbo GM et al 1994 Passive smoking as a determinant of bronchial responsiveness in children. Am J Respir Crit Care Med 149:365–370

Friede A, Baldwin W, Rhodes PH et al 1987 Young maternal age and infant mortality: the role of low birth weight. Public Health Rep 102:192–199

Halonen M, Stern D, Taussig LM, Wright AL, Ray CG, Martinez FD 1992 The predictive relationship between serum IgE levels at birth and subsequent incidences of lower respiratory illnesses and eczema in infants. Am Rev Respir Dis 146:866–870

Jones FA, Green V, Drauss DR 1980 Maternal responsiveness of primiparous mothers during the post-partum period: age differences. Pediatrics 65:579–584

Kida K, Thurlbeck WM 1980 Lack of recovery of lung structure and function after the administration of beta-amino-propionitrile in the postnatal period. Am Rev Respir Dis 122:467–475

Lewis S, Richards D, Bynner J, Butler N, Britton J 1995 Prospective study of risk factors for early and persistent wheezing in childhood. Eur Respir J 8:349–356

Lin H, Mosmann TR, Guilbert L, Tuntipopipat S, Wegmann TG 1993 Synthesis of T helper 2-type cytokines at the maternal–fetal interface. J Immunol 151:4562–4573

Martinez FD, Antognoni G, Macri F et al 1988 Parental smoking enhances bronchial responsiveness in nine year old children. Am Rev Respir Dis 138:518–523

Martinez FD, Wright AL, Holberg CJ, Morgan WJ, Taussig LM 1992a Maternal age as a risk factor for wheezing lower respiratory illnesses in the first year of life. Am J Epidemiol 136:1258–1268

Martinez FD, Cline MG, Burrows B 1992b Increased incidence of asthma in children of smoking mothers. Pediatrics 89:21–26

Martinez FD, Wright AL, Taussig LM et al 1995 Asthma and wheezing in the first six years of life. N Engl J Med 332:133–138

McAnarney ER, Lawrence RA, Aten MJ, Iker HP 1984 Adolescent mothers and their infants. Pediatrics 73:358–362

McAnarney ER, Lawrence RA, Ricciuti HN, Polley J, Szilagyi M 1986 Interactions of adolescent mothers and their one-year-old children. Pediatrics 78:585–590

Morrison SL, Heady JA, Morris JN 1959 Social and biological factors in infant mortality. VIII. Mortality in the postneonatal period. Arch Dis Child 34:101–114

Murray AB, Morrison BJ 1989 Passive smoking by asthmatics: its greater effect on boys than on girls and on older than on younger children. Pediatrics 84:451–459

Naeye RL 1981 Teenaged and pre-teenaged pregnancies: consequences of the fetal–maternal competition for nutrients. Pediatrics 67:146–150

Schwartz J, Gold D, Dockery DW, Weiss ST, Speizer FE 1990 Predictors of asthma and persistent wheeze in a national sample of children in the United States. Association with social class, perinatal events, and race. Am Rev Respir Dis 142:555–562

Soyseth V, Kongerud J, Boe J 1995 Postnatal maternal smoking increases the prevalence of asthma but not of bronchial hyperresponsiveness or atopy in their children. Chest 107:389–394

Strachan DP, Jarvis MJ, Feyerabend C 1990 The relationship of salivary cotinine to respiratory symptoms, spirometry, and exercise-induced bronchospasm in seven-year-old children. Am Rev Respir Dis 142:147–151

Strachan DP, Butland BK, Anderson HR 1996 Incidence and prognosis of asthma and wheezing illness from early childhood to age 33 in a national British cohort. Br Med J 312:1195–1200

Tager IB, Ngo L, Hanrahan JP 1995 Maternal smoking during pregnancy. Effects on lung function during the first 18 months of life. Am J Respir Crit Care Med 152:997–983

Taussig LM, Wright AL, Morgan WJ, Harrison HR, Ray CG 1989 The Tucson Children's Respiratory Study. I. Design and implementation of a prospective study of acute and chronic respiratory illness in children. Am J Epidemiol 129:1219–1231

United States Environmental Protection Agency 1995 Respiratory health effects of passive smoking: lung cancer and other disorders

von Hoegen P, Sarin S, Krowka JF 1995 Deficiency in T cell responses of human fetal lymph node cells: a lack of accessory cells. Immunol Cell Biol 73:353–361

Weitzman M, Gortmaker S, Klein Walker D, Sobol A 1990 Maternal smoking and childhood asthma. Pediatrics 85:505–511

DISCUSSION

Britton: How much of the relationship between maternal age and infant IgE or asthma can be explained by the levels of maternal IgE?

Martinez: I cannot answer this at the moment, but there is a relationship between the positive skin tests in the mother and asthma. If one corrects for the levels of maternal IgE that relationship is still present.

Britton: But do younger mothers have higher levels of IgE?

Martinez: There's no relationship between maternal age and IgE.

Corris: Some of the atopic asthmatic mothers in your study were symptomatic during their pregnancy. Are there any data suggesting that the way in which the asthma behaves in the mother has an influence on the development of asthma in the child? The severity of asthma in the mother may be a surrogate marker for allergen challenge throughout critical periods of the child's development.

Martinez: I'm not aware of any. This is certainly an important issue because if it were true one would suspect certain dose–response relationships such that more severe asthmatic mothers would have an increased likelihood of having children with asthma.

Weiss: We are currently looking at the effects of maternal asthma on fetal growth and development. Generally, we have found that mild maternal asthma has virtually no influence on birth weight or the development of asthma in the fetus. What seems to be the major confounding variable in these studies is maternal cigarette smoking. Once you correct for this, then asthma itself seems to have little effect.

Holt: One of the issues that you have mentioned previously at a recent workshop on early childhood asthma and that is pertinent to this discussion is the relationship between the time of onset of the first wheeze and the final outcome of the disease at eight, nine or 10 years of age. Can you bring us up-to-date on this issue?

Martinez: We have found that early-onset asthma, when associated with atopic markers, such as skin test reactivity to allergens, and a maternal history of asthma, is also strongly associated with the risk of persistent symptoms beyond the age of five or six years. Indeed, in our study children who are asthmatic at age 11 are those who start wheezing early in life and whose mothers have asthma. Unfortunately, other cross-sectional studies are confounded by the observation that two-thirds of children who wheeze early in life have a good prognosis — they stop wheezing by the age of six and they're not wheezing by the age of 11.

Holt: What's the difference between those who stop wheezing and those who don't.

Martinez: The main difference between the two groups is probably the presence or absence of all the risk factors for the development of early atopic sensitization.

Strachan: Our experience with the large national British cohort we've been following is that an increased incidence of wheezing illnesses, particularly in the earlier years, is associated with maternal smoking (Strachan et al 1996). However, this group has a relatively benign prognosis, and maternal smoking is one of the few factors we can find that influences the prognosis of early wheezing into adolescence and adult life. Therefore, our assessment is rather the contrary to what you were suggesting, i.e. those children whose mothers smoke have relatively benign occasional early attacks and are not going to develop the more persistent atopic asthma. I would like to pick up on your findings relating maternal smoking to allergic sensitization because there are a number of studies — including one of yours in collaboration with Erika von Mutius, in Bavaria (von Mutius et al 1994) and our own studies — which suggest that there is a reduced prevalence of sensitization amongst the offspring of smoking mothers. It is probably true to state that there is currently no consensus in the literature on the association between maternal smoking and subsequent allergic sensitization. It is not clear that it is a risk factor, and it could equally be a protective factor.

Martinez: One of the factors influencing these results is probably the degree of exposure. For example, Forastiere et al (1994) have shown that there is an association between hyper-responsiveness and exposure to smoke only in certain areas of Italy where many of the houses are small, and in which, presumably, there are higher concentrations of cigarette smoke. I am aware of those studies that have different results, so I agree that this area is still debatable. However, maternal smoking is clearly not a protective factor for the development of asthma later in life.

Weiss: It's important to distinguish in the longitudinal data the relationship between environmental tobacco smoke exposure and the incidence of asthma. The data suggest that in older children with asthma, parental smoking makes the asthma worse.

Holt: There are also Swedish data on allergic sensitization, which show that if the population is stratified in terms of risk due to family history, it is the high risk group who are selected by the environmental smoke exposure effects, and also by the effects of other respiratory irritants (Björkstén 1994).

Weiss: This is an extremely important point because if the data relating environmental tobacco smoke to asthma in early life are stratified according to family history of allergy/asthma the relationship between exposure to environmental tobacco smoke and asthma incidence in early childhood changes from about two in the general population to about four in the atopics. This suggests that a gene–environment interaction is occurring.

Paré: What is the effect of maternal age on asthma compared with maternal smoking and early wheezing?

Martinez: In my presentation I showed that there was a strong association between maternal age and wheezing in early life and that there was a weaker association between maternal age and asthma at age six. We didn't find any association between maternal age and any of the IgE-related markers of allergic sensitization. We found an association between maternal age and lung function levels as measured both during the first year of life and at age six. Therefore, it seems that maternal age affects lung development more than it affects factors involved with IgE reactivity.

Paré: Are the effect of maternal age and smoking additive?

Martinez: Yes. The effects of maternal age are independent of those caused by maternal smoking.

Holgate: That is most interesting because there has been a steady increase in maternal smoking over the last 20 years.

Britton: We've looked at the prevalence of asthma in the 1958 and 1970 British birth cohorts and found that there was a 70% increase in asthma at age 16 over that period, of which 5% was accounted for by a decrease in average maternal age and virtually none by increased maternal smoking (Lewis et al 1996).

Weiss: Part of the problem with trying to look for simple relationships with environmental exposures is that, in addition to causing small airways and lungs at birth, they may produce many other different effects which complicate the story enormously.

Busse: Passive exposure to cigarette smoke also causes an increase in eosinophil count. Is there any evidence that cigarette smoke can influence lymphocyte or other cell functions, and thus cause a switch to a T helper 2 (Th2)-like cytokine pattern?

Martinez: Smokers also have increased levels of eosinophils compared to those who do not smoke. There has been much work on the factors that mediate the association (Kauffmann et al 1986); however, the meaning of this still needs to be worked out. It's possible that an effect on the Th cell phenotype is involved.

Holgate: In the over 60-year-old age group cigarette smoking is associated with high IgE levels in the circulation. Both smoking *per se* and elevated IgE levels in the serum are independently associated with a more rapid decline in baseline pulmonary function and bronchial hyper-responsiveness, with a greater than additive interaction between the two (Dow et al 1992, Villar et al 1995). These observations suggest that smoking is able to drive a Th2-like response in certain individuals, with elevated levels of IgE in the serum being accounted for by enhanced interleukin (IL)-4 expression by T cells (Byron et al 1994).

Warner: There is clear evidence that normally T cell responses are down-regulated towards full-term in pregnancy. However, this down-regulation does not occur in smokers, and indeed they often have a raised T cell response.

Weiss: We have looked at circulating cytokines in the peripheral blood of adult cigarette smokers and found elevated levels of soluble IL-2 receptor, which were not associated with airway responsiveness or atopy.

Platts-Mills: Did you observe a low incidence of positive skin tests in adults in Tucson, Arizona who were not exposed to passive smoke?

Martinez: No, we have never found any significant effects of passive smoking on allergic sensitization in Tucson.

Platts-Mills: I ask this because in the USA many educated middle-class families have given up smoking. In Los Alamos, which may be the highest intellectual group that's been studied, very few of the population were exposed to passive smoke and we found an extraordinarily high incidence of positive skin tests in children (Sporik et al 1995). This suggests that the idea that passive smoking is associated with a lower incidence of positive skin tests is not a general phenomenon.

Brostoff: Others have shown a biphasic effect of smoking on IgE levels, such that a certain threshold of exposure results in a marked increase in IgE levels with higher exposure leading to suppression of IgE.

Holt: I have a mechanistic comment about all these environmental effects. It's difficult to tease these out immunologically because the magnitude of the effects of individual agents may depend on the background levels of inflammation in the airways at the time of exposure at that stage. Therefore, the effects of passive smoking in healthy, well-nourished people from clean environments such as Los Alamos may be qualitatively and quantitatively different to the effects of passive smoking on individuals from lower socioeconomic groups, who live in polluted environments and have low standards of hygiene.

Martinez: I would like to ask Harold Nelson to comment on the studies performed on cohorts of children regarding the relationship between maternal psychosocial factors and the development of asthma in their children.

Nelson: David Mrazek and Mary Klinnert followed 150 children whose mothers had asthma (personal communication 1996). They visited their homes at three weeks of age to assess the psychosocial situation. They then followed the development of infectious wheezing and classic asthma. In this way, they found three strong predictors for the onset of classic asthma for the children by age three years: (1) poor parenting, including maternal depression, single motherhood and other stresses within the family at the time of the three-week visit; (2) frequent infections in the first year; and (3) a raised level of IgE at six months. However, in six-year-old children the effects of poor parenting had disappeared and only the latter two remained strong predictors.

Holgate: There is also a study of inner-city New York showing that maternal depression and psychosocial factors in the family had a remarkable effect in enhancing the clinical effects of childhood asthma (McLean et al 1996).

Weiss: We have looked at a birth cohort through the first five years of life and we found specific behavioural correlates between maternal stresses and asthma: mothers who were highly stressed had higher allergen levels in their home. Therefore, one of the problems of looking at psychosocial variables is that maternal stresses may in fact be an indicator of high allergen loads.

References

Björkstén B 1994 Risk factors in early childhood for the development of atopic diseases. Allergy 49:400–407

Byron KA, Varigos GA, Wootton AM 1994 Interleukin-4 production is increased in cigarette smokers. Clin Exp Immunol 95:333–336

Dow L, Coggon D, Campbell MJ, Holgate ST 1992 The interaction between immunoglobulin E and smoking in airflow obstruction in the elderly. Am Rev Respir Dis 146:402–407

Forastiere F, Agabiti N, Corbo GM et al 1994 Passive smoking as a determinant of bronchial responsiveness in children. Am J Respir Crit Care Med 149:365–370

Kauffmann F, Neukirch F, Korobaeff M, Marne MJ, Claude JR, Lellouch J 1986 Eosinophils, smoking, and lung function: an epidemiologic survey among 912 working men. Am Rev Respir Dis 134:1172–1175

Lewis S, Butland B, Strachan D et al 1996 Study of the aetiology of wheezing illness at age 16 in two national British cohorts. Thorax 51:670–676

McLean DE, Findley SE, Arcensas M 1996 Determinants of asthma prevalence in Harlem. Am J Respir Crit Care Med 153:255A

Sporik R, Ingram JM, Price W, Sussman HJ, Honsinger RW, Platts-Mills TAE 1995 Association of asthma with serum IgE and skin test reactivity to allergens among children living at high altitude: tickling the dragon's breath. Am J Respir Crit Care Med 151:1388–1392

Strachan DP, Butland BK, Anderson HR 1996 The incidence and prognosis of asthma and wheezing illness for early childhood to age 33 in a national British cohort. Br Med J 312:1195–1199

Villar MTA, Dow L, Coggon D, Lampe FC, Holgate ST 1995 The influence of increased bronchial responsiveness, atopy and serum IgE on decline in FEV$_1$. A longitudinal study in the elderly. Am J Respir Crit Care Med 151:656–662

von Mutius E, Martinez FD, Fritzsch C, Nicolai T, Reitmar P, Thiemann HH 1994 Skin test reactivity and number of siblings. Br Med J 308:692–695

Diet as a risk factor for asthma

Scott T. Weiss

Channing Laboratory, Department of Medicine, Harvard University Medical School, Brigham & Women's Hospital, 180 Longwood Avenue, Boston, MA 02115, USA

Abstract. Asthma prevalence and morbidity have increased in the past 10 years in the face of improved knowledge about pathophysiology and treatment. Changing patterns and interactions among asthma risk factors may contribute to these disease trends. Diet is a newly recognized potential risk factor for asthma occurrence. This chapter focuses on the methodological issues in the assessment of diet as a risk factor for asthma and the available data linking diet to asthma, airway inflammation and airway responsiveness, and it concludes with a consideration of research needs and future directions. Four types of dietary constituents are considered: breast feeding and food avoidance in infancy; antioxidant vitamins, specifically vitamin C; dietary cations, specifically sodium and magnesium; and N3–N6 fatty acids. At present, available data are insufficient to implicate any dietary constituent as a causal risk factor for asthma. Data are strongest for vitamin C, which is associated with protective effects of airway responsiveness, lung function and asthma symptoms. Prospective cohort studies of the effects of early childhood diet on the development of asthma in children (birth to age six years) are needed to assess diet as a risk factor for early childhood asthma and its interrelationship with other risk factors.

1997 The rising trends in asthma. Wiley, Chichester (Ciba Foundation Symposium 206) p 244–257

Asthma is a clinical syndrome defined by airway inflammation, increased airway responsiveness and reversible airflow obstruction. Asthma prevalence and morbidity are increasing in western countries. This increase is occurring in spite of increased knowledge and better treatment of the disease, and it is thought to be due to factors associated with a western lifestyle. Inflammation is a central problem in asthma and this inflammation is thought to be primarily IgE mediated. Factors thought to decrease inflammation might inhibit the physiological consequences of inflammation, such as decreased lung function, airway responsiveness and respiratory symptoms. Western diet has changed dramatically over the past 30 years, with an increase in saturated fat and processed foods, and a decrease in fresh fruits, vegetables and fish. It is perfectly plausible that changes in diet may be contributing to changes in asthma prevalence and morbidity. This chapter will examine four areas of diet thought to be important in asthma: (1) breast feeding/food avoidance; (2) dietary antioxidants; (3) cations; and (4) polyunsaturated fatty acids.

Methods of diet assessment and clinical research

Assessment of human diet as a risk factor for disease is difficult because there is a limited range of variation in diet in western populations and an inevitable measurement error in measuring its intake. In addition, the expected association between dietary factors and asthma is relatively weak with relative risks in the range of 0.5–2.0. The major methodological tool for dietary assessment is the food frequency questionnaire. The rationale for this approach is that the average long-term diet over months and years is the relevant exposure rather than short-term intake. The major problem with this tool is recall bias leading to misclassification of exposure, which will tend to be a null bias in positive studies. Serum levels of micronutrients are also a useful exposure measurement tool. Because of the low relative risks and the degree of error associated with dietary assessment, relatively large sample sizes are required to demonstrate associations in epidemiological studies of diet and disease.

Breast feeding/food avoidance

Despite multiple studies, the role of breast feeding and food avoidance as mechanisms to prevent asthma in early infancy remains controversial. There are as many positive as negative studies (Zeiger 1988). The bulk of these studies are non-randomized and are thus subject to a number of potential biases: lack of blinding; absence of confirmation of compliance; high drop out rates; small sample size; brief duration of breast feeding; and lack of control of maternal diet. The theoretical benefits of breast feeding include the passive acquisition by the infant of maternal antibodies (especially IgG, IgM and IgA), immune-competent cells (such as macrophages and leukocytes) and, depending on the maternal diet, lack of exposure to food antigens. Unfortunately, the infant is exposed to a variety of antigens if the mother does not control her diet and exposures. These include: cotinine; cows milk; eggs; wheat; maternal IgE; and sensitized lymphocytes from the mother.

Recently, Zeiger et al (1989) reported on a randomized trial of breast feeding and food avoidance in the mother and their effects on the development of allergy and asthma in the first three years of life. The sample was infants of atopic parents. Each treatment group and control consisted of approximately 150 infants and mothers. The treatment group consisted of control of maternal diet from the third trimester, breast feeding, supplemental hypoallergenic formula and food avoidance in the child. The result was a reduction of eczema at three years but no change in asthma or allergic rhinitis. Current ongoing trials will try to assess this issue further.

Antioxidants

Free radicals are reactive chemical species, derived from oxygen, that are chemically unstable. Oxygen-free radicals are capable of damaging cellular components, and thus contributing to inflammation. Chemical oxidants can be derived from cigarette smoke, viral infections or allergen exposure — the three most important environmental exposures for asthma. Antioxidant vitamins are the first line of defence against oxidant injury.

Vitamin C

Vitamin C is a water-soluble, free radical scavenger of singular oxygen, superoxide anion and peroxyl-free radicals (Anderson et al 1987). Vitamin C also functions as a coenzyme in the biosynthesis of collagen, and may thus contribute to lung repair (Levine 1986). Vitamin C may also play a role in immune function. It is transported into neutrophils (Washko et al 1989) and lymphocytes (Bergsten et al 1990). The correlation between serum vitamin C levels and vitamin C intake as assessed by food frequency questionnaire is in the order of 0.4 (Willett et al 1987).

The long-term epidemiological data are relatively consistent. At least two studies have not measured vitamin C directly, but have examined intake of fresh fruit and vegetables, foods high in vitamin C. The Zutphen Study found that food intake is inversely related to the incidence of asthma, bronchitis and emphysema, higher fresh fruit and vegetable intake being associated with about a 25% reduction in disease risk (odds ratio 0.73, 95% confidence interval 0.53–0.99) (Miedema et al 1993). No specific effect of vitamin C was seen in this study. Strachan et al (1991) studied a random population in the UK and found that subjects who consumed low levels of fresh fruits had an FEV_1 (forced expiratory volume in one second) 80 ml lower on average than those who were regular consumers. Again, vitamin C was not assessed in this cross-sectional investigation.

Three studies have assessed the relationship of vitamin C intake to the occurrence of wheeze or asthma. Schwartz & Weiss found an inverse association between serum vitamin C levels, but not dietary intake of vitamin C, as measured by 24 h recall and the prevalence of wheezing within the past year. These data are from the National Health and Nutrition Examination Survey II (NHANES II) (Schwartz & Weiss 1990). The investigators found a 30% decrease in wheezing (odds ratio 0.71, 95% confidence interval 0.858–0.88) for a two standard deviation increase in vitamin C, adjusting for age, gender, race, socioeconomic status, cigarette smoking and total energy intake. Troisi et al (1995) examined the effect of vitamin C intake on the subsequent development of asthma among women in the Nurses Health Study, as described above. They could find no relationship between vitamin C intake and the development of asthma in adult women. Thus, of the three studies that have looked at the relationship of vitamin C to wheeze symptoms, two have found an association with lower levels of vitamin C being associated with wheeze or asthma. The one study that found no relationship (The Nurses Health Study) looked at food frequency data and adult incident asthma as the outcome. This at least raises the question as to whether misclassification accounts for the lack of the association in the Nurses Health Study data. An alternative might be that this adult-onset disease is different from disease in childhood.

A series of small case-control studies have examined serum levels of vitamin C in asthma patients and controls (Mohsenin et al 1983, Ogilvy et al 1981, Powell et al 1994, Schwartz & Weiss 1994a). These studies, by virtue of their design, are unable to address the question of whether the low plasma vitamin C levels are the cause or the consequence of airway inflammation.

With regard to lung function outcomes, Schwartz & Weiss (1994b) found a relationship between low levels of vitamin C, as assessed by 24 h recall and a food frequency questionnaire, and low levels of FEV_1 in the NHANES I subjects. This positive correlation is such that the difference between the first and the third tertile in terms of vitamin C intake was associated with an approximate 20 ml difference in FEV_1. These findings were confirmed by Britton et al (1995) in the Nottingham cohort. They estimated that the standard deviation increase in vitamin C was approximately equivalent to the adverse effects of smoking five packets of cigarettes per year on FEV_1. These papers adjusted for age, gender, cigarette smoking, total calories, vitamin E intake, race and socioeconomic status. To date, there are no longitudinal studies on the relationship of vitamin C intake and decline in lung function, nor are there studies that have examined more specific asthma-related outcomes, such as airway reactivity.

In summary, of all antioxidant vitamins, the data linking vitamin C with respiratory outcomes seem the strongest. Short-term clinical trials in asthma patients in general show modest effects on lung function and airway responsiveness. The relationship to lung function is consistent in cross-sectional epidemiological studies. There are, however, no data conclusively linking vitamin C levels to asthma onset.

N3–N6 fatty acids

Horrobin (1987) hypothesized that the low prevalence of asthma among Greenland Eskimos was due to their high intake of eicosapentaenoic acid. These omega 3 fatty acids are essential for cell membranes. N3 and N6 fatty acids are believed to shunt the eicosinoid production away from the arachidonic acid pathway and toward the prostanoic pathway, thus decreasing the production of broncho-constrictive leukotrienes. In vitro studies and studies of small groups of human asthmatic subjects supplemented with doses of eicosapentaenoic acid show that the generation of leukotrienes by neutrophils and mononuclear leukocytes was decreased of eicosapentaenoic acid supplements in the diet (Payon et al 1986). Schwartz & Weiss (1994b) reported on the relationship between dietary fish intake and level of pulmonary function in the NHANES I study. In this investigation, in which over 30 000 individuals representative of the USA population were studied, there was about an 80 ml difference between subjects who regularly consumed fish versus those who did not. This analysis controlled for age, race, gender and smoking, but did not effectively control for social class. In addition, the analysis was cross-sectional, although this is unlikely to have introduced a bias because it is unlikely that subjects knew of the association between fish and pulmonary function. No specific analysis was done to look at asthmatics.

Two separate studies of Australian school children also support the protective association of fish oil and asthma. Peat et al (1992) included a question on fish intake in one of four communities studied as part of a population survey of asthma risk factors. Regular fish intake was associated with a 50% reduction in prevalence of increased airway responsiveness (defined as $PD_{20} < 3.9$ mmoles, where PD_{20} represents the provocation dose of histamine leading to a 20% decrease in pulmonary function as measured by FEV_1) compared with those who did not eat fish. This report did not differentiate type of fish intake or adjust for social class. In a follow-up investigation these investigators utilized a validated food frequency questionnaire to assess the effect of fish intake on asthma (Hodge et al 1996). They found that children whose parents reported eating fresh oily fish had significantly less asthma (odds ratio 0.26, 95% confidence interval 0.09–0.72).

These data suggest, but do not confirm, that a relationship exists between fish oil, or other polyunsaturated fatty acids, and asthma. The confounding effects of social class remain a concern, as does the design of these studies, which remains cross-sectional. These investigations indicate the need for further investigations.

Urinary cations: sodium, potassium and magnesium

Sodium and potassium

Few areas in the relationship of diet to asthma are as confusing and as complex as the relationship of sodium and potassium to asthma. Burney (1987) hypothesized, on the basis of ecological data, that salt intake might be related to asthma. Following this initial report, Burney et al (1986) conducted an observational study examining urinary sodium excretion and its relationship to inhaled histamine among asthmatic patients, and they found a significant relationship. This report was followed by a paper by Javaid et al (1988), in which a small number of asthmatic subjects were followed for one month in a randomized controlled trial, and they found that the PC_{20} (i.e. provocation concentration of histamine leading to a 20% decrease in pulmonary function as measured by FEV_1) to histamine increased with increased sodium intake. Medici et al (1993) performed a similar study on 14 asthmatics using a randomized controlled trial over a nine-week period, comparing salt loading to placebo, and found a worsening of symptoms with salt loading, but there was no effect on PD_{20} to methacholine. Burney et al (1989) subsequently performed a large randomized controlled trial of a low sodium diet versus a high fibre diet in 201 asthmatics, followed at one, two, and three months, looking at daily variation in peak flow as the outcome. They found that there was a 15% improvement in diurnal peak flow in the low salt group. It is important to note that all of these studies were performed in asthmatic patients, most of them young asthmatic patients.

In summary, short-term randomized controlled trials consistently demonstrate a relationship between salt intake and a variety of parameters of asthma functioning. The population-based data are, however, less convincing. Sparrow et al (1991) studied 273 subjects in the Normative Aging Study. The mean age of these subjects was 60 years, and the prevalence of asthma was low. They compared 24 h urinary sodium and potassium levels with methacholine airway responsiveness, and found that there was no significant relationship for urinary sodium, although there was a positive relationship between urinary potassium and airway responsiveness. Pistelli et al (1993) studied the personal salt use (measured using a food frequency questionnaire) and untimed morning urine samples of 2593 subjects between the ages of nine and 16 in Italy. They found that symptoms were related to personal salt use only in boys, and that the PD_{20} was not related to salt use, but to urinary excretion of potassium. Finally, Britton et al (1994a) studied the 24 h urinary sodium and potassium levels of 1702 adults aged 18 to 70 in Nottingham England. Airway responsiveness to methacholine was the outcome variable, and no relationship of responsiveness to urinary sodium was observed, although there was a weak relationship between urinary sodium and skin test reactivity. It is important to consider the potential mechanisms by which sodium might be involved in increasing airway responsiveness in asthma.

Recently, Burney and co-workers examined this issue and found that incubation of human leukocytes in serum from men with hyper-responsive airways leads to increased intracellular sodium levels, probably in part through increased sodium influx into cells (Tribe et al 1994). This influx is independent of sodium chloride cotransport and sodium–hydrogen ion exchange. It is also independent of serum IgE and dietary sodium levels. Dietary sodium, as measured by urinary sodium excretion, had additional independent effects on airway responsiveness in these studies. This study did not measure sodium potassium ATPase activity directly and, hence, cannot definitively answer questions related to mechanisms of this physiological effect. A series of studies has demonstrated that furosemide is an effective treatment for asthma, again supporting the idea that excess sodium may be an important determinant of airway responsiveness (Lockhart & Slutsky 1994).

There is a striking difference between the results of the clinical studies and those of the epidemiological investigations: the clinical studies have focused on asthma patients, whereas the epidemiological studies have focused on general population samples. It should be noted that a single 24 h urine test is a very insensitive method for reflecting chronic dietary sodium intake. There is substantial intra-individual variability with regard to sodium intake, and a food frequency questionnaire is not optimal to assess dietary sodium. Low power may also be a problem, as most of the epidemiological studies are relatively small. Finally, there may be negative confounding by other cationic variables, such as potassium and/or magnesium (see below). Other possible explanations include the fact that bronchial responsiveness has been linked to increased sodium/potassium ATPase activity in rat models (Spivey et al 1990), as well as the increased extracellular potassium in smooth muscle contraction. Control of potassium homeostasis is through the adrenergic system. This control is impaired in asthmatic subjects. High levels of potassium in those subjects with increased airway responsiveness to methacholine may simply reflect this abnormal adrenergic control. This would then be a consequence rather than a cause of the problem. An additional complicating factor besides low power and negative confounding is the possibility that other dietary constituents could influence these relationships. Urinary and dietary sodium are known to be linked to dietary fat intake, and antioxidant intake may also affect transport of anions across cell membranes.

Magnesium

Magnesium is an essential divalent cation that is responsible for the maintenance of electrical potential across cell membranes and, therefore, bronchomotor tone. Additional biological functions of magnesium include its role as an essential cofactor for ATP-requiring enzymes (Del Certillo & Engbeeck 1954). Finally, magnesium is involved in DNA and RNA synthesis and replication. On a functional level, magnesium can relax airway smooth muscle *in vitro* (Matthew & Altuma 1988). Magnesium can also inhibit cholinergic neuromuscular transmission and stabilize mast cell membranes to prevent the release of histamine (Bois 1963). Excess magnesium will block the actions of calcium, whereas magnesium deficiency will potentiate the actions of calcium (Nadler et al 1987). Magnesium is involved in the physiological regulation of calcium influx through cell membranes, and therefore an excess or deficiency will influence sodium and potassium metabolism. Finally, magnesium can influence the stabilization of mast cells (Kemp et al 1994) and stimulate the generation of prostacyclin (Wei & Franz 1990) and nitric oxide (Britton et al 1994b). Magnesium in the diet is obtained principally from green vegetables, unprocessed grains and dairy products. Magnesium is leeched from food during the cooking process; therefore, refined or processed foods are likely to be lower in magnesium. Studies in pigs have suggested that magnesium deficiency may potentiate histamine release in animals exposed to antigen (Britton et al 1994a).

Britton et al (1994a) have investigated the relationships among dietary magnesium (measured using a food frequency questionnaire) FEV_1, airway reactivity to methacholine and self-reported wheezing in the past 12 months in 2633 adults aged 18–70 from Nottingham, England. They observed an association between 100 mg per day or higher magnesium intake and both a 27.7 ml higher FEV_1 (95% confidence interval 11.9–43.5) and a reduction in the relative odds of airway hyper-responsiveness of 0.82 (95% confidence interval 0.72–0.93). The same 100 mg increase in dietary magnesium was associated with a reduction in wheeze symptoms (odds ratio 0.85, 95% confidence interval 0.76–0.95). These analyses were adjusted for age, gender, height, effects of atopy and cigarette smoking, and caloric intake. Although this was a cross-sectional study, the consistency of these results is quite striking. In other words, not only was dietary magnesium intake associated with a decrease in symptoms, but it was also associated with improved lung function and decreased airway reactivity. These findings need to be replicated in a longitudinal study. Britton speculates that the interrelationship of magnesium with potassium and sodium may mean that low levels of dietary magnesium could potentially confound or confuse an interrelationship of sodium or potassium with asthma or airway responsiveness. This hypothesis will require further investigation.

Summary

The study of diet as a risk factor and a potential modifier of the effect of other environmental exposures on asthma is in its infancy. To date, the number of large-scale epidemiological investigations are small, most are cross-sectional, and most are focused on adults. It would appear that, based on existing data, the relationship of vitamin C to asthma is the strongest. What appears to be needed are prospective investigations in children, particularly children between birth and aged 10. It is estimated that over half of all asthma cases are diagnosed by age six; therefore, the identification of the role of dietary factors in the development of asthma would appear to require studies that focus on younger subjects. This will require the use of serum levels to measure exposure or new methodological developments to assess dietary intake in children, as the food frequency approach has not been validated for children this young. Taken as a whole, the existing data are suggestive of important associations, and therefore this is an area that demands further investigation in the future.

Acknowledgements

I thank Linda Bustin for help with the preparation of this chapter. This work has been supported in part by grants HL34695, HL19170 and HL5084 from the lung division of the National Heart and Blood Institute, National Institutes of Health, Bethesda, MD, USA.

References

Anderson R, Theron AJ, Ras GJ 1987 Regulation by the antioxidants ascorbate, cysteine, and dapsone of the increased extracellular and intracellular generation of reactive oxidants by activated phagocytes from cigarette smokers. Am Rev Respir Dis 135:1027–1032

Bergsten P, Amitai G, Kehrl J, Dhairwal DR, Klein A, Levine M 1990 Millimolar concentrations of ascorbic acid in purified human nonnuclear leukocytes: depletion and reaccumulation. J Biol Chem 265:2584–2587

Bois P 1963 Effect of magnesium deficiency on mast cells and urinary histamine in rats. Br J Exp Path 44:151–155

Britton J, Pavord I, Wisniewski A et al 1994a Dietary magnesium, lung function, wheezing, and airway hyperreactivity in a random adult opulation. Lancet 344:357–362

Britton J, Pavord I, Richards K 1994b Dietary sodium intake and the risk of airway hyperreactivity in a random adult population. Thorax 49:875–880

Britton JR, Pavord ID, Richards KA et al 1995 Dietary antioxidant vitamin intake and lung function in the general population. Am J Respir Crit Care Med 151:1383–1387

Burney PGJ 1987 A diet rich in sodium may potentiate asthma: epidemiological evidence for a new hypothesis. Chest 91:1435–1485

Burney PGJ, Britton JR, Chinn S et al 1986 Response to histamine and 24-hour sodium excretion. Br Med J 292:1483–1486

Burney PGJ, Neild JE, Twort CHC et al 1989 Effect of changing dietary sodium on the airway response to histamine. Thorax 44:36–41

Del Certillo J, Engbeeck L 1954 The nature of the neuromuscular block produced by magnesium. J Physiol 124:370–384

Hodge L, Salome CM, Peat JK, Haby MM, Wei XA, Woolcock AJ 1996 Consumption of oily fish and childhood asthma risk. Med J Austr 164:137–140

Horrobin DF 1987 Low prevalences of coronary heart disease (CHD), boriasis, asthma, and rheumatoid arthritis in Eskimos: are they caused by high dietary intake of eicosapentaenaic acid (EPA), a genetic variation of essential fatty acid (EFA), metabolism, or a combination of both? Medical Hypotheses 22:421–428

Javaid A, Cushley MJ, Bone MF 1988 Effect of dietary salt on bronchial reactivity to histamine in asthma. Br Med J 297:454

Kemp PA, Gardine SM, March JE, Bennett T, Rubin PC 1994 The effects of NG-Nitro-L-Arginine methyl ether on regional neurodynamic responses to MgSO$_4$ in conscious rats. Br J Pharmacol 111:325–331

Levine M 1986 New concepts in the biology and biochemistry of ascorbic acid. N Engl J Med 314:892–902

Levine BS, Coburn JW 1984 Magnesium: the mimic/antagonist of calcium. N Engl J Med 310:1253–1255

Lockhart A, Slutsky AS 1994 Furosemide and loop diuretics in human asthma. Chest 106: 244–249

Matthew R, Altuma BM 1988 Magnesium and the lungs. Magnesium 7:173–187

Medici TS, Schmidt AZ, Hacki M, Vetter W 1993 Are asthmatics salt sensitive? Chest 104: 1138–1143

Miedema I, Feskens EJM, Heederik D, Kromhout D 1993 Dietary determinants of long term incidence of chronic nonspecific lung disease. Am J Epidemiol 138:37–45

Mohsenin V, DuBois AB, Douglas JS 1983 Effect of ascorbic acid on response to methacholine challenge in asthmatic subjects. Am Rev Respir Dis 127:143–147

Nadler JL, Goodson S, Rude RK 1987 Evidence that prostacyclin mediates the vascular action of magnesium in humans. Hypertension 9:379–383

Ogilvy CS, DuBois AB, Douglas JS 1981 Effects of ascorbic acid and indomethacin on the airways of healthy male subjects with and without induced bronchoconstriction. J Allergy Clin Immunol 67:363–367

Payon DG, Wong MY, Chernou-Rogan T et al 1986 Alterations in human leukocyte function induced by ingestion of eicosapentaenoic acid. J Clin Immunol 6:402–410

Peat JK, Salome CM, Woolcock AJ 1992 Factors associated with bronchial hyperresponsiveness in Australian adults and children. Eur Respir J 5:921–929

Pistelli R, Forastiere F, Corbo GM et al 1993 Respiratory symptoms and bronchial responsiveness are related to dietary salt intake and urinary potassium excretion in male children. Eur Respir J 6:517–522

Powell CV, Nash AA, Powers HJ, Primhak RA 1994 Antioxidant status in asthma. Ped Pulmonol 18:34–38

Schwartz J, Weiss ST 1990 Dietary factors and their relationship to respiratory symptoms: the second National Health and Nutrition Examination Survey. Am J Epidemiol 132:67–76

Schwartz J, Weiss ST 1994a Relationship between dietary vitamin C intake and pulmonary function in the first National Health and Nutrition Examination Survey (NHANES I). Am J Clin Nutr 59:110–114

Schwartz J, Weiss ST 1994b The relationship of dietary fish intake to level of pulmonary function in the First National Health and Nutrition Examination Survey (NHANES I). Eur Respir J 7:1821–1824

Sparrow D, O'Connor GT, Rosner B, Weiss ST 1991 Methacholine airway responsiveness and 24-hour urine excretion of sodium and potassium. Am Rev Respir Dis 144:722–725

Spivey WH, Skobeloff EM, Levin RM 1990 The effect of magnesium chloride on rabbit bronchial smooth muscle. Ann Emerg Med 19:1107–1112

Strachan DP, Cox BD, Erzinclioglu SW, Walters DE, Whichelow MJ 1991 Ventilatory function and winter fresh fruit consumption in a random sample of British adults. Thorax 46:624–629

Tribe RM, Barton JR, Poston L, Burney PGJ 1994 Dietary sodium intake, airway responsiveness and cellular sodium transport. Am J Respir Crit Care Med 149:1426–1433

Troisi RJ, Willet WC, Weiss ST, Trichopoulos D, Rosner B, Speizer FE 1995 A prospective study of diet and adult onset asthma. Am J Respir Crit Care Med 151:1401–1408

Washko P, Rotrosen D, Levine M 1989 Ascorbic acid transport and accumulation in human neutrophils. J Biol Chem 204:18996–19002

Wei W, Franz KB 1990 A synergism of antigen challenge and severe magnesium deficiency on blood and urinary histamine levels in rats. J Am Coll Nutr 9:616–622

Willett WC, Reynolds RD, Cottrell-Hoehner S, Sampson L, Browne ML 1987 Validation of a semiquantitative food frequency questionnaire: comparison with a one-year diet record. J Am Diet Assoc 87:43–47

Zeiger RS 1988 Development and prevention of allergic disease in childhood. In: Middleton E, Reed CE, Ellis E, Adkinson NF Jr, Yunginer JW (eds) Allergy. Mosby, St Louis, MO, p 930–968

Zeiger RS, Heller S, Mellon MH et al 1989 Effect of infant food-allergen avoidance on development of atopy in early infancy: a randomized study. J Allergy Clin Immunol 84:72–89

DISCUSSION

Heusser: Has anyone looked at vitamin A? Because vitamin A acts on various nuclear factors and has been shown in mice to change a T helper (Th) 1 response into a Th2 response (Racke et al 1995). Furthermore, *in vitro* it induces the production of interleukin (IL)-4 and IL-5 and inhibits the expression of γ-interferon from T cells.

Weiss: There was one study of the relationship between vitamin A and chronic obstructive lung disease which demonstrated a small potential protective effect (Morabia et al 1989). Vitamin A deficiency is probably going to become important with regard to respiratory infections in early life, and therefore it is something that we should start investigating.

Busse: If you take peripheral blood cells from people who take vitamin C and evaluate their eosinophil functions, do you find that these cells are less likely to generate an inflammatory response?

Weiss: I'm not aware that anyone has looked at this.

Potter: Is there any evidence that chronic exposure to sulfites used as preservatives in foods or beverages are contributing to the rising trends in asthma?

Weiss: I haven't looked at that specifically, but Richard Schwartzstein in our group has suggested that it is not a major factor.

Woolcock: Jenny Peat has recently found in her children's dietary questionnaire (personal communication 1996) that salt intake in boys, but not girls, is associated with hyper-responsiveness. Do you have any information regarding these gender differences?

Burney: No. Research into the effects of sodium and other electrolytes on asthma was a fruitful area of research in the 1920s and 1930s but people lost interest in the early 1940s, possibly because of the introduction of steroids. Unfortunately, many of the early studies were not as well designed as they would be now. It seems to be a fairly consistent result that there are differences between the sexes, but we haven't yet performed the necessary studies to determine why. We have tried to look at the physiology of this, but our studies were only of men (Tribe et al 1994). Although men apparently have this extra risk factor, i.e. that they respond badly if they have a high sodium intake, the paradox is that women tend to have more severe asthma. I suspect that for some reason women are already naturally stimulated in this way, i.e. the sodium leak in men is already compromised in women, but we haven't yet looked at this.

Holt: It has been suggested that red wine has a possible protective effect in relation to cardiovascular disease via its antioxidant activity. Are there any similar protective effects of red wine intake on asthma?

Weiss: We have not looked at this.

Holgate: There is some literature on alcohol in both human asthma and in animal models in which the causative factor is thought to be the production of acetaldehyde (Wilson et al 1996, Trenga et al 1996).

Platts-Mills: In the hypertension literature there are consistent data on people who respond to sodium and people who don't. Would it be possible to look for a similar response to sodium in relation to bronchial activity?

Weiss: Looking at the sodium and potassium literature on mechanisms is complicated. It has also been established that African Americans are more salt sensitive than Caucasians (Sowers et al 1988, Simon et al 1994, Falkner et al 1986, 1992).

Platts-Mills: Is a high salt diet in African Americans really a new phenomenon?

Boushey: The major difference may not be as much in sodium intake as in potassium intake. The average potassium intake in African Americans is 50% lower than in white Americans, possible because of a lower intake of fresh fruits and vegetables. Fresh vegetables may be relatively expensive in developed urban economics, but are available across the economic scale in rural economies. Diets in westernized societies are generally lower in potassium, but we have not evolved to crave potassium as we do sodium, possibly because potassium was so rich in the foods eaten by our evolutionary ancestors.

Weiss: There are two aspects of a westernized diet that are important: the increased salt and saturated fat intakes; and the decreased intake of fresh fruit and vegetables, which are rich sources of vitamin C and potassium. The published data did not examine vitamin C *per se* but fresh fruit and vegetable intake and its relationship to asthma. There are clearly numerous dietary factors involved.

Potter: Africans living in cities, in our experience, suffer from more severe asthma, hypertension and heart muscle diseases. We've never compared salt intake in rural and urban environments, but it is important that we do so.

Britton: Of the different potential aetiologies we've been discussing at this symposium, diet is the only one that's changed in the right direction, i.e. for the worse, to explain the rising trends in asthma. Therefore, it may be a better candidate than some of the other factors that we've looked at.

Secondly, there may be important distinctions between the effects of diet on lung function/risk of emphysema and the risk of asthma. For example, antioxidants may protect lung function but there is no strong evidence that they protect against asthma. The consistent finding is that the electrolyte balance across cell membranes is somehow likely to be involved. One point that may be relevant is that we have just finished analysing the expansion study of low versus high magnesium intake in asthmatic patients, and there is some evidence that their symptoms and their use of β-agonist decrease when they are given magnesium supplements.

Beasley: Results that favour the antioxidant theory are those which have examined the relationship between selenium status and asthma. There are many cross-sectional studies in different countries that have linked low levels of selenium and reduced glutathione peroxidase activity with an increased risk of asthma (Beasley et al 1991). More recently, there was a small longitudinal study of children in New Zealand which reported that asthma was more common in children with low levels of selenium in serum taken eight years earlier (Shaw et al 1994).

Weiss: I regard the potential importance of antioxidants with regard to asthma as modulators of immune function and also because they may influence the activities of other co-factors such as cytokines and regulatory proteins. These are relatively unexplored areas.

Britton: There is evidence that vitamin C suppresses respiratory inflammatory cell activation, and there is substantial literature reporting the effect of antioxidants on inflammatory cells in asthma. However, I can't believe that the suppression of minor parts of the asthmatic inflammatory response will have a major effect on the disease. In contrast, antioxidant damage is a major player in the development of emphysema.

Holgate: Molecules that are over-expressed in asthma — the chemokines, some of the Th2 cell cytokines and adhesion molecules — are under the control of the transcription factor NFκB, which is activated by the intracellular accumulation of reactive oxygen intermediates (Manning et al 1994). There is some evidence that antioxidants can protect against this — for example, the inflammatory effects of ozone on acquired bronchial hyper-responsiveness (Trenga et al 1996). Therefore, there is at least one plausible mechanism relating to inflammation in which dietary antioxidants could have an effect.

Brostoff: I could not let a session on dietary risk factors in asthma go by without a discussion of *post hoc* factors. It is quite clear from the data we have published that some asthmatics respond to an elimination diet, i.e. the ingestion of the foods by those people produces an asthmatic response (Brostoff et al 1979). What is not known is what proportion of asthmatics with chronic asthma would benefit from dietary elimination.

Holgate: Perhaps we need better markers of the response to dietary interventions; for example, markers of airway inflammation.

H. R. Anderson: Most of the data in relation to diet seem to suggest that diet can worsen asthma, and there are fewer data suggesting that diet can initiate asthma. Trends in asthma over time are more likely to reflect a change in initiating factors, so although the dietary hypothesis has some attractions because diet has changed, I doubt whether it can explain the upward trend in asthma incidence.

Weiss: That's a fair comment. Unfortunately, relative to coronary disease, the study of diet in relation to asthma is in its infancy. Almost all of these data are cross-sectional and don't even address the issue of temporal relationships. All one can really do at present is to marry long-term trends in asthma prevalence with long-term dietary trends.

Burney: The distinction between initiation and exacerbation is not necessarily appropriate in this case. An atopic individual who does not have clinical asthma could easily be made symptomatic by a change in diet. Is this initiation or exacerbation? A change in diet could lead to an apparent change in prevalence.

Weiss: The first studies of cholesterol and coronary heart disease looked at similar factors to what we're looking at here. When these initial studies were completed, they realized that small differences in cholesterol could produce a large population effect. We don't yet have the data, all we have is the suggestion that something should be studied.

References

Beasley R, Thomson C, Pearce N 1991 Selenium, glutathione peroxidase and asthma. Clin Exp Allergy 21:157–159

Brostoff J, Carini C, Wraith DG, Johns P 1979 Production of IgE complexes by allergen challenge in atopic patients and the effect of sodium cromoglycate. Lancet I:1268–1270

Falkner B, Kushner HH, Khalsa DK, Canessa M, Katz S 1986 Sodium sensitivity, growth and family history of hypertension in young Blacks. J Hypertens (suppl) 4:381S–383S

Falkner B, Hhulman S, Kushner H 1992 Hyperinsulinemia and blood pressure sensitivity to sodium in young Blacks. J Am Soc Nephrol 3:940–946

Manning AM, Anderson DC, Bristol JA 1994 Transcription factor NF-κB. An emerging regulation of inflammation. Ann Rep Med Chem. Academic Press, San Diego p 235–244

Morabia A, Sorenson A, Kumenyika SK, Abbey H, Cohen BH, Chee E 1989 Vitamin A, cigarette smoking and airway obstruction. Am J Respir Dis 140:1312–1313

Racke MK, Burnett D, Pak S-H et al 1995 Retinoid treatment of experimental allergic encephalomyelitis: IL-4 production correlates with improved disease course. J Immunol 154:450–458

Shaw R, Woodman K, Crane J, Moyes C, Kennedy J, Pearce N 1994 Risk factors for asthma symptoms in Kawerau children. NZ Med J 107:387–391

Simon JA, Obarzanek E, Daniels SR, Frederick MM 1994 Dietary cation intake and blood pressure in black girls and white girls. Am J Epidemiol 139:130–140

Sowers JR, Zemel MB, Zemel P, Beck FW, Walsh MF, Zawada ET 1988 Salt sensitivity in Blacks: salt intake and natriuretic substances. Hypertension 12:485–490

Trenga CA, Williams DV, Koenig JO 1996 Dietary antioxidants and ozone-induced bronchial hyperresponsiveness. Am J Respir Crit Care Med 153:305A

Tribe RM, Barton JR, Poston L, Burney PGJ 1994 Dietary sodium intake, airway responsiveness and cellular sodium transport. Am J Respir Crit Care Med 149:1426–1433

Wilson SJ, Manning AM, Anderson DC, Holgate ST 1996 The role of NF-κB in the allergic inflammatory response. Am J Respir Crit Care Med 153:227 (abstr)

Summary

Stephen T. Holgate

School of Medicine, University of Southampton, Level D, Centre Block, Southampton General Hospital, Tremona Road, Southampton SO16 6YD, UK

When I first thought about the possibility of suggesting a symposium on asthma I was motivated by pathogenesis and how our new-found knowledge could be linked to any changes in asthma prevalence and severity. The Ciba Foundation study group, who discussed the identification of asthma in 1971, were largely physiologists, whereas many of those present at this symposium are epidemiologists. It is clear that epidemiology — genetic and environmental — has much to offer when it comes to elucidating aetiology. The members of the 1971 study group decided that asthma could not be defined on the basis of the information available at that time. They recommended that patients with asthma should be studied over a considerable period of time to look for definable patterns. While it is clear that we have made considerable progress in understanding the cellular and mediator basis of asthma, and have identified some of the factors in the environment that initiate the disease, it is disappointing that almost nothing is known about the natural history of asthma, which not infrequently is a lifetime disease. That allergens are important in initiating the inflammatory response of the airways is without dispute. Moreover, it seems probable that changes in the time of exposure, the level of exposure or even the range of allergens contribute, at least in part, to the increase in asthma prevalence reported in some parts of the world. However, it seems unlikely that this is the entire explanation. To draw together possible contributing factors, it is probably helpful to review the working definition of asthma.

The best description of asthma, which encapsulates the 1959 description and some of the more important epidemiological studies that have been completed, is the one that Ann Woolcock used during her presentation, i.e. that asthma is a state of the airways which makes them prone to narrow too much and too easily in response to provoking stimuli.

I would like to run through each presentation to highlight the key points that were raised. In my introduction I wanted to make the point that the factors which initiate asthma may not be the same factors involved in the persistence of asthma or in its progression over the years. For example, I was persuaded by some of the data presented by Paul Cullinan on occupational asthma that, after a critical period of exposure to a sensitizing agent and the withdrawal of the agent, asthma may progress relentlessly for years without further exposure. A similar situation may exist for asthma

258

of the more ordinary type. It appears that the resident, constitutive or structural cells in the airways contribute towards the development of the asthma phenotype as the disease matures into a chronic form. This process may have three components: remodelling the airways by adding structural proteins and other substances including proteoglycans to the airway wall; addition of functional cells (such as nerve cells and those comprising smooth muscle and blood vessels) to the airway; and a positive contribution of the constitutive cells in the airway (such as the epithelium, smooth muscle cells, fibroblasts and the endothelium) to supporting the inflammatory process itself involving mediator and cytokine secretion, which is distinct from an immune response. Although we have largely accepted the T helper (Th) 2 cell paradigm for the induction of asthma, other signals from the immune system, particularly the superimposition of a Th1-like response (on top of an established Th2 response), may contribute to disease progression. One example of this is the effect of respiratory virus infection in provoking the deterioration of asthma over many weeks in which cytotoxic, $CD8^+$ or Th1-like cells are recruited.

Pat Holt gave a clear account of the current knowledge of mucosal immunology as it relates to asthma. Asthma is a disease of the immune system, at least in its initiation, with allergen sensitization being the key event. Those who progress to sensitization are those who select T cells to particular allergens relevant to that early event. He discussed the concept of a 'window of opportunity' when events were changing rapidly, not only in terms of the systemic and local immune response, but also in terms of lung growth and maturation, thereby providing special opportunities for interventions.

In discussing the primary immune response, the pivotal role of the dendritic cell was stressed. This professional antigen-processing and antigen-presenting cell is found in abundance in the bronchial epithelium and submucosa, and its number and level of activation appear enhanced in asthma. The cell originates from a $CD34^+$ precursor in the circulation and, once in the airways, matures in the presence of a number of key cytokines — specifically granulocyte macrophage colony-stimulating factor, interleukin (IL)-4 and IL-13 — with the resultant acquisition of the cell surface marker CD1a, together with both low and high affinity receptors for IgE. The mature dendritic cell has the role of signalling to the T cell (which involves major histocompatibility complex class II as well as a number of accessory adhesion molecules) what the repertoire of cytokines should be in future immune responses. The concept is that dendritic cells promote T cell differentiation along the Th2 pathway in genetically at-risk individuals.

Pat Holt also emphasized the potential role of micro-organisms in subverting this response. Much of the evidence presented argued in favour of infections exerting a negative influence on the allergic phenotype, i.e. that a bacterial or viral infection stimulates a Th1-like response in early life, possibly through IL-12, which serves to inhibit a Th2 response that may be initiated by simultaneous allergen exposure. This is an interesting concept because it is a potential area for therapeutic development and possible vaccine development, with the objective of deliberately inducing a Th1 response in those at risk of developing asthma. The concept was extended from pathogens to commensals, the early life pattern of which may also influence the development of a Th2-like response.

In building upon the concept that asthma is a disease of the mucosal immune response, Barry Kay covered the area of T cell biology. Available evidence in mild to moderate asthma emphasizes the importance of Th2 skewing in fully developed allergic asthma. In dissecting out the individual contributions made by cytokines of the IL-4 gene cluster on chromosome 5, he suggested that IL-4 was more a marker of allergy, whereas IL-5 was a marker of asthma. I am not sure that met with universal agreement, particularly when one considered that IL-4 knockout mice fail to develop an eosinophil-mediated airway response despite the availability of IL-5. Nevertheless, the Th2 cytokine repertoire is undoubtedly implicated as the major factor driving the eosinophil response, at least in the development of asthma and in early disease. The second point to be extracted from his presentation was the concept of what constitutes non-allergic, or intrinsic, asthma. It is possible that in both extrinsic asthma, for which there is a known environmental sensitizing agent, and intrinsic asthma one is dealing with a common mechanism, the only difference being that in more classical asthma there are peripheral readouts of the IgE signal through skin tests or circulating IgE, whereas in patients with the 'intrinsic' form of the disease, who are usually older, sensitization may be restricted to the airways and not reflected in the peripheral circulation as elevated IgE or positive skin tests. In animal models local sensitization without systemic responses can exist and in those forms of asthma that are 'non-allergic' this is clearly a testable hypothesis that should be pursued even if the offending antigen(s) is not known.

Peter Paré picked up on the area of chronic asthma and airway wall remodelling. Based on careful morphological analysis of post-mortem material, he presented some convincing results demonstrating thickening of the submucosa and the adventitia outside the smooth muscle. This occurs by the accumulation of either cells or new proteins, glycoproteins or proteoglycans, and it results in changes in the mechanical behaviour of the airway wall. He drew our attention to the macromolecule versican, which is a molecule that has a role in supporting the proteoglycan matrix within the airway wall, and he indicated that smooth muscle may also contribute to providing this altered matrix. Making the airways stiffer may be a natural protective mechanism, although if excessive it could lead to progressive loss of bronchodilator responsiveness. The greater the number of epithelial folds present in the small airways, the stiffer the airways become.

Gene Bleecker was our token geneticist, not because asthma genetics is not an important field, but because we were assembled to discuss the rising trends of asthma, which are most likely due to environmental factors. However, it would have been inappropriate not to have had some reference to the genetics of asthma since this field is progressing rapidly and any environmental or pharmacological interventions might best be targeted to genetically at-risk individuals if they could be identified. The main points relevant to the environmental epidemiologists in his presentation were the multifactorial nature of the asthma trait and the concept of genetic heterogeneity, such that in different populations it is highly likely that genes interact in different ways to produce a final common phenotype. The asthma phenotype was debated at length. The genetic epidemiologists are particular about the identification of well-defined disease markers against which they can undertake their linkage or association studies. In this respect, possible new markers were discussed, including induced sputum as a new marker for inflammation, adenosine challenge as a marker of mast cell priming and nitric oxide as a marker of epithelial cell activation. Those in the group who are environmental epidemiologists felt that constraining asthma, with its many forms of presentation into predetermined phenotypes, was not that helpful and they suggested that more emphasis should be placed on dissecting which components best identified asthma in different studies. Particular mention was made of specific regions of interest on the human genome that have arisen from a number of separate studies using different analytical techniques. One of these regions is on 5q, which contains most of the genes encoding cytokines secreted by Th2-like cells (as well as mast cells, eosinophils and basophils), the β2-adrenoceptor, the corticosteroid receptor, leukotriene C4 synthase and an interferon (IFN) regulatory factor. Another area of interest is located on the long arm of chromosome 12, which contains the genes encoding IFN-γ, nitric oxide synthase and a mast cell growth factor. Clearly one of the most enthralling areas of science to emerge over the next 10 years in asthma research will be the study of the genetic–environmental interface. Largely due to lack of information and the appropriate cellular and molecular tools, epidemiologists presently have little contact with those concerned in the genetic regulation of complex diseases. Possibly, over the next 20 years, these two disparate, but equally important, fields of research will converge to create extremely exciting and important developments.

Peter Burney questioned some of the basic principles of the methods used by genetic epidemiologists to search for phenotypic markers. He reminded us that the members of the Ciba Foundation guest symposium on asthma in 1958 described asthma in terms of labile airways. In particular, he considered that looking for the ideal phenotype is a waste of time because of the natural variations in responses even in monogenic disorders. He also made the point, which genetic epidemiologists would probably agree with, that the standardization of techniques used to measure particular phenotypic markers was more important than their validation. This becomes particularly important when trying to compare the findings from one centre with those of another, both within and between countries. Currently, genetic epidemiologists are running into problems because they are using different methods to measure various indices of asthma, including skin tests and airway hyper-responsiveness, and because numerous questionnaires are being used to capture the symptoms. One illustration of how a question can be fairly robust across different countries was identifying 'waking up at night with shortness of breath'. This seemed to be easily and widely understood irrespective of which language it was translated into. It was apparent to the group that better markers in questionnaires were needed to identify asthma severity and chronicity.

There has recently been much concern and publicity on trends in asthma mortality. Richard Beasley gave us an overview of a complicated area. While by no means unanimous, some clear points have emerged; namely, that with one or two exceptions (e.g. the Barcelona soybean epidemic) asthma mortality seemed to be linked more to health care management than to any environmental factors important in disease severity or progression. In areas with poor health care management, for example the inner cities of the USA, increased asthma mortality has become a serious health, as well as political, issue. Both in the 1960s and in New Zealand in the 1970s increased asthma mortality was probably linked to excess use of non-selective β-adrenoceptor agonists coupled with inadequate use of anti-inflammatory drugs and plans for managing asthma across the primary–secondary care interface. While on the subject of β2-agonists, genetic epidemiologists are beginning to identify polymorphisms of the β2-adrenoceptor, in particular polymorphisms at amino acids 16 and 27, that are linked to asthma severity. It is possible that this is the first example of genetic studies that inform broader epidemiological issues in asthma.

An important point was made about the difficulties in interpreting mortality data between different countries. Peter Burney's questionnaire on asthma mortality that was sent to investigators in several countries produced wide-ranging and often contradictory responses, which gives a good reason for the wide-ranging mortality figures between and even within countries. Therefore, until common methodology is agreed, mortality statistics should be treated with a considerable degree of caution, especially when used for comparative purposes.

Contrary to popular opinion, the overall trend of asthma mortality is decreasing in most parts of the world, probably due to natural variations in disease severity but also to the increasing awareness of asthma management guidelines and better use of health care resources. One exception to this is the high asthma mortality and morbidity in the inner-city areas of the United States, where there are still considerable problems with the delivery of health care. This is a problem that may have its solution more embedded in politics than in science. When considering how asthma mortality data are interpreted, the point was made that it is necessary to correct statistics for the disease prevalence in the region or country for which the term 'case fatality' might be used.

Although it seems clear that allergens encountered in the indoor environment, especially in domestic housing, influence the onset of asthma in those genetically at risk, it was recognized that outdoor allergens also play a role. This applies not only to 'epidemics' of asthma after thunderstorms or under exceptional circumstances, such as that of the Barcelona epidemic, but also in driving seasonal asthma where allergens from tree and grass pollens and fungi are important. Where the levels of indoor and outdoor allergens are high, the risks of asthma seem particularly great.

Ann Woolcock delivered one of the main points of this symposium, i.e. the evidence for a worldwide increase in asthma prevalence. The general conclusion from analysing a large number of time-trend studies including those from her own group was that, although there were some methodological problems in some of the studies, there has been a rising trend in asthma over the last 20 years. The magnitude of the increase and the time over which it has occurred were less easily defined, but in most countries it was in the order of a doubling in prevalence over 15–20 years. In some countries the increase was 10-fold or more. One difficulty that introduced less precision into deriving comparative figures between countries was the different methods used to assess asthma prevalence, whether using questionnaires and/or objective measures of airway function. One observation was that countries and continents in the Southern hemisphere, Southeast Asia and some of the Pacific Islands seemed to have markedly higher figures than countries in the Northern hemisphere. A possible explanation suggested by Ann Woolcock was that good hygiene was associated with the rising trends in asthma and that, at least in Australia and New Zealand, the increased appearance in the disease appeared to parallel the increase in life quality being experienced by these populations. Under such circumstances, reduced exposure to factors that initiate or maintain a Th1 cell response might lead to allergen-driven Th2 responses. However, Ann Woolcock also considered that there was a requirement for additional factor(s) that interact with the Th2-mediated IgE, mast cell and eosinophil responses. One possibility was an alteration in the way the actin and myosin interacted in the airway smooth muscle (the 'latch' factor). Alternatively, there may be other factors that have not yet been identified which in some way magnify the effects of airway inflammation on the final airway response. A number of known risk factors to account for the rising trends were identified. These include: early expression of atopy; maternal smoking; allergen load (particularly in the domestic environment); infection in early infants; diet; and low birth weight. It was felt that atopy alone was insufficient to account for the rising trends in asthma even though it is likely to be a major factor. One idea which was put forward was that low and persistent allergen exposure drives sensitization in individuals who are especially genetically susceptible. Thus, in isolated populations where extensive inbreeding has occurred there could be a selection of 'asthma genes' of minor effect overall but, when over expressed, they could lead to greatly enhanced responses to relatively low levels of allergen stimulation in the environment. In larger more heterogeneous populations genetic epidemiology studies suggest the existence of several genes of major effect together with minor genes. Whatever the answer, it would appear that genes which increase the susceptibility to sensitization with only low levels of exposure are those which will attract most interest.

Occupational asthma is a useful paradigm for studying a single sensitizing agent. Paul Cullinan highlighted the opportunities in occupational asthma from both epidemiological and pathological points of view to understand how aetiological factors interacted with pathogenetic mechanisms, especially when looking at disease induction and the factors that accelerate disease progression. Work on gene–environment interactions would seem to be a particularly productive area when applied to occupational asthma, especially if there were efforts to extrapolate methodology from studying simple reactive chemicals to some of the more complex proteins (such as the mouse and rat urine proteins) that are well-recognized and characterized occupational sensitizing agents. Sensitization to these substances reaches a maximum within the first one or two years of exposure, which again suggests the idea of a 'window of opportunity' at which to direct interventions. Thus, removing individuals from the workplace who were becoming sensitized within the first year of exposure may help prevent the development of occupational sensitization, whereas if exposure continued beyond two years then the risks of asthma developing were much greater, particularly if they smoked cigarettes or had some other attendant risk factor. Another interesting aspect of occupational asthma is that, unlike childhood-onset asthma, there are measurements of exposure. Indeed, the IgE response to platinum salts and to acid anhydrides relates strongly to the intensity and persistence of the exposure. Smoking seems to be a well-identified adjuvant factor for increased sensitization in the work place, although no clear mechanisms have yet been shown. An important feature that can be learnt from occupational asthma is that disease progression may not only extend beyond the period when the person leaves the workplace, but also beyond the period when immunological markers indicative of sensitization have disappeared. This brings us back to the concept of airway remodelling and the recruitment of additional local factors that may be important in disease progression. It is also possible that some clinical substances in our environment may be responsible for some of the 'non-allergic' (intrinsic) asthmatics that have a later onset of disease but no identifiable external causative agents.

Thomas Platts-Mills emphasized that house dust mite, cat, cockroach and *Alternaria* antigens were the primary antigens important in asthma, as opposed to other allergic diseases. These dominated the allergen repertoire in most of the studies. Although they play a role, it is paradoxical that pollens, which are ubiquitous and powerful allergens, do not seem to be strongly associated with asthma. Whether there is something special about the allergen itself, in addition to the period of time in life when exposure on a regular basis is encountered, is an important question that needs to be answered. Although there is now good evidence that the level of exposure, as well as the duration, influences the process of sensitization, once sensitized there is a lack of any relationship between the level of exposure to the particular allergen and the presence of symptoms. In established asthmatics an interaction between allergen exposure and viruses is considered important for the acute exacerbation of asthma, although the mechanism of this interaction still requires elucidation. On a more controversial note, Thomas Platts-Mills also suggested that children are becoming increasingly exposed and sensitized to allergens in the domestic environment because they are spending much more time indoors watching television. Harold Nelson tempered this suggestion by referring to the importance of other psychosocial factors that may equally be as important.

Ross Anderson provided evidence from epidemiological as well as chamber studies which indicated that outdoor air pollution was unlikely to explain the new cases of asthma, although further studies need to be done on this to be absolutely certain. It was almost certain that air pollution could make asthma worse in individuals who already had the disease by interacting with already inflamed airways, but this will depend very much on the intensity of the pollution in different parts of the world.

There was some discussion on the interaction of allergens with pollutants, not only in terms of the way that the allergen may be induced to 'leak' their allergenic proteins but also the attachment of allergens to chemical particulates, such as PM10 or PM2.5, which may augment sensitization. This area of 'allergotoxicology' requires a critical analysis of the possible relationships between air pollution and allergen exposure. David Strachan made an important point, not only for chemical air pollutants but also for allergens, that much better personal exposure data are needed for many of these environmental measures because it is not known what components of the environment are critical for sensitization and later augmentation of established asthma — possibilities included pulses or continuous exposure or a combination of both.

William Busse provided an overview of the role of viruses in asthma, a complicated area in many respects because of the confusion between virus exacerbations of asthma and virus-induced augmentation or protection of sensitization. He mentioned the possible roles of viruses either in augmenting or in protecting against allergen sensitization. There is much work to be done on the clarification of the roles of viruses in early life, a field judged to be of great importance because therapeutic strategies could emerge from it. One point which was established was that viruses could augment allergen-induced inflammatory responses and that these are linked to the development of both late-phase allergic inflammatory reactions in the airways and bronchial hyper-responsiveness. The human rhinovirus accounts for most of the virus infections that cause the worsening of asthma in adults and children, and it could therefore account for a large proportion of asthma exacerbations that result in the admission of asthmatics to hospitals. Thus, viruses play a major role in disrupting the life quality of patients with asthma. Some mechanistic aspects of virus-induced asthma were discussed with two particular areas of interest emerging. The first was the key role played by the epithelium in asthma, the bronchial epithelium being particularly receptive to colonization by viruses; and the second was the role of the T lymphocyte in converting the response into an eosinophil-mediated inflammatory reaction involving combinations of cytokines and chemokines.

Throughout the symposium there was general agreement that early life was a key period for the initiation of asthma. Jill Warner emphasized that the process may start earlier, i.e. in pregnancy when the immune responses in the fetus are still developing. She suggested that immune responses to allergens which reach the fetus can occur as early as 22 weeks in pregnancy. This has clear implications for allergen-avoidance strategies. She also emphasized the possible dysregulation of cytokine networks and, in particular, the role of IFN-γ in controlling immune responses in the intra-uterine environment. The interesting idea was advanced that the maternal feed response is normally a Th2 response and that, in the critical period of development, this may be augmented or inhibited by various maternal factors, including cigarette smoking and presentation of allergens across the placenta. While it was recognized that T cells in cord blood could be shown to respond to a range of allergens (including aeroallergens) by proliferating, little is known about how this could occur and, in particular, in what form and where the allergen presentation takes place.

Fernando Martinez continued to build on the idea of early life being important and made the point that asthma and respiratory infections in early infancy were inversely related to maternal age. The observation that disadvantaged mothers are tending to have children at a younger age may be an important social factor in contributing to the rising trends in asthma in developed as well as developing countries. Maternal, as opposed to paternal, atopy and asthma had a greater influence on the development of allergy and asthma in the child, at least in the first six years of life, and it highlighted the importance of early maternal interactions with the fetus. Maternal smoking both in pregnancy and after pregnancy, and in particular the effect of cigarette smoking on the retardation of lung development both *in vitro* and in the first two years of life, was further emphasized as being detrimental. Smoking in pregnancy also influenced the direction of the T cell response towards the generation of IgE and the appearance of the atopic phenotype.

One factor that has changed over the last 20 years and is especially linked to the western lifestyle is diet. Scott Weiss presented data showing that antioxidants, a number of electrolytes (sodium, potassium and magnesium), dietary protein and fatty acids could, under certain circumstances, lead to the worsening of asthma in those who already have the disease. What was not known, however, was how diet could influence the development of new asthma. A number of recent studies have suggested that maternal diet could, through placental programming of the fetus, influence various disease phenotypes occurring later in life. Maternal nutrition (possibly overnutrition) and its influence on the processes linked to the development of asthma is an important area for future research since this presents opportunities for interventions.

Homer A Boushey

Department of Medicine, University of California, PO Box 0130, 505 Parnassus Avenue, San Francisco, CA 94143, USA

The trends in asthma have certainly risen over the past 20 or 30 years, and the problem now is to identify what has caused this rise. Is it due to some change in the environment or to some change in the people exposed to the environment? We have much to learn from the studies of immigrants, since increases in the prevalence of asthma have been observed in Jews returning to Jerusalem after more than 2000 years of the Babylonian captivity, Kenyans moving from rural villages to Nairobi and African Americans moving from rural Georgia to Atlanta. What changes in the environment are likely causes? Are they increases in the materials or events that favour allergenic sensitization of the airways, or decreases in materials or events that inhibit allergenic sensitization of airways? That is, is it more of the 'bad' indoor allergens or is it less of the 'good' air pollutants and viral infections? Has something about the host changed? It seems impossible that a genetic shift could have occurred so abruptly, but it does not seem impossible that the response to aeroallergens has changed as a secondary consequence of some other change in the environment, starting as early as in fetal life. This question is important because we must have a clear idea of the cause of the rising trends in asthma before concluding that bold and expensive interventions would be worthwhile. We need to be extremely careful, for example, in recommending as public policy measures to reduce exposure to domestic allergens. Studies such as those in Los Alamos, where asthma is not uncommon even though house dust mite levels are low and few cats are kept as pets, suggest that there may be something about the host that simply favours sensitization to whatever allergen is around. If this is true, elimination of domestic allergens may have a low yield. Should we instead consider another bold and expensive intervention, i.e. stimulating Th1 activity in people prone to asthma by virtue of their lineage? Should we restore a particular pollutant? Does a reduction in the frequency of viral respiratory infections or other illnesses explain the rising trends in asthma? If so, should we seriously entertain the idea of using an attenuated virus, or some other much better and safer way, to promote Th1 activity? Finally, is it possible that changes in diet or activity from those of rural life to those of urban life alter the ease of allergic sensitization or its consequences? We thus have much to study and much to learn before we can consider the broad changes in public policy or public education to reverse the consequences of the trends in asthma over the past 30 years.

Ann Woolcock

Institute of Respiratory Medicine, Royal Prince Alfred Hospital, Camperdown, Sydney, NSW 2050, Australia

There are a number of questions that could be addressed by epidemiologists working together with immunologists. An important one is: what are the environmental factors that determine symptoms of asthma after the age of four years in children who are predisposed because they have a Th2-type response? It is estimated that about 30% of four-year-old children in our societies have the Th2-type pattern identified by specific IgE responses to the common inhalant allergens. We would like to determine the environmental factors that influence whether the IgE response is lost as the individual gets older, whether the IgE response remains but the individual does not develop symptoms or whether the IgE response stays high and the individual develops asthmatic symptoms. The evidence presented at this symposium indicates that the following would be documented: parental asthma, allergens (i.e. type and load) diet and infections. There are additional lifestyle factors, such as the lack of exercise due to the number of hours watching television and the level of hygiene, that are more difficult to quantitate. This would be a cohort study, which should be performed in two communities: one with a high and one with a low level of asthma. We would have to choose the populations carefully to ensure stability because of the problems of population migration and of changing environments. Each year we would conduct radioallergosorbent and skin prick tests, measure lung function and airway hyper-responsiveness, and give subjects a diet questionnaire and a diary to list their infections and treatments for asthma. We would also cryopreserve samples of nasal secretions and blood so that we could later decide whether they had a Th1- or Th2-type response and look at the DNA. We could also measure the levels of IL-4, IL-5 and specific IgE responses in these samples to determine if they had been infected by viruses, and we could look for possible genetic markers.

Index of contributors

Non-participating co-authors are indicated by asterisks. Entries in bold type indicate papers; other entries refer to discussion contributions.

Indexes compiled by Liza Weinkove

Subject index

Other Ciba Foundation Symposia:

No. 195 **T cell subsets in infectious and autoimmune diseases**
Chairman: N. A. Mitchison
1995 ISBN 0 471 95720 8

No. 204 **The molecular basis of cellular defence mechanism**
Chairman: Sir Gustav Nossal
1997 ISBN 0 471 96567 7

No. 207 **Antibiotic resistance: origins, evolution, selection and spread**
Chairman: Stuart Levy
1997 ISBN 0 471 97105 7